Public Policy Challenges in Rethinking Public Health

Comparative Perspectives

World Scientific Series in Global Health Economics and Public Policy

ISSN: 2010-2089

Series Editor-in-Chief: Peter Berman *(The University of British Columbia, Canada & Harvard University, USA)*

The World Scientific Series in Global Health Economics and Public Policy, under the leadership of Professor Peter Berman, a renowned healthcare economist, public policy specialist and researcher in this field, seeks to fill this gap. It strives to publish high-quality scientific works, including monographs, edited volumes, references, handbooks, etc., which address subjects of primary scientific importance on the global scale, as related to international economic policies in healthcare, social capital and healthcare economics in different global markets, etc. The titles in this series appeal to researchers, graduate students, policy makers, practitioners and commercial businesses, dealing with healthcare economics worldwide.

Published:

More information on this series can also be found at
https://www.worldscientific.com/series/wssghepp

(Continued at end of book)

World Scientific Series in Global Health Economics and Public Policy – Vol. 10

Public Policy Challenges in Rethinking Public Health

Comparative Perspectives

Edited by

Katherine A Fierlbeck

Dalhousie University, Canada

World Scientific

NEW JERSEY • LONDON • SINGAPORE • BEIJING • SHANGHAI • HONG KONG • TAIPEI • CHENNAI • TOKYO

Published by

World Scientific Publishing Co. Pte. Ltd.

5 Toh Tuck Link, Singapore 596224

USA office: 27 Warren Street, Suite 401-402, Hackensack, NJ 07601

UK office: 57 Shelton Street, Covent Garden, London WC2H 9HE

Library of Congress Control Number: 2024024825

British Library Cataloguing-in-Publication Data
A catalogue record for this book is available from the British Library.

World Scientific Series in Global Health Economics and Public Policy — Vol. 10
PUBLIC POLICY CHALLENGES IN RETHINKING PUBLIC HEALTH
Comparative Perspectives

ISBN 978-981-12-9629-1 (hardcover)
ISBN 978-981-12-9630-7 (ebook for institutions)
ISBN 978-981-12-9631-4 (ebook for individuals)

For any available supplementary material, please visit
https://www.worldscientific.com/worldscibooks/10.1142/13934#t=aboutBook

Desk Editors: Sanjay Varadharajan/Claire Lum/Kura Sunaina

Typeset by Stallion Press
Email: enquiries@stallionpress.com

About the Editor

Katherine Fierlbeck is a McCulloch Research Professor and Chair of the Department of Political Science at Dalhousie University, with a cross-appointment in Community Health and Epidemiology. She was the Director of the Jean Monnet Network for Health Law and Politics, funded by the European Union's Erasmus+ program, from 2017 to 2022. Dr. Fierlbeck focuses on the politics of health policy. She has a particular interest in issues of governance and mechanisms of accountability. Some of her recent books include *Health Care in Canada* (2011), *Canadian Health Care Federalism* (2013), *Comparative Health Care Federalism* (2015), *Health System Profiles: Nova Scotia* (2018), *Transparency, Power, and Influence in the Pharmaceutical Industry* (2021), *Health Law and Policy from East to West: Analytical Perspectives and Comparative Case Studies* (2022), and *The Boundaries of Medicare: Public Health Care Beyond the Canada Health Act* (2022).

About the Contributors

Ollie Bartlett is an Assistant Professor of Law in the School of Law and Criminology at Maynooth University, Ireland. His research focuses on public health law and policy. He has built particular expertise in alcohol control, the right to health, European Union (EU) health policy, public health governance tools, and public health ethics. Ollie has worked on a variety of interdisciplinary public health projects, for example, on the impact of the EU's Better Regulation agenda on EU health policy, on the ethics of sugar tax policies, and on the control of health misinformation. Ollie regularly collaborates on alcohol policy projects with the World Health Organization as well as Irish and European non-governmental organizations (NGOs) and has co-authored reports on, for example, the regulation of digital alcohol marketing and minimum unit pricing.

Peter Berman is a Professor Emeritus at the University of British Columbia School of Population and a Public Health and Adjunct Professor of Global Health at the Harvard T. H. Chan School of Public Health. He is a health economist with over 40 years of experience conducting research aimed at developing primary care systems, strengthening service delivery, and improving healthcare financing. He has worked extensively in India, Ethiopia, Indonesia, and Malaysia, and he has also worked with the World Bank as Lead Economist in Health, Nutrition and Population in the New Delhi office and in Washington D.C. with the World Bank's Health Systems

Global Expert Team. Dr. Berman is the author or editor of 5 books and more than 50 academic articles.

Evelyne de Leeuw holds a Canadian Excellence in Research Chair (CERC), in "One Urban Health" at the Université de Montréal, and is a Professor of urban health and policy at the University of New South Wales, Sydney. With Patrick Harris she is Editor-in-Chief of Oxford University Press's (OUP's) Oxford Open Infrastructure and Health, and with Patrick Fafard of the Palgrave Studies in Public Health Policy Research book series. She is a strong proponent of "health political science" and has used hundreds of "Healthy Cities" as field studies and opportunities to invest in better health, urban planning, and good governance.

Thibaud Deruelle is a public policy scholar with specific research interests in health policy within the EU, the role of experts, and bureaucratic reputations. He currently is a Senior Researcher on the Swiss National Foundation for Science project "Condominio Europe" at the University of Geneva, where he works on third countries' participation in EU agencies. His work is featured in *European Policy Analysis*, *Health Economics, Policy, and Law*, *West European Politics*, and *Big Data and Society*.

Birger C. Forsberg is an Associate Professor (Docent) in International Health at Karolinska Institutet. He is a medical doctor specializing in Social Medicine. His main fields of work have been health planning, evaluation, and health economics both in Sweden and internationally. He held a position as överläkare (senior physician) at Region Stockholm from 2001 to 2022. Over the years, he has had various leadership positions. He has work experience as a staff member and consultant with the WHO, the World Bank, UNICEF, and various bilateral development agencies. His research focuses on communicable diseases, child health, and health system issues, particularly in the interaction between the public and private sectors. He has many years of experience in the teaching and supervision of students. He is also the author of a textbook in Swedish on Health Planning and has some 100 publications in the scientific literature.

My Fridell is a PhD student at Karolinska Institutet, where she is currently researching the concept of health system resilience and lessons learned from COVID-19. Her specific aim is to assess regional preparedness plans in Sweden. Prior to her PhD, she worked as a management consultant, providing support to both public and private healthcare clients throughout Scandinavia. My Fridell holds a bachelor's degree in public health and a master's degree in health economics, policy, and management.

Scott L. Greer is a Political Scientist who researches the ways in which political systems operate and shape health policy decisions. He has done extensive research on a variety of topics including COVID-19 policy response, health governance, strategic purchasing in healthcare, the politics of public health and disaster response, federalism, science policy, and European integration. He conducts research on the European Union, the United Kingdom, and the United States in particular. He is also a Senior Expert Advisor on Health Governance to the European Observatory on Health Systems and Policies.

Patrick Harris is a public health social scientist focused on healthy public policy. His work crosses sectors and disciplines while retaining a core focus on health and equity. His research is pioneering the connections between health, political science and critical theory, and he has particular interest in institutions and power. His sectoral policy expertise spans urban and regional planning systems, infrastructure, and impact assessment. He is the founding co-editor-in-chief of the new Oxford University Press flagship open access journal *Infrastructure and Health*. His book, *Illuminating policy for health*, has recently been published by Palgrave.

Margitta Mätzke is a Professor of Politics and Social Policy at the Johannes Kepler University of Linz, Austria. She has a PhD in Political Science from Northwestern University (2005). Her research focuses on decision-making and institutional dynamics in the development of Western welfare states, and she is especially interested in family policy, health policy, and public health. Her articles are published in the *Journal of Policy History*, the *Journal of Public Policy, Social Policy &*

Administration, the German-language journal *Leviathan*, and the *Journal of European Social Policy* (where she co-edited a Special Issue on *Recent Change in European Family Policies*).

Miriam Mosesson works within the area of research communication at the Department of Global Public Health at the Karolinska Institutet. She obtained her bachelor's degree in Linguistics from the University of Amsterdam, where she specialized in sociolinguistics. Her master's degree in communication and information focused on rhetoric and argumentation theory, including argumentation and communication in health care and science.

Pavitra Paul is an Economist working at the intersection of health and wellbeing, and sustainable development. He provides consulting services to multilateral development organisations for the analysis of policy coherence, social cost-value analysis, equity embedded cost-effectiveness analysis, and on the related themes within the framework of economics for population health development. He is a research professor (adjunct) in the Faculty of Economics and Business Administration, Babeş-Bolyai University, Cluj-Napoca, Romania. His research focuses on equity in health policies, choice modelling for health care services, and measuring health systems performance. At present, he is working on "Contributions to Decision Making in Health Economics" for his Habilitation à Diriger des Recherches (HDR), at the Institut du Management, Ecole des Hautes Etudes en Santé Publique (EHESP), 35043 Rennes, France. He was an Academy of Finland scholar for the study on the welfare effect of choice in the compulsory insurance-based healthcare system in the Russian Federation. He has published in *Applied Economics, International Journal of Health Economics and Management*, and so on.

Glen Ramos is a public health policy consultant with 30 years of experience in healthcare policy and advocacy as a senior executive and director. He has initiated and influenced public inquiries, judicial inquiries, and legislative changes at state and commonwealth levels resulting in policy change improvements to injury and communicable disease prevention, access to mental health services, access to specialist medical services, and tort law reform. Currently based within the Centre for Health Equity Training, Research, and Evaluation at UNSW Sydney he is undertaking a PhD in Public Health on pandemic preparedness and management. He has interests in health promotion, healthy cities, epidemiology, and health political science and currently serves on the boards of numerous peak health organisations including the Australian Health Promotion Association, Australasian Epidemiological Association, Public Health Association (NSW), Australian Thyroid Foundation, and Australian and New Zealand Head and Neck Cancer Society. He is also a Fellow of Australasian College of Health Service Management; Royal Society for Public Health, Royal Society of Medicine, Governance Institute of Australia, and Institute of Managers and Leaders Australia and New Zealand.

Candice Ruck is a Global Health Researcher at the University of British Columbia. She has worked on research projects analyzing the policy responses to COVID-19 in numerous countries. including Canada, South Korea, Taiwan, Australia, and New Zealand. She has a master's in Experimental Medicine and has previously conducted research assessing the vaccine responses of HIV-exposed infants in South Africa.

Tomislav Sokol obtained his PhD in 2014 at KU Leuven on the topic of free movement of cross-border healthcare services in the European Union. He is an Assistant Professor at the Catholic University of Croatia where he teaches health law. Sokol was an Assistant Minister of Science and Education in Croatia, as well as a Member of the Croatian Parliament. To date, he has published around 20 papers and a book on issues related to health in the context of EU law, including several articles in leading European journals, such as *Common Market Law Review*, *European Law Review*, and the *European Law Journal*. He is currently a Member of the European Parliament and the European People's Party Coordinator in the Committee on Public Health (SANT).

Göran Tomson is a Professor Emeritus in International Health Systems Research in the Department of Learning, Informatics, Management, and Ethics at the Karolinska Institutet in Stockholm, Sweden. He is a Distinguished Fellow at the George Institute of Global Health, Sydney, and an Honorary Visiting Professor at Shandong University, China. He is a member of the Swedish Research Council on strategic research in viruses and pandemics and has co-founded four international networks, including ReAct to contain antimicrobial resistance (AMR). He has served in scientific committees including the Alliance for Health Policy Systems Research at the World Health Organization (WHO) as well as in global health research councils in the Netherlands, Norway, and Sweden. Universal health coverage in resource-poor settings and preparedness for health are major research interests. Ongoing work includes human and planetary health, systems thinking and climate change, and conflict and COVID-19. With 234 peer-reviewed publications, he has recently initiated the Nobel Forum meeting at the KI on EU's new Global Health Strategy.

Contents

Chapter 1

Introduction:
Themes and Choices

Katherine Fierlbeck and Peter Berman

1.1 Stepping Back

COVID-19 focused public attention on public health as never before. Ordinary people began to think about how public health was organized, funded, and executed; how it connected both to clinical pathways and to broader social practices; and how the evidence it was based on (or not) was collected, interpreted, applied, and explained. People also became aware of the political, ethical, and economic costs and tradeoffs public health responses required during the pandemic. Throughout the pandemic, "public health" was proposed and used to frame our approaches to COVID-19. But COVID-19 also gives us a better opportunity to examine the nature of "public health" itself. The post-pandemic forensic evaluations of each jurisdiction's handling of COVID-19 are useful in addressing identifiable gaps, conflicts, or errors in pandemic management, and the contributions in this volume cover the intricacies of pandemic management in some detail. However, the larger question is what COVID-19 has brought to light regarding the nature of "public health" itself.

The objectives of this volume are twofold. First, it provides a series of jurisdictional evaluations assessing how well each unit was able to manage the challenges posed by the pandemic, and it identifies the variables that either facilitated or obstructed good public health management in each jurisdiction. More profoundly, and perhaps more importantly, it leads us to examine how (and whether) the lessons learned throughout the pandemic are shaping the practice of public health across these jurisdictions. If clinical or organizational insights were gained from the experience of COVID-19, to what extent do the institutional, political, and organizational contexts within which public health actions are embedded provide a sufficiently malleable environment to incorporate these insights?

The starting point for this volume, then, is the observation that "public health" is an entity that must be viewed from multiple vantage points. Facilitated by the Jean Monnet Network for Health Law and Policy (2017–2020), we have drawn together not only public health experts but also health lawyers, health economists, and health policy analysts to provide a robust and nuanced understanding of why disparate jurisdictions undertook particular measures, the degree to which they can be considered successful, and the extent to which COVID-19 has shaped the nature of public health.

The enormous breadth and diversity of policy responses to COVID-19 cannot be overstated. Despite the consistently articulated claim that public health directives were "science-based," the range of policy measures diverged considerably. This is why it is so critical to understand the wider sociopolitical context within which public health systems operate. The pandemic put enormous political pressure on administrations to "do something," but the choices they made were determined not only by the pathogen itself but also by the legal institutions within which they operated, their economic and clinical capacity, their organizational structures, the evidence they chose to use, the social support for specific measures, and the tradeoffs they were willing to make. Given the potential rigidity of some of these variables, it is not inconceivable that disadvantageous measures taken in response to COVID-19 could be repeated yet again in a future crisis. Our confidence in the aspirational assertions that "we must do better next time" would be greater if we could develop a more lucid understanding of why desirable health policy strategies so often fail to materialize.

Nonetheless, broader and more focused insights can be gleaned from these chapters. There are four overarching themes that emerge from this volume. Those looking for quick solutions that can be applied to public health systems, such as new laboratories or new training programs, will be disappointed in the complexity conveyed here. Each theme involves a tension between a set of competing choices, each with its own narrative of justification. Each of these themes is discussed in more detail in Section 1.3, with reference to the contributors' case studies.

The first theme addresses the temporal aspect of pandemic management. One of the most pervasive difficulties that states had was the tendency to conceptualize the pandemic (and pandemic management) as a single coherent event, rather than as a complex, sustained phenomenon where the contours were continually shifting. Traditional responses to pandemic management, based on models of infectious disease outbreaks, are generally undertaken in a command-and-control mode with its roots in military conflict. Where time is of the essence, messaging must be clear, and lines of accountability must be apparent: in such cases, a linear, top-down form of management is highly useful to achieve timely and effective control. Over time, however, this rigid vertical system of decision-making tends to get in the way of the nimbleness and responsiveness needed to address the shifting nature of this pandemic, with its rapidly evolving infectious agent, and public responses to it.

The second theme focuses on the extent to which jurisdictions chose to see the pandemic exclusively as a medical event rather than as a socio-political one. The immediate response of most states was to "flatten the curve" and to implement immediate strategies to dampen demand on clinical facilities to free up capacity to treat the sick. The focus was mainly on masking, testing, vaccination, and the strict regulation of public spaces. For many states, containing the spread of the COVID-19 pathogen was the only important public health objective. For others (and, over time, almost everywhere), the wider effects of the consequences of COVID-19 management demanded to be taken more into account, including social isolation, economic consequences, educational outcomes, the consequences of limiting or postponing clinical interventions, and potentially even the iatrogenic effects of treatments themselves.

The third, and related, theme was the narrative of health equity and the place of more vulnerable populations in pandemic management. The issue of health equity is a familiar one within public health discourse. It emphasizes a focus on equal health provision, as in current calls for universal health coverage (https://www.uhc2030.org/un-hlm-2023/). Is this sufficient for effective pandemic control, or should we be targeting policies and strategies toward more vulnerable groups in society whose needs are more pronounced? This tension within public health is of course highly political, as it involves the distribution of critical but limited resources, and it incorporates the wider non-medical determinants of health (including income, education, employment, race, and geography) into the discussion. That societies are only as safe as their most vulnerable populations are healthy pushed health equity more forcefully onto the table, and the highly contagious nature of COVID-19 confronted the invisible tendency to ghettoize some marginalized groups, as decision-makers became aware that the spread of disease in some sub-communities could have a very real impact upon the overall well-being of the larger population.

The fourth theme addresses the way in which data underlying pandemic policy responses were gathered, selected, defended, and made transparent (or not). Each state was adamant that it was "following the science," yet these "science-driven" strategies seemed to diverge enormously even when based on the same evidence resources. Since scientific discourse legitimized policy directives, the question of what "scientific" really means, and how it is understood by citizens, is worth pursuing. Given that "science" connotes an objective set of processes and principles, it is ironic that this was perhaps the most politically contentious aspect of pandemic management. While some states had formal provisions requiring the state to justify its public health activity, or to ensure that it was "based on science and proven experience," the scientific discourse in other jurisdictions was deliberately curtailed. Again, decision-making within the context of a pandemic is informed by an uncomfortable tension between open scientific debate and the desire to keep the public calm and on-side with official public health strategies regardless of data that may be incomplete, ambiguous, or conflicting.

1.2 Framing the Discussion: About "Comparative Public Health"

What concepts and methods are useful and appropriate for comparing "public health systems" and their responses to COVID-19? The rich literature on health systems more broadly includes a robust discussion of how to categorize and understand healthcare systems across states. Is it possible to develop a similar kind of analytical system for public health, encompassing the entities involved in public health response and how they may or may not be "systems"?

Health systems writ large, at the most basic level, have often been classified according to the way in which they are funded: thus, the most simple schema will categorize a system according to whether its healthcare funding is largely based on private market-based funding (US), general taxation (UK), or social insurance (Germany). But the focus on funding ignores the way in which services are delivered; by combining the two variables, we now have a conceptual quadrant where healthcare can be funded and provided in any combination of "public" and "private." A major confounder here is that the imposition of different specific regulatory frameworks can importantly make public funding models behave more like private ones (e.g. managed competition) or privately funded models act more like public ones (e.g. sickness funds). And, as Wendt *et al.* (2008) argue, we must not only consider these three dimensions of healthcare — funding, service provision, and regulation — but also identify which actor is responsible for each task. Thus, "when connecting state, non-governmental and market influences with the dimensions of financing, service provision and regulation, 27 combinations emerge ($3 \times 3 \times 3$)" (p. 71).

However, Böhm *et al.* (2013) have argued that one of these dimensions — regulation — must be considered more a fundamental organizing principle, and that when it is given priority of consideration, "the superior dimension restricts the nature of the subordinate dimensions" (p. 258) such that the number of "theoretically plausible types" is limited to ten (only five of which exist in practice). This framework is interesting insofar as states that are normally considered within the same category are, under this new typography, placed in different ones. So, for example, while both

Canada and the UK have universal coverage financed through general revenue tax-based sources, Canada (like Australia and New Zealand) significantly utilizes a system of provider payment where payment is made to physicians as private contractors largely on a fee-for-service basis; the UK, in contrast, makes greater use of capitated payment methods to primary care physicians, who are also private contractors but with funding other than insurance reimbursement. Similarly, while both France and Germany ground healthcare provision on a model of social insurance, Böhm *et al.* classify France (along with Belgium) as an "etatist" social health insurance system because the state plays a greater role in regulating the sickness funds. In Germany (as with Austria and Luxembourg), in contrast, private actors have more autonomous authority in implementing the scope and nature of the social insurance model; they are thus considered "social health insurance systems" more properly in their classification.

Yet there is no clear reason why the categorization of health systems must be limited to only these three defining characteristics (funding, delivery, and regulation). Marchildon (2022), for example, argues that many healthcare systems exist within a federal structure and that the distribution of taxation capacity and regulatory functions between federal jurisdictions also have a considerable effect on the way in which their respective health systems function. He notes, in addition, that the scope and depth of coverage of healthcare services (which services are covered, which individuals are covered, and the percentage of costs of each service provided by the state) is yet another important metric providing a vantage point from which to compare and assess healthcare systems and that this can vary between jurisdictions in the same country as is the case in Canada and others.

What seemed like a straightforward classification rubric for healthcare systems begins to appear, on deeper examination, to be a more arbitrary exercise depending upon the variables one presumes to be most important. Yet even focusing upon three basic criteria — funding, provision, and regulation — is much more problematic when one delves into a more detailed analysis of national healthcare systems. In practice, those states paying private healthcare contractors through social insurance also tend to have some healthcare workers employed directly by the state, while others may be remunerated privately. Models of healthcare classification tend to focus on whether the *preponderance* of funding, delivery, or regulation manifests in a particular way, but as each state in the hard light of reality is a complicated combination of numerous elements of these "pure" models, the utility of placing them into one discrete category diminishes as one begins to see how each healthcare system becomes, in effect, its own idiosyncratic "model."

It is important to set out the conceptual issues and limitations underlying the discussion over how to go about comparing *healthcare* systems because these same kinds of intellectual problems could inform the comparative analysis of *public health* systems. From what vantage point, and using which metrics, should we evaluate the performance of public health systems in pandemic management, and the way in which public health systems have been reorganized or reconceptualized (if at all) in the wake of COVID-19? The insight gleaned from the attempt to categorize healthcare systems is that, from a birds-eye view, we can privilege certain features in order to provide a certain intellectual order. Yet there may not be consensus on which characteristics of a system are the relevant ones and, as one recognizes the complex interplay of components comprising each state's healthcare system, each must, at a certain point, simply become *sui generis*.

This insight could also inform the comparative analysis of public health systems. But there is a deeper problem in pursuing this goal that demands more urgent attention. The domain of action for "healthcare" may be more easily understood and, as such, can be applied to help us focus on the dimension of the healthcare system. In contrast, the domain of action of "public health," and consequently, the actors and the scope of their actions, is much less clear and often contested.

Some would like to categorize "public health" as a specialized branch within diverse healthcare systems, treating it as a less complex and more functionally homogeneous body, and thus more amendable to comparative evaluation. As Greer and Mätzke argue in the following chapter, however, this assumes a "misplaced concreteness" that effectively distorts our understanding of its nature and function. This needs consideration if we are to attempt an analysis of public health systems.

They suggest a number of possible conceptual lenses (or "frames") from which to view public health. The literature on classification schemes for healthcare systems writ large generally focuses less on the "what" (as in what is the health system) and more on the question of which factors affect its actions and performance. For public health, the "what" (is public health) is still an important question. The vantage point one chooses to answer that question will influence the way in which one chooses to analyze public health systems.

The most obvious way of conceptualizing public health, as Greer and Mätzke note, is by listing its expected activities. As they illustrate, there is no consensus on these activities; each complex grouping of public health bodies may provide its own account of what is (and is not) properly under its ambit. A second approach is to identify the actors involved in the public health arena. Again, the categories become blurred the more sharply one examines them. Public health, when organized as a branch of medicine, is to a large extent consultative and advisory: public health officials do not "do" medicine as much as they recommend particular courses of action to key decision-makers (Litvak *et al.*, 2020). Moreover, as above, there is little consistency in *who* does public health: to the extent to which public health functions are ambiguous, as noted earlier, so too will public health actors vary across states. For example, monitoring and addressing safe water supply may be performed by actors located in departments of environment, while the safety of the beef supply may rest in departments of agriculture.

A third way of conceptualizing "public health," as Greer and Mätzke astutely recognize, involves applying a more normative lens. A "public health approach" is generally understood to look beyond acute clinical conditions and to incorporate non-medical determinants of health. This is a distinct and unique perspective within the traditional field of medicine. As a discipline, medicine is generally premised on the specific needs and well-being of each individual; in public health, individual need is eclipsed by a focus on populations — public welfare writ large. This tension between individual and collective well-being, which became very apparent throughout COVID-19, contributes to the highly political nature which arises in applying these different framings.

Greer and Mätzke suggest that a fourth approach to understanding public health is through an institutional and organizational lens. This frame, they note, has the advantage of being the easiest to grapple with from an empirical perspective, as the legal framework and the organizational structure for public health systems, though subject to change, can generally be identified and described quite clearly. That is why it is the starting point for each of the case studies in this volume. Each chapter provides a description of the legal and organizational basis of public health in each respective jurisdiction and includes an organogram setting out the flow of function and responsibility to complement this discussion. But, as Greer and Mätzke warn, the disadvantage of the institutional-organizational approach is that it risks "nominative determinism" insofar as the formal institutional titles or flowcharts may or may not represent the way in which public health systems actually operated during COVID-19. For this reason, the contributors to this volume go beyond the formal articulation of what institutions were expected to do and also provide a qualitative and interpretive analysis of how and why public health strategies took the shape they did.

Finally, argue Greer and Mätzke, public health can be understood conceptually from a functionalist perspective as "the field that addresses collective causes of avoidable morbidity and mortality." This creates considerable epistemological difficulty in circumscribing the field — the list of what influences avoidable morbidity and mortality is extensive — but, as this volume describes in detail, the proper scope of public health was exceptionally relevant during COVID-19 as it was a highly political issue that dominated public discourse across jurisdictions.

"Comparative public health" is a subdiscipline in its infancy; it does not have the depth or breadth of literature enjoyed by comparative health systems. The COVID-19 pandemic has brought the question of "how ought we to compare public health systems" to the fore. Unsurprisingly, the nascent field of "comparative public health" has been largely informed by the intellectual context of public health rather than by comparative health policy (see, e.g. Wang and Mao, 2021). There is certainly a utility in comparing public health systems within a vernacular with which participants are familiar and comfortable, one that discusses policies, metrics, and outcomes.

Initially, this volume was not specifically directed to these larger questions of "comparative public health," but the work of its contributors led us to these questions. The chapters collected here provide new insights into these topics, while accommodating the epidemiological focus (what strategies were undertaken? On what basis? What were the outcomes?) within a wider health policy perspective (why were some choices made rather than others? Whose voices prevailed? What is the relationship between policy and power?). The contributors begin with a description of the formal legal/institutional context and then engage in a more qualitative analysis of why particular policy choices were made, whose interests they represented, what the political and organizational difficulties were, and, ultimately, whether the disruption of pandemic governance resulted in significant rethinking of public health in each jurisdiction, or whether the entrenched institutional and political variables within each country have neutralized substantive reform.

1.3 What Do Comparative COVID-19 Case Studies Tell Us About the State and Nature of Public Health?

How does the global experience with COVID-19 help us to think more clearly about the policy challenges we need to face to improve public health? Many jurisdictions have already engaged in forensic analyses of pandemic management. In these cases, the attempt has mostly been to examine in a more technical sense where the problems arose, and how to "fix" them, especially with an eye to the possibility that another pandemic event may arise in the foreseeable future. This volume takes a slightly different approach. Rather than assuming that what is needed are specific additional material investments — "staff, stuff, and space" in a formula made well-known by Dr. Paul Farmer — that can be applied to fix public health systems, the contributors look more closely at the underlying social and institutional context of public health to understand what happened during COVID-19 — Farmer's fourth "s" systems — and whether a simple fix to the problems that arose is even tenable.

Rather, this volume begins with the assumption that there is often a clear reason why undesirable outcomes arose and that this reason is not simply grounded in a lack of attention, or foresight, or the technical aspects of "preparedness" (as the poor correlation between COVID outcomes and the 2019 Global Health Security Index demonstrated).

Doing public health *differently* often comes with a cost attached (economic, but more often political), and the cost involved in rethinking public health may simply be unpalatable. As many of the chapters here explain, there are distinct institutional, political, and organizational structures within which public health is embedded which significantly determine the parameters of policy response. And reforming these structures — laws, organizations, and the power relations ensconced in them — can require an immense degree of political capital and economic investment. As is often the case after significant public health crises in federal states, for example, a window of opportunity exists to rethink and rebuild the way that public health is structured. In response to COVID-19, both Australia and Russia declared a commitment to establish a federal public health body that could coordinate pandemic management. This is similar to Canada's establishment of the Public Health Agency of Canada (PHAC) after a brief but frightening experience with Sudden Acute Respiratory Syndrome (SARS) in 2003. But the simple construction of a new organization simply relocates power relations to a different sphere rather than solving organizational problems altogether. While the existence of PHAC in Canada when COVID-19 arose mitigated the worst problems experienced in 2003, it was subsequently weakened through federal politics and did not prevent the same kind of problem that Canada had experienced from other public health crises from occurring yet again.

Public policy change, in this account, is a more complex sphere of winners and losers, where aspirational declarations that "we must do better" are rarely executed into substantive policy outcomes. But it would be wrong to imply that clear improvements are simply stymied by opportunistic political players. Rather, the key issues arose during COVID-19 because there was tension between competing but defensible choices. Committing to one beneficial outcome can involve costs that others (not unjustly) will censure. Thus, rather than thinking about public health reform as a set of "patches" or "fixes" that improve the entire system, our analyses see the public policy challenges in rethinking public health as tensions or competing choices that lead to negative externalities as well as improvements and galvanize interests to condemn or resist policy directions.

As described in the previous section, the tricky aspect of comparing causal outcomes across political regimes is in determining whether they are similar enough to merit comparison. Are we comparing apples to apples, or apples to refrigerators — and, if the former, why do similar regimes exhibit different outcomes? The starting point for this volume is that COVID-19 produced the same kinds of policy tensions in each jurisdiction but because of the specific institutional and organizational architecture (or "scaffolding"), sociopolitical context, and level of economic or technological capacity, different (and sometimes contradictory) policy choices were made. Conceptually, we situate comparative public health policy within a similar set of competing tensions and then try to understand how each regime addressed these tensions through a more granular analysis. We have selected a diverse group of states in order to provide a wide range of political and institutional contexts, including various regions within the European Union (EU) (Sweden, France, and Croatia/Slovenia), directly outside the EU (the UK and Russia), and the EU itself (which, as a political player, both coordinated a response to the pandemic but also benefitted from the role which it played). Complementing the focus on Europe are case studies from Australia and Canada, two seemingly comparable states that nonetheless exist a world apart and that face quite distinct structural and contextual realities.

The following are the key tensions that structured public policy challenges during COVID-19 identified in this volume. How have they informed states' attempts to restructure their public health systems?

1.3.1 *Temporal tensions*

The first of these tensions, as noted earlier, was between the need to present a coherent, rapid, and accountable response to COVID-19 that, over time, obstructed the flexibility and nimbleness needed to adapt to shifting epidemiological realities and social responses. This tension is also ingrained more deeply within public health itself, where infectious disease management, once a pathogen arrives, can be addressed more effectively within an outbreak-focused command-and-control structure.

Nonetheless, the day-to-day work of keeping communities healthy outside pandemic conditions can require an extensive fascia of public health officials working with local populations, doing public health from the ground up rather than the top down. It may benefit from a "health in all policies" approach built on a horizontal model of governance rather than a vertical one. More decentralized systems can also have a greater challenge in responding to pandemic-level crises; the experiences of both Australia and Canada here are illustrative of that point. The devolved structure of the UK's health system is also indicative of this organizational challenge: as Bartlett explains, some public health measures were determined centrally across the UK, while others were the responsibility of devolved public health bodies in Scotland, Wales, and Northern Ireland. But, because England's public health strategy was governed only by the central UK public health authorities, confusion arose regarding what public health measures were meant only for England, and which applied across the UK. (The Hallett inquiry has also cast light on these structural issues, including the fact that Northern Ireland's public health office only had observer status at the UK public health table.).

At the same time, an underlying command-and-control structure in and of itself can be problematic insofar as it limits the voices involved in public health management and poses a barrier to transparency in decision-making. This is most glaringly the case of Russia, as Paul describes, but also applies to France, where formal public health bodies found themselves relegated to observer status only.

Yet the issue is not simply one of whether vertical or horizontal management models are superior; a more difficult tension is that a model that is well-suited to one stage of pandemic management may not work well in subsequent stages or such a long-term and all-of-society event. A major public health crisis cannot be understood as a single point in time; it is an evolving situation where a rigid structure that cannot respond nimbly to change can become a liability. Very few pandemic plans conceptualize the temporality of pandemic management well (to the extent that it can be done well at all). What works effectively at the outset can become an obstacle when circumstances change, yet decision-makers are loath to relinquish strategies that have worked well for them.

1.3.2 *The tension between narrow clinical outcomes and wider sociopolitical outcomes*

One of the most fascinating aspects of comparative public health management during COVID-19 was the way in which states framed the nature of the problem. Many jurisdictions formally saw the pandemic primarily in terms of clinical outcomes, where the only important variable was the prevalence and severity of the pathogen. As the Australian authors note, a pandemic management report published only three months before COVID-19 did not foresee "larger social disruptions" as a policy problem to be addressed even in a worst-case scenario. As in other states (including Canada and the UK), the conceptualization of the severity of the pandemic was measured only in clinical data focusing largely on hospitalization and mortality due to COVID-19.

The most remarkable contrast to this is the pandemic strategy taken by Sweden where, as the Swedish authors note, there was no mandatory quarantine and little employment of contact tracing. While classroom size was reduced, schools were not closed, and remote work was not mandatory. Rather than demanding that people stay indoors, outdoor activity was strongly encouraged. Domestic travel was not restricted, international travelers were not quarantined, and mask mandates were limited only to public transport. And yet, as the authors point out, the mortality indicators for Sweden were moderate and certainly lower than those for countries that had imposed more rigorous measures, including the UK, Spain, Austria, and Italy. The perplexing issue of excess non-COVID mortality is also relatively low in Sweden in comparison to many other countries.

Why did Sweden choose an independent path, despite considerable international opprobrium? From the very beginning, Sweden had decided to make a considered attempt to balance clinical outcomes with wider sociopolitical ones. Institutionally, its Communicable Disease Act even stipulates that any containment measures *must* be both proportionate and "based on science and proven experience." This required public health authorities publicly to acknowledge the costs and disadvantages of exceptional public health measures. It also expected them to justify these measures with reference to high-quality scientific studies — which, when COVID-19 began, were quite limited in scope and depth. The reason that masking was so limited was because the clinical evidence for widely encompassing mask mandates was negligible (and those that existed were of poor quality). Given the poor quality of the available data, such large-scale intrusive public health strategies simply could not be coherently justified.

Sweden's willingness to understand pandemic management from a much wider perspective is also comprehendible as an aspect of Sweden's well-documented practice of viewing "health" within the parameters of the larger social determinants of health. But this was not the only variable that influenced countries' unwillingness to impose protracted public health restrictions. Smaller countries heavily dependent on tourist dollars, for example, (such as Croatia), were quite cognizant that strict public health measures, especially as widespread immunity grew, had to be balanced against the pressing economic need to reestablish tourism, a critical economic industry for the region.

1.3.3 *Tensions between equity and universality*

A related, but even more inherently political, tension is the question of how marginalized populations should be addressed in systems that already pride themselves in offering universal healthcare. The question of how widely to distribute limited healthcare resources — a perennially political issue — became exacerbated during the pandemic when the well-being of the better-off became more closely dependent on the well-being of the most marginalized. Vulnerable groups, by definition, are more susceptible to highly contagious diseases. Yet political resistance to measures focusing on these groups arises not only because resources are limited but also because of a worry that engaging these groups may institutionalize their political influence over the longer term. One might also be concerned that well-intentioned efforts to protect vulnerable groups from discrimination perversely led to insufficient attention to their higher risks.

One key focus resulting from COVID-19 was on long-term care facilities, many of which had inadequate ventilation and poor infection control. That these facilities were sub-optimal was not unknown; they simply were not a priority. The conditions within long-term care facilities were exacerbated by labor force policies that utilized casual and part-time employees to keep costs down, resulting in a cadre of support workers who regularly worked across multiple institutions, providing an efficient vector of infection. Industries such as meat processing were also disproportionately affected by COVID-19 morbidity due to close proximity in the workspace, especially in countries such as Canada (which depends on temporary foreign workers in this area), and the close living quarters workers were given compounded this susceptibility to transmission. Communities of discrete ethnic communities, often wary of public authority, were also more susceptible to the spread of COVID-19, especially if inhabitants were highly engaged in public-facing service jobs that increased their exposure to the virus.

Pandemic reports in many countries have identified these vulnerable areas, although few seem committed to invest the funds and political capital to make any real change. Australia has formally noted the importance of equity concerns in addressing pandemic management, although there is no clear evidence of how these aspirations will be operationalized. The UK, likewise, has recognized the increased vulnerability of marginalized populations but focuses on a strategy of changing individual behavior rather than on a strategy of structural reform. Unsurprisingly, the jurisdiction most articulate in the need to better focus on equity as a public health strategy — Sweden — is already one of the leaders in that area. Perhaps the most intriguing post-pandemic equity challenge will be the EU itself. Despite substantial regulatory powers, the EU has little capacity to redistribute economic resources from wealthier to poorer regions on a scale similar to any of its member states. Notwithstanding an initial haphazard response of *sauve qui peut*, the EU has, as Greer describes, taken advantage of the pandemic to become a more forceful player in the public health arena. Whether the EU is able to capitalize on this shift to achieve a more emphatic redistribution of funds — possibly through a strategy of debt mutualization — is now a question worth considering.

1.3.4 *Crisis management and open scientific discourse*

Finally, political choices must be understood within the context of larger epistemological issues surrounding the nature of science and scientific discourse. Regardless of the highly disparate selection of public health and related policy instruments employed by the jurisdictions in this volume, they were always taken with reference to "following the science." Exactly what "science" was, and who would be the arbiter of that, was left unsaid. The tension here is quite clear: especially at the outset, pandemic management may involve invasive social actions that must be performed immediately and comprehensively. The public health messaging must be clear and convincing. Those subject to restrictions must understand exactly what is expected of them and why. They must be given reassurance that the policy-making process is in good hands. The problem, of course, is that (especially at the outset of a major event) solid and reliable data are limited. There is a strong political imperative for governments to be seen to be "doing something," and judgment calls must be made.

Yet "science" in its truest form is an iterative process of challenge and debate. As the Australian chapter notes, in many cases, there was a perception that "the battle was more important than the evidence" and that the evidence could be chosen selectively to support a particular policy strategy. Few jurisdictions were completely transparent about how the "scientific evidence" on which policy choices were made was selected. Was there a scientific council? Who chose the council? Was any such council limited to responding to specific questions put to it by decision-makers, or did it have the ability to articulate best practices independently? If there was no clear scientific council, who gave advice to the chief public health officer? And to what extent was this advice taken or rejected by policy-makers?

As the pandemic lengthened, and the evidence base kept increasing, scientific voices themselves became more fractured as they disagreed over the relevance or integrity of studies and statistics. The disagreement between public health officials, and the influence this had on formal public health advisory groups, is a recurring theme in these case studies. In Slovenia, for example, the government-appointed expert group was dissolved in 2022, and its function was taken over by the National Institute of Public Health, led by an epidemiologist who had left the former advisory group (twice) due to his lack of confidence in its advice. The French government bypassed formal public health bodies and instead set up selective *ad hoc* groups of clinical practitioners to provide advice. In the UK, the Scientific Advisory Group for Emergencies (SAGE) was expected to communicate advice to government "within the political frame in which it was requested," leading to an "independent SAGE" that declared itself free of the political whip and financial conflicts of interest. And, in Canada, where public health policy-making was significantly decentralized, 13 jurisdictions pursued quite different (and sometimes conflicting) pandemic management strategies over the course of COVID-19 — all based, of course, on science.

Another aspect of this tension was the level of tolerance (or intolerance) for medical and scientific voices which were uneasy with the quality of scientific evidence underlying public health policies (such as the main mode of disease transmission, the lack of data and rapid authorization mechanisms for novel vaccines and antivirals, the incidence of severe adverse events resulting from them, or the utility of masking school-age children during the Omicron phase). The need to keep formal public health messaging "clear" by censoring scientific opinion that challenged it, in the long run, only served to deepen public distrust in "scientific" messaging across the board.

But there were notable exceptions. In December 2021, Croatia's Constitutional Court declared that public health decisions delivered by the government's Civil Protection Headquarters had to contain reasoning that would justify the measures undertaken (including clear metrics and reference to public health measures taken in other jurisdictions). In Sweden, as noted earlier, the Communicable Disease Act requires disease containment to be based on measures that are both proportionate and "based on science and proven experience." Tellingly, as the Swedish analysis describes, public support for the country's public health strategy remained high, in sharp contrast to the high level of public disillusionment and distrust in other states as the pandemic continued.

1.4 Conclusion

The COVID-19 pandemic was not an unanticipated event. WHO had in place a clear set of obligations on its member states through the International Health Regulations and a formal process of review and planning for improvement (Kandel *et al.*, 2020). All jurisdictions included in this volume had some form of public health crisis plan in place: the pandemic planning document in Russia was produced six months before COVID-19 appeared, while Australia's report was published a mere three months prior to COVID-19. And yet, as the authors in this volume observe, Australia's report spent little time discussing the interventions that ultimately played the greatest role in pandemic management, including lockdown, better ventilation, and masking policies. No doubt more reports will be produced across countries asking why so many gaps and failures occurred despite all the pandemic readiness plans that had been dutifully compiled.

This volume suggests that any forensic analyses that do not thoughtfully consider the wider structural and contextual factors within which public health is embedded will be no more useful than the fix-it reports that get filed away after every public health crisis each state encounters. The legal frameworks, the organizational structure of public health, the political culture of a state, and even the nature of the broader healthcare system will influence not only the explanation of what went wrong but also the possibility that things will ever be otherwise.

The overarching political structure of a state is the most obvious hard constraint. Federal or decentralized states do have a more difficult time during public health crises, as the requirement to establish clear channels of communication and to have a precise delineation of roles and responsibilities under heightened governance conditions can be daunting. The case studies of both Australia and Canada illustrate the difficulty of implementing an effective national pandemic management strategy when the political authority for so many public health functions rests with discrete regional units, and exhortations that federal states must simply try harder to coordinate at a national level show a poor understanding of the political dynamics involved. Even Sweden has reflected on whether its more decentralized governance structure in relation to other Nordic states might have contributed to its poorer pandemic metrics. The effect of COVID-19, like earlier public health crises, will lead more federal states to establish national institutions that can help coordinate public health measures, especially in emergency conditions, but even this (as Canada illustrates) is not a sufficient solution to the challenge of developing effective multilevel response relationships.

At the same time, however, devolved authority certainly has its advantages for public health. Especially with larger geographical states, the ability of disparate regions to be able to tailor public health responses more specifically to discrete populations can be effective not only from a public health perspective but also in terms of local populations accepting or "owning" the measures imposed on them.

But multilevel governance is not the only structural limitation shaping effective public health reform. As Sokal observes in his study of Croatia and Slovenia, a more fragmented political system — one that is built on a shifting coalition of several political parties — rarely has the ability to push through sweeping policy reform, especially compared to majoritarian parliamentary governments.

Another structural variable that will have an effect on a state's public health response during a crisis, as well as its willingness to rethink public health management in the wake of the crisis, is its relationship to political entities beyond its borders. The role of the EU is particularly evident in these case studies. As the Hallett inquiry has shown, "Brexit distraction" played a role in poor pandemic preparedness in the UK. The drive by the EU to provide various forms of public health assistance for its member states — facilitated by key players such as France — not only mitigated the worst effects of the pandemic for some of these states, but it also served to reinforce the relevance of the EU itself. And the lure of EU funding is especially influential for smaller member states in their willingness to rethink public health and public healthcare structures in light of vulnerabilities exposed by the pandemic. The current debates around a new "pandemic treaty" being formulated through the United Nations is another example of these challenges of public health policy-making within an international context.

Beyond the intractable realities of the way in which states are politically structured, and the wider political context within which they are embedded, it is important to acknowledge the role that national institutions play not only in considering what kinds of solutions are possible but also the roles that they played in impeding or facilitating pandemic management. In Croatia, for example, where most primary care is performed by private physicians, there was considerable resistance by general practitioners in shouldering public health functions, such as the administration of testing. This tension was not evident in Slovenia, where primary care is largely provided publicly.

The pairing of Croatia and Slovenia also provides an excellent lesson in the role that courts played throughout the pandemic. In contrast to Croatia, where the Constitutional Court's interpretation of emergency public health measures undertaken by the government was generally supportive, the Constitutional Court of Slovenia refused to sanction a blanket emergency authorization law, requiring any emergency measures to be clearly and strictly circumscribed with reference to their specific function.

Finally, the pairing of Russia and Sweden also brings into sharp contrast the more inchoate but still potent role of political culture in attempting to establish an effective public health system. Notwithstanding the structural challenges confronting such a large and variegated country as Russia, there is also, as Paul describes, a general sense that a strong central authority is necessary for effective public administration and that "without this top-down pressure, the lower layers of the governance hierarchy do not invest enough effort for the effective implementation of state policies." This wide acceptance of a strong vertical hierarchy can, he notes, severely constrain the ability of policy entrepreneurs to make thoughtful improvements to public health systems. In Sweden, too, it is arguable that the underlying political culture played an important role in the country's pandemic response. As Forsberg and colleagues explain, the unique path undertaken by Sweden during the pandemic was perhaps influenced by a widespread sociocultural view that "a functioning economy is a prerequisite for people's well-being and health." The unwillingness of Sweden to impose restrictive public health measures was also supported by the knowledge that Swedes have a considerable level of social trust — even compared to other Nordic states — and would be more willing to follow advice suggested by public health authorities.

One legacy of COVID-19 has been an interest in comparing public health systems across jurisdictions. This volume suggests that such a task should be undertaken carefully with explicit attention to the perspectives of different disciplines and explicit and thoughtful examination of how their theories and concepts intersect (Wu *et al.*, 2022). The plasticity of the concept "public health" makes it quite difficult to cleanly categorize these systems on organizational or functional grounds. The purpose of this volume is to dig more deeply into the nature of public health systems and to understand them as products of distinct and diverse contexts. These embedded contexts can, frustratingly, mean that many policy solutions cannot simply be expected to produce effective results and that initiatives that work well in one state may not work well in others. Yet a deeper understanding of what can work in any particular jurisdiction (and what probably won't) is a useful starting point in attempting to rethink public health systems. A more systematic approach to thinking about public health systems is offered by Berman and Ruck in this volume. By having a better appreciation of the upstream factors that shape public health systems, they argue, we are better placed to understand why certain kinds of policies work, and others do not. Aspirational exhortations about how public health systems *ought* to work are useful as ideal models, but a richer understanding of the constraints on policy change may, in the longer run, produce more substantive results.

References

Böhm, K., Schmidt, A., Götze, R., Landwehr, C., and Rothgang, H. (2013). Five types of OECD healthcare systems: Empirical results of a deductive classification. *Health Policy*, *113*(3), 258–269. http://dx.doi.org/10.1016/j.healthpol.2013.09.003.

Kandel, N., Chungong, S., Omaar, A., and Xing, J. (2020). Health security capacities in the context of COVID-19 outbreak: An analysis of International Health Regulations annual report data from 182 countries. *Lancet, 395*, 1047–1053. https://doi.org/10.1016/S0140-6736(20)30553-5.

Litvak, E., Dufour, R., Leblanc, E., Kaiser, D., Mervure, S.-A., Tuong Nguyen, C., and Thibeault, L. (2020). Making sense of what exactly public health does: A typology of public health interventions. *Canadian Journal of Public Health, 111*, 65–71. https://doi.org/10.17269/s41997-00268-3.

Marchildon, G. P. (2022). Comparative healthcare systems in North America and Europe: Similarities and differences. In K. Fierlbeck and J. Cayón-de las Cuevas (Eds.), *Health Law and Policy from East to West: Analytical Perspectives and Comparative Case Studies* (pp. 37–54). Pamplona: Thomson Reuters/Editorial Aranzadi S.A.U.

Wang, D. and Mao, Z. (2021). A comparative study of public health and social measures of COVID-19 advocated in different countries. *Health Policy, 125*(8), 957–971. DOI: 10.1016/j.healthpol.2021.05.016.

Wendt, C., Frisina, L., and Rothgang, H. (2009). Healthcare system types: A conceptual framework for comparison. *Social Policy & Administration, 43*(1), 70–90. DOI: 10.1111/j.1467-9515.2008.00647.x

Wu, A., Khanna, S., Keidar, S., Berman, P., and Brubacher, L. J. (2022). How have researchers defined institutions, politics, organizations, and governance in research related to epidemic and pandemic response? A scoping review to map current concepts. *Health Policy and Planning 2022.* DOI: 10.1093/heapol/czac091.

© 2025 The Author(s)
https://doi.org/10.1142/9789811296307_0002

Chapter 2

What is Public Health? Problems of Definition and Conceptualization

Scott L. Greer and Margitta Mätzke

2.1 Introduction: The Swear Jar

It does not take long in and around public health discussions to hear the use of "public health" as if it were a unitary body: "Public health should" or "Public health does." It is easy to nod along with it, as if there were a single body with agency named "public health." But to do so is to contribute to the conceptual confusion that surrounds debates about the topic of public health and its politics, and thereby make it still harder to develop a political science in or of public health (Fafard *et al.*, 2023).

We propose the creation of a "swear jar" in all discussions of public health. A "swear jar" is a physical jar into which anybody who uses a forbidden word must put some money. In our proposal, anybody who uses the phrase "public health" without either scare quotes or a noun attached (e.g. public health advocates, agencies, researchers, approach, politics, policymakers, and discussions) should be obligated to put a unit of the local currency such as a dollar, euro, or pound into the jar.

This chapter makes the case for a swear jar, explains the problems revealed by speaking of "public health" as a person or unitary actor, and proposes some conceptualizations of the phenomena that make up "public health." It does not propose a final conclusion to the debate or even argue that there should be a conclusive conceptualization. Nor does it propose a use for the money accumulated in the swear jar, which (if implemented correctly) might be quite substantial.

2.2 Misplaced Concreteness in Public Health

"Misplaced concreteness" occurs when an abstract category or concept, such as "markets," "medicine," or "public health," is given too much concreteness in policy discussion, as in "markets decided," "public health is committed to equity," or "medicine treats the individual" (Brown, 1983). In each of these common phrases, there is an analytically problematic carelessness. In each case, misplaced concreteness naturalizes the phenomenon (e.g. hiding the ways in which markets are socially and politically constructed), implies intentional agency (as if public health were a single person with one mind and code of ethics), and disguises the internal diversity and fuzzy borders of the field (e.g. hiding the people in and near medicine who do not think in purely individualistic terms).

The reason for objecting to misplaced concreteness in general is that specifying the nature of variables — independent or dependent — is necessary for advancing a research agenda. In broader welfare state literature, for example, there is a long history of debate and work by political scientists and sociologists who specified the broad categories of welfare state programs (such as pensions, healthcare insurance, and disability insurance), basic functions of welfare states (such as insuring against old age and disability or investing in human capital), and a variety of indicators for outcomes and trajectories (such as replacement rates, catastrophic healthcare costs, or health indicators). While scholars constantly debate all of these issues, they are doing so within a framework crowded with existing variables and with a well-known set of basic ideas available.

Public health scholarship has many well-established technical concepts, especially in epidemiology, but none of that tacit agreement on what it is or does, and definitional debates (such as reviewed in (ASPHER, 2018)) are often abstract. Different concepts of public health will almost necessarily drive different kinds of analysis. It is also problematic and difficult because imprecision around the nature of the variable "public health" is in some sense unavoidable.

In this chapter, we present several different concepts, or perhaps better frames, for the phenomena of "public health," in order to illustrate different approaches. Our hope is to perhaps refine the conceptualizations and to show the stakes and possible advantages of different research approaches to different concepts. The study of public health might be impaired by the lack of an agreed-upon conceptual vocabulary with clear empirical utility, but a clean slate is by no means bad, and some debate about what "public health" actually should be seen as is a useful opportunity to clarify the purpose of studying public health and its politics.

2.3 Conceptualizations of Public Health

2.3.1 *Activities*

Important public health agencies, including the World Health Organization (WHO) and the US Centers for Disease Control and Prevention (CDC), have definitions of public health and what it does, and accreditors of public health education programs tend to mandate that students be taught these frameworks (Box 1).

Box 1. Defining public health by functions.

WHO Essential Public Health Functions (WHO, 2022)

(1) Monitoring and evaluating the population's health status, health service utilization and surveillance of risk factors and threats to health.
(2) Public health emergency management.
(3) Assuring effective public health governance, regulation and legislation.
(4) Supporting efficient and effective health systems and multisectoral planning, financing and management for population health.

(Continued)

(Continued)

(5) Protecting populations against health threats, including environment and occupational hazards, communicable disease threats, food safety, chemical and radiation hazards.

(6) Promoting prevention and early detection of diseases, including noncommunicable and communicable diseases.

(7) Promoting health and well-being and actions to address the wider determinants of health and inequity.

(8) Ensuring community engagement, participation and social mobilization for health and well-being.

(9) Ensuring adequate quantity and quality of public health workforce.

(10) Assuring quality of and access to health services.

(11) Advancing public health research.

(12) Ensuring equitable access to and rational use of essential medicines and other health technologies.

US CDC Essential Public Health Operations (*Centers for Disease Control and Prevention*, 2020)

(1) Assess and monitor population health status, factors that influence health, and community needs and assets.

(2) Investigate, diagnose, and address health problems and hazards affecting the population.

(3) Communicate effectively to inform and educate people about health, factors that influence it, and how to improve it.

(4) Strengthen, support, and mobilize communities and partnerships to improve health.

(5) Create, champion, and implement policies, plans, and laws that impact health.

(6) Utilize legal and regulatory actions designed to improve and protect the public's health.

(7) Assure an effective system that enables equitable access to the individual services and care needed to be healthy.

(8) Build and support a diverse and skilled public health workforce.

(9) Improve and innovate public health functions through ongoing evaluation, research, and continuous quality improvement.

(10) Build and maintain a strong organizational infrastructure for public health.

The status of these frameworks, regardless of their practical usefulness, is oddly ambiguous. It is not clear whether they mean that public health, to be public health, should have all these activities, or whether anybody performing those activities is somehow in public health whether they know and intend it or not, or whether it is simply a set of things that public health agencies really ought to do. In practice, they give students a rough sense of what is done, and they open up opportunities to conduct gap analyses and lobby for more responsibilities or resources in order to better fulfill these functions. Public health agencies advocating for new roles or additional resources need not be too concerned with the nature of public health or its explanation, and students who will find their own ways in the field of public health need landmarks more than a definition.

What can scholars empirically do to understand public health through this lens? Perhaps it would be possible to study its social construction and evolution since these lists were formulated in concrete meetings with minutes and known participants. Their evolution might be interesting, from the first time the need for such a list was perceived to the inclusion or removal of particular activities. Comparing and contrasting the two influential examples in Box 1 is already interesting. Such a study would teach us what key public health agencies and scholars worldwide regard as the key activities of public health and how such determinations are made, but it is an open question how much that explains or changes public health on the ground. As a guide to studying the broader politics and position of public health agencies or activities, it seems limited.

2.3.2 *Actors*

The second conceptualization of "public health" is as an actor — probably the most common source of violations of the rule that public health should be an adjectival phrase that comes with a noun. In this concept of public health, there are broadly two types of thoughts. One is that public health is a profession with education, credentials, and a measure of professional self-governance that allows it to act on its members and in broader political environments. The problem with this perspective is that it is at best a "minor profession," in Glazer's terminology (Glazer, 1974). Viewed as a profession, public health has very limited control over an intellectual domain, a strong tendency to lose out in contests with other professions (especially its near neighbor and perhaps landlord, clinical medicine), limited closure, and very weak self-government (since a public health qualification usually does not entitle its bearers to do restricted activities in the same way as a social work or medical qualification) (Abbott, 1994). The COVID-19 pandemic, in particular, showed that public health professionals' control over even a restricted domain such as infectious disease prevention, surveillance, and control is very limited. Government after government around the world sidelined public health agencies and managed the pandemic through *ad hoc* committees with representation from all sorts of experts and actors, such as modelers, virologists, and doctors, who had no professional public health affiliations (Greer *et al.*, 2022c).

The second approach is more explicitly political and normative and portrays public health as an activist cause, with an obligation for true public health practitioners to speak out against and work to change causes of avoidable mortality and morbidity, in particular unjust ones such as the consequences of class inequality or environmental racism. This approach is most often articulated precisely within internal conversations among self-identified public health practitioners between those whose aspiration is a profession and those whose aspiration looks more like a political actor. It is not necessarily common among working public health professionals, most of whom are, after all, government employees.

There are possibly syntheses. In particular, to claim that public health is a profession with a moral obligation to campaign is a longstanding move since at least Rudolf Virchow's work at the dawn of both microbiology and public health (Mackenbach, 2009; Taylor & Rieger, 1985). It is one with echoes across public health and medical history. Professional organizations and individual professions can and do campaign, and the resources and visibility of an organized profession are an excellent platform for advocates. There is nonetheless a tension here since it presumes something that cannot be presumed, which is that the normative commitments of the advocates and the findings of scientific inquiry will always be aligned. Nobody is capable of purely apolitical scientific inquiry, but there will always be a temptation to focus on results and studies that agree with authors' preferences about the world. In "normal science," there are a great many mechanisms that allow scientists to arbitrate findings regardless of the personalities and politics [reviewed in (Strevens, 2020)]. A field committed to advocacy risks losing that self-regulation.

Furthermore, professions' political activity always tends to come with tensions. The resources and visibility of an organized profession such as medicine tend to come about because of a deeply entrenched position in society, one with an agreed-upon function and many sources of support (a strong profession combines reputational uniqueness and political multiplicity to adapt Carpenter's formulation) (Carpenter, 2001). That position can be eroded to the extent that political actors, citizens, or their own members view its political campaigns as divisive or unhelpful. Picking sides in — or starting — political debates might not be helpful for a profession that depends on the state for other functions it performs (such as credentialling members, advocating for larger budgets, or providing advice). Interest groups of any kind that become part of a partisan coalition can gain when their party is in power but can lose credibility, autonomy, and policy influence if they are seen to be part of a political coalition.

Finally, the ability to define the public health field as a profession is limited and made problematic by the sheer diversity of things done in public health organizations. In particular, there is something of a tension between elite public health, made up of often well-funded and high-status researchers, and public health organizations on the ground, which are often concerned with low-status activities (restaurant inspection, water quality monitoring, or pest control) or target populations that are low-status, minoritized, and vulnerable (sex workers, poor people, or undocumented migrants). To the extent that public health as a profession means sexual health outreach or food service inspection, it loses status since professions get their status from their clients. To the extent that it is redefined as an elite activity based in universities and the top of government, it starts to look less and less like a profession, loses even more policy tools, and starts to resemble an academic discipline comparable to economics or criminology.

Much of the effort put into presenting public health as a profession or activist cause takes the form of institution-building or exhortation. The impact of such activities can be studied empirically. A more sophisticated research approach that takes these claims seriously, albeit one with measurement and data-gathering problems, would be to model public health as a network, presumably with professional organizations, universities, civil society organizations, and government agencies as major nodes. Pursued a bit further, the advocacy coalition framework for public policy or similar might be a good way to document and conceptualize public health as an actor.

2.3.3 Perspectives

The third approach to public health fundamentally views it as a perspective, worldview, or approach. In this perspective, there is a distinctive "public health approach" to understanding and addressing problems. The public health approach, in this definition, has a number of clearly repeated attributes: epidemiological reasoning, population-based thinking, prevention, harm reduction, and in many cases, community engagement and empowerment or an equity focus (just search on "public health approach" in any scholarly database). In particular contexts, this perspective-based approach has quite clear implications. For example, defining illegal drug use or illegal sex work as a public health problem rather than a moral problem or a criminal problem forecloses some approaches (police sweeps or shaming communication strategies) and opens up others (needle exchanges or demarcated safe places for sex workers). Whether that is the right approach is obviously a highly political question, but the choice of a public health approach to these questions brings along a clear set of commitments and policy tools.

By the same token, a public health approach to COVID-19 meant prevention, first non-pharmaceutical interventions and then vaccinations, in contrast to defeatism (e.g. herd immunity or denialist approaches), misplaced individualism (e.g. viewing masks as personal protection rather than source control of infection), or the common one of viewing the pandemic as a problem for the healthcare sector (seen in the logic of "flattening the curve" or the focus of so many politicians on hospital occupancy rather than infections) (Jarman, 2021).

The advantage of seeing public health as a perspective is that it can identify people who think in a similar way and might form advocacy coalitions across institutions to promote their views (Jenkins-Smith & Sabatier,

1994), as well as a style of reasoning that can be adopted by policymakers who have no formal affiliation with public health, in the same way that Popp Berman traced the "economic style of reasoning" across people and institutions with limited roles for formally trained economists (and the way that the spread of that style of reasoning, encouraged by trained economists, led to the hiring and empowering of economists in government) (Berman, 2022; Helgadóttir, 2016).

2.3.4 *Institutions*

The fourth approach is to focus on the instructional and organizational structures of public health, particularly in the context of government and law. In this approach, public health is essentially what governments and related large institutions say it is, with some modifications to local political language and laws. Thus, in most rich countries, public health would mean the public health departments in the local and regional government, the central public health agency, the academic research and teaching enterprise called public health, some NGOs with clear public health missions as accepted by the named parts of government, and a few parts of central government that are named as and clearly involved in the same activities. That would be the field of public health.

This approach is perhaps the easiest target for empirical research and has some important advantages. It creates some comparability and generally does produce cross-national agreement on the core components of a public health body (such as surveillance, field epidemiology, advice, communications, and health education campaigns). It does not require that investigators specify *a priori* what public health should mean, which removes a major possible source of bias. Thus, for example, nominalism allows us, in the European Union (EU), to watch the public health policy space slowly incorporate (or at least start to overlay) other policy areas by watching the increasing use of the public health treaty article (168 TFEU) as a treaty base or the functions of the relevant Directorate-General (Greer & Jarman, 2021; Greer *et al.*, 2022b).

Bodies such as the EU and WHO define public health agencies (including the functions listed in Box 1) and oblige member states to nominate agencies and people as representatives, which creates more isomorphism: the notifying bodies of the European Centre for Disease Prevention and Control (ECDC) network are, in the EU, the presumptive center of each member states' public health undertakings, and they have indeed been getting more organizationally homogeneous since the creation of the ECDC. Compare the situation today with the far more diverse situation recorded in (Elliott *et al.*, 2012).

That increased European organizational homogeneity reflects a broader argument that is enabled by this approach. It takes advantage of, and allows us to study, the social construction of a transnational field and category (Meyer & Rowan, 1991; Scott & Meyer, 1991). There is clear institutional isomorphism in the tendency of agencies around the world to include the initials "CDC" in their English-language names. For those who find isomorphism arguments too disembodied, there are also a host of funding schemes, associations, and how-to books for the creation and extension of specific kinds of public health agencies (consult IANPHI, the International Association of National Public Health Institutes, for example).

This approach risks nominative determinism, in which names rather than substance determine activities and formal competence becomes confused with real competence (Mätzke, 2012). Is restaurant inspection part of public health? Not in England after 1974, where it is part of environmental health because "public health" was split off and integrated into the National Health Service (NHS), leaving former areas of public health jurisdiction such as environmental health and social work in local government (the public health function was "returned" to local government in 2014, but it remains a separate funding stream to local governments).

In short, institutionalist approaches have many advantages but they probably must be used pragmatically to avoid nominative determinism, and too much pragmatism can simply reopen all the debates about the nature of public health.

2.3.5 *Functions*

Fifth and finally, there is functionalist reasoning: by its manifest and latent activities in society shall you know it. Functionalist reasoning is hardly popular in the contemporary social sciences, (and for good reasons) but there is functionalism to be found in any kind of social argument. In particular, there is a sensible enough argument that public health should be understood as "addressing a problem" and evaluated as such. In public health classrooms, this can often be stated in a definition of public health as the field that addresses collective causes of avoidable morbidity and mortality. If it collectively reduces avoidable mortality, it is "public health" regardless of whether it is a vaccination mandate, parental leave, a needle exchange, or a drainage ditch that stops mosquitos breeding.

By that standard, the field of public health, and the standing to intervene in the policy of those who claim to speak for public health, is immense: not just inserting "health in all policies" into education or transport debates but potentially viewing nuclear war as a public health problem because it would undeniably be a major source of avoidable mortality. This view, at the extreme, is obviously nonsense. A public health degree does not confirm expertise or power in education or transport or grand strategy, and somebody who claims it does is likely to be laughed out of politics (Fox, 2003) (Greer *et al.*, 2018). Hence, the focus of the "Health in All Policies" or "Health for All Policies" literature is on politics, coalition-building, and advocacy with other sectors (Greer *et al.*, 2022a). Notably, the role of public health agencies and the topics of public health researchers in the 2022 Russian invasion of Ukraine, one of the biggest land wars since World War II, did not address the justice or strategy of Russia and Ukraine. Agencies' behavior and scholars' response alike focused on target populations and problems well known to them, such as sex work and human trafficking, refugee health, and communicable diseases. Those were far from the biggest sources of avoidable mortality associated with the invasion of Ukraine, but there was a tacit acceptance that the generals did not need to hear about strategy from the epidemiologists.

While Russia's invasion of Ukraine showed the limits of public health claims in the face of vast and needless suffering, the COVID-19 pandemic showed how common it is to adopt a rough and ready functionalist definition of public health that evaluates its success by its ability to control infectious disease. This is what is happening whenever the success or failure of a country's "public health" is evaluated by reference to COVID-19 cases, COVID-19-attributed mortality, or excess mortality. The equation is problematic on both sides. On the outcome side, measures of the damage of COVID-19 are variable, subject to vast and political measurement error, and in many countries, unavailable. But on the other side, it is unclear that COVID-19 outcomes tested public health as an actor, institution, or approach since nowhere did public health agencies or scholars make up the whole response and, in most cases, they did not lead it in any meaningful sense.

2.4 Conclusion: From Lamentation and Misplaced Concreteness to Political Science

If misplaced concreteness often starts a public health conversation, then the end is frequently lamentation. Conversations in public health scholarship, conventions, and agencies often focus on the weakness, poor resourcing, and low status of their field relative to rivals (notably healthcare), the problems public health faces, or the scale of government enterprise. Cost-effective and equitable public health policies, practitioners, and academics lament are pushed aside in favor of other political priorities, while "health" is widely regarded as the activity of doctors, not those with a Masters of Public Health or public health nursing qualifications. Special interests, lack of political will, the short time horizons of politicians, and other stock concepts of political discussion in public health all play their role. Sometimes the target is the superiority of medicine; sometimes the target is health inequalities; sometimes the target is more political, but the scale of group grievance is hard to miss.

People with many points of view might agree that societies should invest more energy and resources in public health activities, or public health professionals and advocates, or preventative, collective health measures, or policies focused on the reduction of avoidable morbidity and mortality. But as social scientists, there are serious limitations to analysis that starts by asking why one particular interest, however nebulously defined, is not pursued with more vigor. Asking what public health comes to mean and explaining that is a far more productive approach. In the same way, breaking down the welfare state into variables connected with stratification and risks made it easier to understand and measure without cutting off theoretical debate about its nature and explanations.

We provided conceptions of public health found in the literature, with greater or lesser degrees of novelty, articulation, and acceptance. Each of these approaches has advantages and disadvantages, ranging from concordance with public health textbooks to concordance with law to concordance with what we might like to see in society. It might be that advancing on all fronts is the best approach, e.g. try a comparison with a country or pair and see how different they actually are.

Each perspective at least has the advantage of forcing the question: public health what? Public health tasks, actors, perspectives, institutions, or functions? Research focused on the dissemination of public health perspectives or the growth of public health institutions might produce different explanations, but they will be explanations of defined variables rather than phenomena. The explanations might be less likely to adopt teleologies of autonomous professionalism, a Center for Disease Control, the transformation of capitalism, or something else. In doing so, they would also create new ways to understand public health and public health politics, even at the price of a lighter swear jar over time.

Acknowledgment

We would like to thank Rachel Kulikoff, Katherine Fierlbeck and Peter Berman, for their comments.

References

Abbott, A. (1994). *The System of Professions: An Essay on the Division of Expert Labor*. Chicago: University of Chicago Press.

Association of Schools of Public Health of the European Region (ASPHER) (2018). ASPHER's European list of core competences for the public health professional. *Scandinavian Journal of Public Health*, *46*(23_suppl), 1–52. DOI: 10.1177/1403494818797072.

Berman, E. P. (2022). *Thinking Like An Economist*. Princeton: Princeton University Press.

Brown, L. D. (1983). *Politics and Health Care Organization: HMOs as Federal Policy*. Washington, DC: Brookings Institution.

Carpenter, D. P. (2001). *The Forging of Bureaucratic Autonomy: Reputations, Networks, and Policy Innovation in Executive Agencies, 1862–1928.* Princeton: Princeton University Press.

Centers for Disease Control and Prevention (2020). 10 Essential public health services. https://www.cdc.gov/publichealthgateway/publichealthservices/essentialhealthservices.html.

Elliott, H., Jones, D. K., and Greer, S. L. (2012). Mapping infectious disease control in the European Union. *Journal of Health Politics, Policy, and Law,* *37*(6), 935–954.

Fafard, P., de Leeuw, E., and Cassola, A. (Eds.). (2022). *Integrating Science and Politics for Public Health.* Cham, Switzerland: Springer.

Fox, D. M. (2003). Population and the law: The changing scope of health policy. *Journal of Law, Medicine and Ethics, 31,* 607–614.

Glazer, N. (1974). The schools of the minor professions. *Minerva, 12*(3), 346–364. DOI: 10.1007/bf01102529.

Greer, S. L., Bekker, M. P. M., Azzopardi-Muscat, N., and McKee, M. (2018). Political analysis in public health: Middle-range concepts to make sense of the politics of health. *European Journal of Public Health, 28*(suppl_3), 3–6. DOI: 10.1093/eurpub/cky159.

Greer, S. L., Falkenbach, M., Siciliani, L., McKee, M., Wismar, M., and Figueras, J. (2022a). From health in all policies to health for all policies. *The Lancet Public Health.* https://doi.org/10.1016/S2468-2667(22)00155-4.

Greer, S. L., Rozenblum, S., Fahy, N., Brooks, E., de Ruijter, A., Palm, W. I., and Wismar, M. (2022b). *Everything you always wanted to know about European Union health policy but were afraid to ask* (3rd, completely revised ed.). Brussels: WHO/European Observatory on Health Systems and Policies.

Greer, S. L., Massard da Fonseca, E., Raj, M., and Willison, C. E. (2022c). Institutions and the politics of agency in COVID-19 response: Federalism, executive power, and public health policy in Brazil, India and the U.S. *Journal of Social Policy.*

Greer, S. L. and Jarman, H. (2021). What is EU public health and why? Explaining the scope and organization of public health in the European Union. *Journal of Health Politics, Policy and Law, 46*(1), 23–47. DOI: 10.1215/03616878-8706591.

Helgadóttir, O. (2016). The Bocconi boys go to Brussels: Italian economic ideas, professional networks and European austerity. *Journal of European Public Policy, 23*(3), 392–409. DOI: 10.1080/13501763.2015.1106573.

Jarman, H. (2021). State responses to the COVID-19 pandemic: Governance, surveillance, coercion and social policy. In S. L. Greer, E. J. King, A. Peralta-Santos, and E. Massard da Fonseca (Eds.), *Coronavirus Politics: The Comparative Politics and Policy of COVID-19*. Ann Arbor, Michigan: University of Michigan Press.

Jenkins-Smith, H. C. and Sabatier, P. (1994). Evaluating the advocacy coalition framework. *Journal of Public Policy, 14*, 175–203.

Mackenbach, J. P. (2009). Politics is nothing but medicine at a larger scale: Reflections on public health's biggest idea. *Journal of Epidemiol Community Health, 63*(3), 181–184. DOI: 10.1136/jech.2008.077032.

Mätzke, M. (2012). Commentary: The institutional resources for communicable disease control in Europe: Diversity across time and place. *Journal of Health Politics, Policy, and Law, 36*(1), 967–976.

Meyer, J. W. and Rowan, B. (1991). Institutionalized organizations: Formal structure as myth and ceremony. In W. W. Powell and P. J. DiMaggio (Eds.), *The New Institutionalism in Organizational Analysis* (pp. 41–62). Chicago: University of Chicago Press.

Scott, W. R. and Meyer, J. W. (1991). The organization of societal sectors: Propositions and early evidence. In W. W. Powell and P. J. DiMaggio (Eds.), *The New Institutionalism in Organizational Analysis* (pp. 108–142). Chicago: University of Chicago Press.

Strevens, M. (2020). *The Knowledge Machine: How Irrationality Created Modern Science*. New York: Liveright Publishing.

Taylor, R. and Rieger, A. (1985). Medicine as social science: Rudolf Virchow on the typhus epidemic in Upper Silesia. *International Journal of Health Services, 15*(4), 547–559.

World Health Organization (WHO). (2022). *21st Century Health Challenges: Can the essential public health functions make a difference? Discussion Paper*. Geneva: WHO. Retrieved from https://www.who.int/teams/integrated-health-services/health-service-resilience/essential-public-health-functions.

Chapter 3

Sweden

Birger C Forsberg, Miriam Mosesson, My Fridell,
and Göran Tomson

3.1 Introduction

Sweden is a country on the Scandinavian peninsula in Northern Europe with a population of 10.5 million (SCB, 2022). The average life span is 84 years for women and 81 years for men. Sweden has proportionally one of Europe's largest elderly populations. About 20% of the Swedish population were 65 years or older in 2019. Most of them (96%) lived at home, of which about 40% lived alone.

The current population growth rate is approximately 1% per year, with immigration contributing around 75% of that growth. Around 20% of the population is "immigrant" in the sense that they were born outside Sweden. Syria has generally been the most common country of origin among immigrants. Other prominent countries of origin are Iraq, Poland, Iran, Somalia, and Afghanistan. However, in total the four Nordic countries other than Sweden are still the most common place of birth for immigrants (SCB Statistikdatabasen, 2023).

The government system in Sweden is characterized by multilevel governance with three levels of vital decision-making: national, regional, and municipal. Each level is ruled by a parliament or a council to which politicians are elected every fourth year. All levels raise taxes to carry out their duties and responsibilities. The politicians are responsible to the electorate in their constituency and not to the other levels. Hence, the Swedish government system is not hierarchical but formed of three levels that have the power and mandate to rule within their jurisdiction.

3.1.1 *Public health organization*

Public health functions in Sweden are distributed among many agencies and actors. The Public Health Agency Folkhälsomyndigheten (FoHM) has the responsibility to provide advice on public health developments and interventions based on available evidence. The agency produces guidelines and advice available to all actors, including the public. The Public Health Agency is responsible for monitoring health developments in the population and regularly reporting on those developments.

The agency does not implement preventive programs; rather, it provides financial support to non-governmental organizations that are active in health promotion and prevention when commissioned to do so by the government. FoHM is the national agency with the authority for communicable disease control.

Regions in Sweden are responsible for financing healthcare services, and they also provide the bulk of those health services. The regions can choose their level of engagement in broader public health prevention. Regions finance antenatal care and child health check-ups. They are also responsible for the implementation of national child vaccination programs. These programs are decided upon by the government at the recommendation of the Public Health Agency and financed by the national government. The regions are legally responsible for communicable disease control within their constituencies.

Municipalities in Sweden have the main responsibility for essential public health functions, such as water, sanitation, and food control. Many municipalities are also, to a varying degree, active in promotion of healthy lifestyles and health-supportive environments (such as safe bicycle routes to school). Preschools and schools are financed by municipalities. Most are also operated by the municipalities, but private schools exist. They operate under agreements with the municipalities and abide by the same rules and regulations as the public actors. Pre-schools and schools have the responsibility for all matters related to teaching children up to the age of 18, and matters related to health are part of that instruction. School health services have the responsibility for national vaccination programs for school-aged children.

Public responsibility for broader societal determinants of health of the population, such as transport systems, housing, food production and markets, and socio-economy, falls under different government agencies and ministries. There is no formal coordination of the work of these agencies with regard to public health. However, the Swedish government has made a strong commitment to the Sustainable Development Goals (SDG) and Agenda 2030. Within that framework, action has been taken to facilitate communication and collaboration between different government agencies.

An organogram summarizing the Swedish government structure for public health is given in Figure 3.1.

Many different laws have implications for the way society acts in relation to public health determinants, but none of them are specific to public health. The Swedish Parliament has adopted a National Public Health Policy which defines eight target areas that are key to public health developments. Qualitative goals are set within each target area (Prop., 2017/18:249). The Public Health Agency has the task to monitor the National Public Health Policy.

Many Swedish non-governmental organizations are active in health promotion. There are organizations addressing the use of drugs, alcohol, tobacco, nicotine, etc. while others are promoting physical activity or supporting mental health. Some NGOs actively provide individual support to people and families who have been hit by mental illness or various life-crisis events. Most of the NGOs receive financial support from the national, regional, or municipality level for their work.

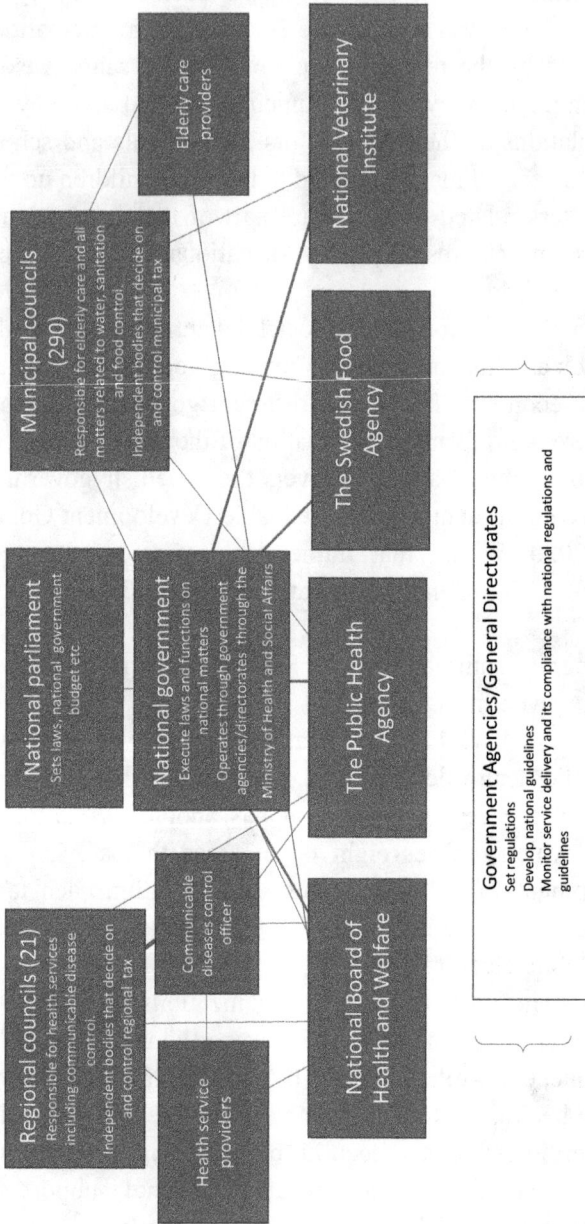

Figure 3.1.   Essential public health functions in the government system in Sweden.

3.1.2 *National-level organization*

Sweden is a constitutional monarchy built on parliamentarianism, meaning that the government is responsible to the Parliament (Riksdagen). The Prime Minister is approved by the Parliament. The Riksdagen sets all laws in the Swedish system. The Parliament also approves the government budget. Traditionally, the national government's main steering tools are decrees or laws. The national level has limited financial power over the operations in the regions and municipalities as their main sources of income are regional or municipal taxes.

The Ministry of Health and Social Affairs is responsible in the country for overall healthcare and social care, including elderly care. However, the Ministry does not have direct power over the regions and municipalities.

Several government agencies and general directorates are responsible for regulating, analyzing, and evaluating health and social services. Foremost among them are

- The National Board of Health and Welfare (Socialstyrelsen — SoS).
- The Medical Products Agency (Läkemedelsverket — LMV).
- The Dental and Pharmaceutical Benefits Agency (Tandvårds-och läkemedelsförmånsverket — TLV).
- The Public Health Agency (Folkhälsomyndigheten — FoHM).
- The Health Care and Social Care Inspectorate (Inspektionen för vård och omsorg — IVO).

The agencies work within their terms of reference as given by the regulations for each respective agency. The government agencies and general directorates provide guidelines for operations. They are in most cases not legally binding. The government agencies monitor and follow up how well services are provided. They also work on investigations given to them by the Ministry of Health and Social Affairs. Such tasks are often linked to on-going needs for the development of services or to service issues brought up in the public debate.

There is little formal coordination between the agencies. Such coordination must go through the ministry.

All five agencies listed earlier became actively involved in the corona pandemic control in various ways. In addition, the Swedish Civil Contingencies Agency (Myndigheten för samhällsskydd och beredskap — MSB) had an important role in actions required in other sectors than the health and social sectors during the pandemic control.

Universities are under the responsibility of the national government. Health professionals are trained at universities. Specialist training is done while working in health services that fall under the authority of the regions. Auxiliary staff, such as assistant nurses and social care assistants, receive their degrees from high schools. High schools fall under the responsibility of municipalities.

3.1.3 *Regional organization*

Sweden is divided into 21 regions. The main responsibility of a region is healthcare. Regions mostly act as purchasers and regulate provision of care through agreements and contracts. Around 12% of public expenditures on healthcare are spent on buying services from private providers. The rest goes to provider units that are owned and operated by the regions. About 46% of visits in primary healthcare, 13% of visits in specialist outpatient care, and 18% of visits in psychiatric ambulatory take place through private services (Vårdföretagarna, 2019).

In general, private providers did not differ from public providers in relation to given tasks or behavior during the COVID-19 pandemic. All providers that had agreements with the regions were compensated for loss of income that followed from heavy reduction of patients coming to the services. This resulted from the recommendation from the authorities to the public not to seek care during the lockdown of the country, other than for emergencies.

There are 7 university hospitals and about 70 smaller hospitals in Sweden. Primary care is organized in approximately 1,200 healthcare centers. Primary care is responsible for basic medical treatment, preventive work, and rehabilitation.

Since 2015, there has been quite a significant growth in digital health services, driven by private investors and new private providers of these services. Digital advice and services are now also provided by public providers. Digital health accelerated during the pandemic. Use of the public sector advisory function on health and healthcare, named 1177, also increased significantly during that period.

3.1.4 *Municipal organization*

There are 290 municipalities in Sweden. In addition to the functions mentioned under 1, they provide basic healthcare below physician's level to patients in ordinary housing and in nursing homes under the leadership of a qualified nurse. They also provide rehabilitation by occupational therapists and physiotherapists. Municipalities do not employ doctors so any matters that require input from a doctor need to be covered by regionally financed health services. Often, there will be agreements between a municipality and a region to arrange for doctor visits on a regular basis to nursing homes.

3.2 The Legal Framework for Health and Social Care Provision

3.2.1 *Healthcare*

The Health and Medical Service Act (HSL) (SFS, 2017:30) regulates all healthcare in Sweden. Under the HSL, healthcare of high quality should be available to all citizens on equal terms (SFS, 2017:30). Municipal responsibility for home healthcare assumes an agreement between the municipality and the region to take over such responsibility (SFS, 2017:30).

In addition to the HSL (SFS, 2017:30), there are several laws that pertain to health services. The *Patient Act* (SFS, 2014:821) aims to strengthen and clarify the patient's position and to promote patient integrity, self-determination, and participation. A patient discharged from inpatient care has the right to receive summary information on the care and treatment provided during the period of care. The *Patient Safety in Health Care Act* (SFS, 2010:659) defines the professional responsibility of healthcare professionals to provide good and safe care. For care providers, there are supplementary provisions on their obligations to conduct systematic patient safety work (HSLF-FS, 2017:40, n.d.).

3.2.2 *Social elderly care in Sweden*

The *Social Services Act* (SFS, 2001:453) gives all citizens the right to claim public services and assistance to support themselves in their day-to-day existence if their needs cannot be met in any other way. The support includes social service, short-term housing, and social care in special housing and in the home (SFS, 2001:453). Special accommodation (Särskilt boende — SÄBO) is defined as an institution providing care around-the-clock, including care from a registered nurse, and resembles what is internationally called nursing homes. To get a place in a special accommodation, a person must have *major* medical and social needs. The needs are assessed by a qualified social care worker at the municipality level who accordingly decides what support the person can receive from the municipality. Some 12% of people over 65 years of age received healthcare and/or social care from the municipalities in 2019, 8% at home, and 4% in special accommodation (Socialstyrelsen, 2021).

Social care is mostly provided by professional staff, such as assistant nurses, but due to shortage of such staff, about 30–40% of the staff are not formally qualified for their tasks (IVO, 2019). Some of them may however have gained significant experience over the years working in the social care services, while others come and go. Additionally, 25% of staff in nursing homes are hourly employees who often work in several residences. This increases the risk of infections spreading from household to household (SOU, 2020:80). The turnover of staff in elderly care services became a much-discussed issue during the pandemic. So was the number of staff involved in visits to a particular person. Home care recipients met an average of 16 different staff during a 14-day period in 2021 (15 staff in 2020) with a variation from 7 to 24 staff among the country's municipalities (Socialstyrelsen, 2022a).

In 2009, a new act enacted by Parliament (the *Act on System of Choice in the Public Sector*, (SFS, 2008:962) gave the municipalities the opportunity to contract out services to private providers. The degree to which the municipalities apply the system of choice varies. In 2018, 19% of the special accommodation for older people and social care at home were privately operated (Vårdföretagarna, 2019).

3.2.3 *Coordination between healthcare and social care*

In 1992, a major reform, known as the Ädelreformen, took place. This changed responsibility for long-term inpatient healthcare and care for the elderly from county councils to municipalities (Anell *et al.*, 2012). As a result of this shift in responsibility, a municipality chief nurse (Medicinskt ansvarig sjuksköterska) was instated in the municipalities with responsibility for maintaining patient safety and quality of care in all the municipal healthcare services (SFS, 2017:30).

As the regions and municipalities enjoy a high degree of self-governance, they may apply different practices depending on the political and service leadership, on the healthcare needs of the residents, and on the healthcare infrastructure in the area (Rechel *et al.*, 2018). This fact was much discussed during the pandemic as there were challenges in making both health services and social care services comply with what was considered the most efficient way to contain the virus, contain its spread, and manage cases.

Better coordination of services from the municipality and the region has been called for, especially for the elderly who suffer from chronic and multiple diseases (SOU, 2020:80). An *Act on Coordinated Discharge* was implemented in 2017 to clarify the responsibilities (SFS, 2017:612). The act aims to promote good quality of healthcare and social service for individuals who, after discharge from inpatient care, need assistance from both regional and municipal services. One obstacle to coordination is the lack of a joint information system.

In 2017, the Health and Social Care Inspectorate (IVO) conducted a national oversight of 38 operations focusing on collaboration between inpatient care, primary care, rehabilitation, and home healthcare, regarding care of older people with comorbidities who were cared for in ordinary living (IVO, 2017). The report pointed to the need for improving staffing and staff continuity. The level of education of the nursing staff in elderly care varied not only in the country but also in the same municipalities. The need for continuous training of staff to adapt to new developments and methods was also called for. The inspection found that there were deficiencies in information transfer and lack of drug handling related to delegation of responsibilities to social care personnel. Overall, it was concluded that care transitions from regional to municipal providers could create unclear responsibilities for involved care professionals.

The challenges arising from inadequate coordination between regions and municipalities were issues raised as a possible reason for the pandemic hitting the elderly particularly hard. IVO made a review of how people in nursing homes were treated during the pandemic. IVO's review of medical records for 847 people diagnosed with COVID-19 in 98 special accommodation facilities showed that in as many as around 20% of those cases, no medical assessment took place at all. In 40% of these cases, there was no individual assessment by a nurse. Furthermore, IVO's review showed that less than 10% of the patients/care recipients received an assessment on-site in the accommodation (SOU, 2020:80).

3.2.4 *Communicable disease control and emergency preparedness*

Communicable disease control in Sweden is regulated by the *Communicable Disease Protection Act* (SFS, 2004:168). It gives the Public Health Agency (FoHM) the responsibility to provide regulations, guidelines, and information on communicable disease control and epidemic control. The agency is also given the task to coordinate communicable disease control at the national level among the government agencies. Furthermore, the Public Health Agency oversees communicable disease surveillance in the country.

The national act stipulates that the national government has the authority to decide on all matters related to which diseases shall be notifiable and the regulations around reporting cases from these diseases. As of February 2023, 27 diseases were classified as notifiable. Furthermore, diseases can be classified as threats to society (samhällsfarlig sjukdom). This allows more urgent measures to be taken to control the spread of the disease. Only three diseases are currently listed as "samhällsfarliga" (ebola, smallpox, and SARS). COVID-19 was classified as such a disease on February 1, 2020 through a government decree (Krisinformation, 2020a) and later through a temporary act adopted on January 10, 2021, the so-called "Pandemilagen" (SFS, 2021:4). A new act declassified COVID-19 as being a "samhällsfarlig sjukdom" from April 1, 2022 (Prop., 2021/22:137).

The decision-making of the government can be delegated to a relevant government agency. In communicable disease control, this is the Public Health Agency. The work at FoHM on epidemic control is coordinated by a State Epidemiologist. As mentioned, municipalities are in charge of food control and control of water sources and sanitation. During the pandemic, all matters related to control of restaurants and public spaces were entrusted to them.

Each region must have an emergency preparedness plan to be updated after each election period (SFS, 2006:544). A new structure for civil defense and emergency preparedness in Sweden was established on October 1, 2022 (SFS, 2022:524). The new regulation defines the preparedness sectors, civilian areas, and sector-responsible authorities. The National Board of Health and Welfare is the sector-responsible authority for preparedness within health and social care. The regions are responsible for provision of care during crises and for implementing their emergency preparedness plans.

3.3 Epidemiology and Control Measures

3.3.1 *Epidemiology of the disease*

The first case of COVID-19 in Sweden was confirmed on January 31, 2020 by the Public Health Agency. The person in question had visited Wuhan in China. The second case was reported on February 26 and five new cases on February 27. After that, the virus spread like wildfire in the population and, within very little time, many got ill and hospitals began to fill up with patients. Later it was proved that viral strains had arrived from many countries, mostly by Swedes going abroad on vacation. Mortality from the disease started to increase in March. There were reports of persons in the productive ages contracting the disease and developing serious symptoms. Soon, attention was directed toward nursing homes, in which many elderly expired. This pushed mortality rates in Sweden high in comparison with other countries, not least the other Scandinavian countries, during the first three months of the pandemic. Researchers debated this at length (King *et al.*, 2020) and public persons criticized the Public Health Agency for being too slow and too relaxed on the urgency of the situation created by the pandemic.

At the time of this writing in early June 2023, Sweden had had 2,710,457 cases (54% women) (Coronavirus Resource Center, 2023), 126,213 hospitalized cases, 10,344 persons treated in intensive care units (ICU) and 24,389 deaths (Table 3.1).

The age distribution of persons hospitalized and the age distribution of deaths are given in Figure 3.2.

As illustrated, deaths were skewed toward higher age groups. Most of the verified cases occurred in the age groups up to 60 years, while most ICU cases were in age groups 50–80 years. Most of the deaths occurred in the age group 70 and around 60% of total deaths were in persons 80 years and older. Hence, the mortality rate from COVID-19 increased considerably with age. Staying in a nursing home was associated with increased mortality risk as compared to living at home. Many of the

Table 3.1. Number of cases, hospitalized, patients treated in ICU, and deaths due to COVID-19 in Sweden from February 24, 2020–May 28, 2023 (Folkhälsomyndigheten, 2023a).

Variable	Number
Cases	2,710,457
Hospitalized	126,213
ICU treated	10,344
Deaths	24,389

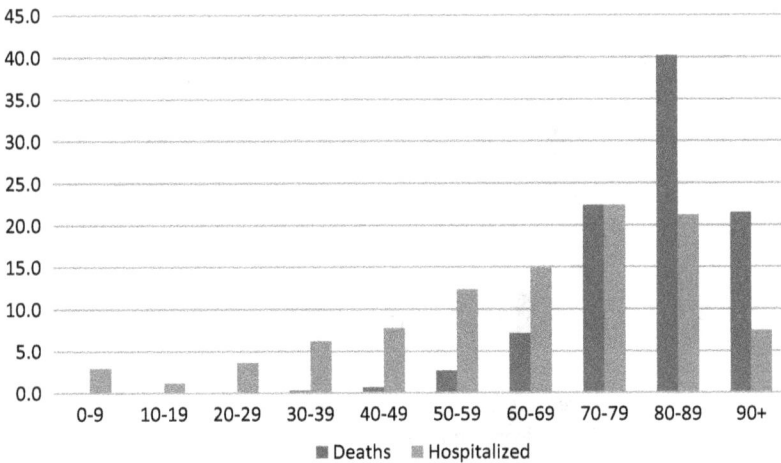

Figure 3.2.   Distribution of hospitalized cases and deaths due to COVID-19 in Sweden from February 24, 2020 to May 28, 2023 (Folkhälsomyndigheten, 2023b).

deaths occurred in nursing homes (44.7% of all) and only 4.1% in private housing. The rest (48.9%) died in hospital (Folkhälsomyndigheten, 2023a).

In addition to age, it was found that being born abroad meant a 20% increased risk of dying from COVID-19 (Socialstyrelsen, 2022b).

Figure 3.3 shows the number of ICU cases per day in Sweden as an illustration of the epidemic. The number of ICU cases peaked in April 2020, in December 2020, and in April 2021. An outbreak in early 2022 did not have as serious consequences in terms of ICU cases and deaths as earlier peaks, most probably reflecting an increased immunity against COVID-19 in the population and possibly less virulent virus strains as a result of vaccinations and natural development of the virus (Folkhälsomyndigheten, 2023a).

In 2020, the lack of testing facilities was reflected in the low number of cases registered that year (Figure 3.4). Also, on April 17, 2020 a national strategy for testing was presented by the Public Health Agency. The strategy aimed at establishing a sustainable capacity for testing. Highest priority was given to staff in health services, elderly care, and institutions for physical and cognitive impairment and to hospitalized

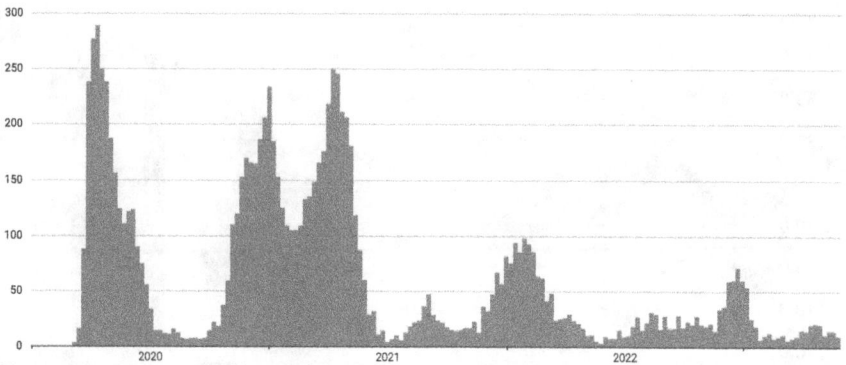

Figure 3.3.   New Intensive Care Unit (ICU) cases per day in Sweden from February 24, 2020 to May 28, 2023 (Folkhälsomyndigheten, 2023b).

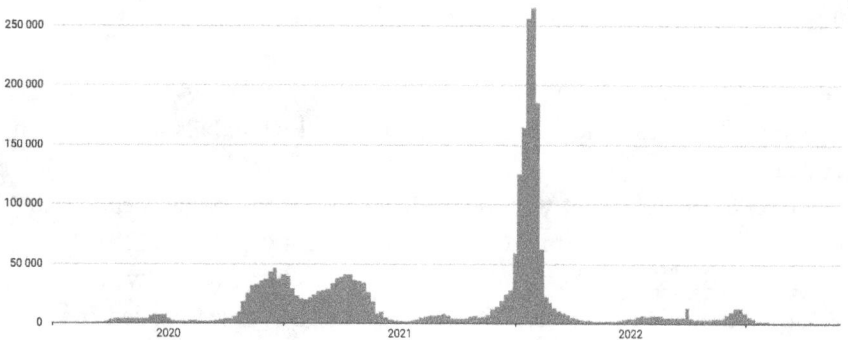

Figure 3.4.   Confirmed cases of COVID-19 in Sweden from February 24, 2020 to May 28, 2023 (Folkhälsomyndigheten, 2023b).

patients who were suspected of having COVID-19 infection (SOU, 2021:89).

The reported cases in the population were many and the disease was then widespread. This was also reflected in the heavy workload on health services from cases with COVID-19 as documented in the ICU chart. In contrast to this initial period of the pandemic, there was a high number of laboratory-confirmed cases in 2022 when testing facilities were well established in health services and rapid test kits were sold at reasonable prices (USD 5–10) in pharmacies and groceries.

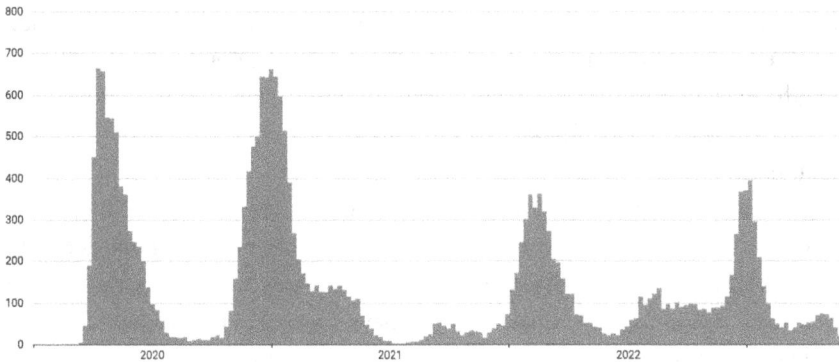

Figure 3.5. Deceased with COVID-19 in Sweden from February 24, 2020 to May 28, 2023 (Folkhälsomyndigheten, 2023b).

While testing was low, the mortality was high, in the first half of 2020 (Figure 3.5).

Sweden had high mortality rates in the second quarter of 2020 in comparison with many other countries. The situation has changed. The overall mortality rate in Sweden in international statistics was set by the Johns Hopkins Coronavirus Resource Center to 202.37 per 100,000 population in March 2023 (Coronavirus Resource Center, 2023). This placed Sweden at place 46 among 193 countries for whom data are shown. Though the international comparison of COVID-19 mortality rates has shortcomings and potential sources of error, Sweden does not stand out as having suffered more than many others from the pandemic. Countries with higher mortality rates are, for instance, Czechia, the USA, Brazil, Poland, Italy, the UK, Belgium, Portugal, Spain, and Austria. The other Scandinavian countries have however had proportionally fewer cases. Norway had in the latest data report a mortality rate of 76.61/100,000 population, Denmark 123.72, Iceland 62.42, and Finland 112.66.

3.3.2 *Control measures*

The first case of COVID-19 in Sweden was reported on January 31. A press release from the Public Health Agency stated that one case did not imply that there was spread of the virus in Sweden. The agency said that they considered the risk of such spread very small based on the experience of other countries (Krisinformation, 2020b). The agency also said that health services had good procedures for taking care of cases like the first one in a proper and safe way. In fact, no spread from that case was ever documented.

Already on February 1 the government had taken a decision to classify coronavirus as an emergency infectious threat to society. This decision was taken to allow the disease control authorities to take extraordinary measures to control the disease. Five days later, FoHM announced that travelers from areas in China from which cases of corona disease had been reported should be watchful for symptoms. However, they were not required to quarantine. On February 11, the Ministry of Foreign Affairs (Utrikesdepartementet — UD) advised people not to visit Hubei and Zhejiang provinces in China. On February 17, all travels to China were discouraged by UD. Soon the travel recommendations were extended to several other Asian countries.

On February 25, the FoHM changed its assessment of the risk of a general spread of the coronavirus in the Swedish population from "very low" to "low" (on a scale with very low, low, modest, high, and very high as grades). On February 26, a new case of COVID-19 disease was reported by the agency. This was a person who had visited northern Italy. Still, the agency, through the State Epidemiologist, stated that healthcare services were well equipped to deal with the case and prevent the spread of the virus. The State Epidemiologist said that it is important to distinguish isolated cases from a community spread of the virus which "we do not have in Sweden" (Krisinformation, 2020c). The day after, the agency reported five new confirmed cases, now from three different regions. The agency said that all cases were related to visits abroad and that there were no signs of transmission of the virus in the population.

After that, developments were quick. On March 2, the agency elevated the risk of community spread to "modest." On the same day, flights from Iran were stopped at the advice of the FoHM and, on March 6, travelers were advised not to visit Italy and South Korea. On March 9, the agency advised people to test themselves for COVID-19. The advice was directed at persons who had visited Tyrol in Northern Italy and who showed symptoms of COVID-19 disease. On March 10, the agency declared for the first time that there were signs of domestic transmission of the virus, meaning that there were cases in Sweden that were not connected to travel abroad. This was 38 days after the first case had been diagnosed in Sweden. The risk assessment of community transmission was changed to "very high." Persons with symptoms were advised to limit their contact with others. This was particularly targeted to persons working in elderly care and relatives of persons living in nursing homes. Only a few days later the government took several measures to limit community spread of the virus and, on March 14, people were advised not to travel abroad. Strong recommendations were also given to keep physical distance of at least 2 meters from other persons. This message and messages on personal hygiene, such as regular hand washing, were from then on communicated intensely through public media campaigns.

A full list of all major measures taken at the national level to control the COVID-19 pandemic is given in Table 3.2. The measures are listed in the order in which they were introduced. The duration of the measure is also given in Table 3.2.

Table 3.2. Measures taken, date of introduction, date of cancellation, and duration of measurement in months. Sorted by start date (European Centre for Disease Prevention and Control and the Joint Research Centre of the European Commission, 2023).

Measures taken	Start date	End date	Duration in months
Quarantine, domestic (General Public, recommendation)	2020-01-27	2022-02-08	24
Contact tracing	2020-01-27	2022-03-31	26
Isolation of cases, persons with confirmed covid should stay at home	2020-02-27	2022-03-31	25
Public gathering restriction for indoor event of over 500 persons	2020-03-12	2021-09-29	6.5
International travel advice, dissuasion from unnecessary travel	2020-03-14	2022-03-31	24.5
Teleworking (work from home)	2020-03-16	2022-03-31	24.5
Higher education (university), closure	2020-03-17	2021-05-31	14.5
Upper secondary school, closure	2020-03-17	2020-06-15	3

(Continued)

Table 3.2. *(Continued)*

Measures taken	Start date	End date	Duration in months
Total border closure, entry ban for individuals other than citizens of the EU, EEA, and United Kingdom	2020-03-17	2022-03-31	12
Visitors to serving establishments must be seated	2020-03-25	2020-07-07	3.5
No events with over 50 people are allowed	2020-03-29	2021-05-31	14
Risk groups (elderly) recommended to stay at home	2020-04-01	2020-10-22	6.5
Travel advice, avoid unnecessary travels within Sweden	2020-04-01	2020-06-12	2
Other (regulates number of customers in shops, payment queues, etc.)	2020-04-01	2020-12-31	9
Temporary legislation giving the municipalities the authority to reduce congestion in restaurants	2020-07-01	2020-12-31	6
Public spaces, restrictions in restaurants	2020-07-01	2021-09-28	4
Possibility to introduce local general restrictions in regions	2020-10-19	2022-03-31	17
Upper secondary school closure	2020-11-13	2020-12-06	1
Visiting restrictions (home for the elderly)	2020-11-19	2022-02-09	15
Private gathering restrictions (max. 8 persons)	2020-11-30	2021-09-29	10
Quarantine, domestic a Asymptomatic children and students living with someone with COVID should stay at home)	2020-12-01	2022-03-31	16
Upper secondary school, closure	2020-12-07	2021-01-06	1
Protective masks voluntary closed space (public transport)	2021-01-07	2021-07-01	6
Public spaces: Restrictions on visiting shops, shopping malls, and gym centers	2021-01-10	2021-05-17	4
Gym sports centers, partial (min. space per person)	2021-01-10	2021-06-01	5
Non-essential shops: Partial (visitors should enter alone)	2021-01-10	2021-05-17	4

Table 3.2.   (*Continued*)

Measures taken	Start date	End date	Duration in months
Upper secondary school, partial distance learning to avoid too many students in schools	2021-01-11	2021-04-01	3
Quarantine for international travelers	2021-01-22	2022-03-31	14
Border screening	2021-02-06	2022-03-31	14
Travel advice, internal	2021-03-01	2022-03-31	13
Public spaces: Restrictions on entertainment venues (amusement parks, zoos, museums, art galleries, etc.)	2021-03-25	2021-05-31	2
Vaccinated are exempted to NPIs	2021-04-16	2021-11-30	7.5
Public transport restrictions, limited number of passengers on long-distance public transport	2021-06-01	2021-07-15	1.5
Public gathering restriction indoor over 500	2021-12-01	2022-02-09	2
Vaccination certificates for public gatherings	2021-12-01	2022-02-09	2
Indoor over 50	2021-12-23	2022-01-18	1
Protective masks voluntary closed space (public transport)	2021-12-23	2022-02-08	1.5
At public gatherings indoors, seated participants required more than 20 participants, vaccination certificate if more than 500	2021-12-23	2022-01-18	1
Higher education (university, high school), partial closure	2022-01-12	2022-02-08	1
Public spaces: Restrictions on restaurants, bars, etc. (close by 23 H, max 8 persons/table)	2022-01-12	2022-02-09	1
Private gathering restrictions (max. 20)	2022-01-19	2022-02-09	1

All special measures against COVID-19 were abolished from April 1, 2022 (Läkartidningen, 2022).

The table provides useful information on the implementation of the pandemic control in Sweden and gives a broad view of control history. Still, there are details in the interventions that are not covered in the table. For instance, quarantine, introduced January 27, 2020, never went beyond a recommendation to people to stay at home and not see other people than the closest family when they had been abroad or fell ill. There was never any mandatory quarantine. Contract tracing was formally established on January 27, 2020 but was never realized much in practice. A major reason, brought up earlier in the paper, was that the regions did not have the capacity to speed up contract tracing with the relatively limited staff they had at hand in their communicable disease control units. The system simply got overwhelmed with COVID-19 cases.

The mandatory measures taken were restrictions on indoor gatherings of more than 500 persons (which hit the sports industry hard), the move to teleworking (working from home), the imposition of border closure, and the closure of high schools and universities, all imposed in March 2020. Teleworking was not compulsory but almost all public organizations followed the recommendation, while compliance varied in private companies. Overall, around 40% of the workforce has been estimated by the Public Health Agency to have worked from home during the pandemic. Pre-school and primary and secondary schools (up to age 16) were never closed, but it was recommended that schools should seek to limit the number of students in the classroom (by, for instance, having half the students work from home every second day).

Domestic travel was strongly discouraged by FoHM, and through agreements with mobile phone operators, the weekly movement of people was monitored and reported. The recommended restrictions on domestic travel were lifted from June 13, 2020. The eight first measures adopted were also the ones to be kept in place the longest. As can be seen from the table, other measures were repeated as the pandemic resurged at the end of 2020 and the beginning of 2021 and for a short period at the end of 2021 into 2022. Only 1 out of 12 measures listed as having been taken from December 1, 2021 was kept for more than 2 months.

As interesting as the information in the list is, what is not on the list is perhaps even more interesting. There are few mask recommendations in the list. The only one is for masks to be worn on public transport (which was introduced as late as July 1, 2021). A reason given for the restrained position of the FoHM with regard to face masks was that the agency did not find sufficient scientific evidence of their effectiveness in reducing viral spread.

Another control measure missing from the list is that schools below the level of high school were never closed. A third is that there were no restrictions on movement outdoor. Everybody was strongly advised to keep a two meters distance, but they were never asked to stay inside or not to meet outside in low numbers. In fact, physical activity was encouraged by the Public Health Agency (Krisinformation, 2020d). There was never any compulsory quarantine on international travelers. Those who arrived from abroad were advised to stay at home in their accommodation of choice for at least five days. If they had no symptoms after that, they were free to move.

Personal protective equipment (PPE) was quickly introduced by the regions for staff in hospital services. In elderly care, the intensity of provision varied significantly with the service providers. This was one of the issues raised when mortality started to increase in nursing homes (SOU, 2020:80). A problem was, as in many other European countries, that there was a shortage of supply of such protective gear (SOU, 2022:10).

Further characteristics of the Swedish pandemic control were the relatively limited testing (Frediksson & Hallberg, 2021) and little contract tracing in Sweden. The more forceful measures were the restrictions on eating places (restaurants, bars, etc.) and on public gatherings, both supported by parliamentary acts. These two measures were criticized by representatives of the restaurant owners and sports clubs. Still, they also expressed understanding for the need to limit the spread of the virus through restricting their activities.

Health services were active in testing patients from early on. This was part of diagnostics and primarily intended to make sure that patients with symptom-free COVID-19 were not placed in wards with other patients. Also, the FoHM recommended on April 17, 2020 that all health staff and staff in elderly care facilities test themselves regularly. On November 17, 2021, the agency recommended that the regions test all persons who were 6 years or older with symptoms of the disease. This was in reaction to the reports that the incidence of COVID-19 disease on the rise in other countries and in Sweden. Testing was recommended for all patients except those who had had confirmed COVID-19 infection in the preceding 6 months.

A complete description of how the Swedish community at large reacted to the pandemic would be exhaustive. Most government and non-governmental organizations took action to adjust their daily operations to the fluctuating situation that the pandemic and control measures created. Many also provided resources and expertise needed to reduce the impact of the pandemic. In the following box, this is illustrated with a description of the comprehensive program that was put in place at the Karolinska Institute to this end. Measures were taken on *ad hoc* basis for short-term support to anything from lab testing to clinical research, but important decisions were also taken on long-term support to a sustainable health crisis management system in Sweden.

Fact Box

A Swedish university's response to the pandemic.

This box is meant to illustrate with an example how the Swedish academic community reacted to the pandemic and its development.

As a university, Karolinska Institutet (KI) is Sweden's single largest center of medical academic research and offers the country's widest range of medical courses and programs. There are some 6,500 students at bachelor's and master's levels at the institute and around 2,100 PhD students. The institute has around 5,400 full-time employees. In addition, a larger number of researchers are affiliated to KI, often with another organization as their main employer. Research at Karolinska Institutet spans the entire medical field, from basic experimental research to patient-oriented and nursing research.

During the pandemic, KI took many structural actions that were influenced by the government's decisions as well as independent scientific and rational thinking within the academic community. Many on-going research activities were kept on hold to allow for resources to focus on research related to the virus and the pandemic. Much effort was put

---

(Continued)

into various aspects on the public health aspects of the pandemic. Other prominent research areas were clinical studies of symptoms and case development, including post-COVID, and essential studies of the virus and immunology studies, including vaccine development. Up to March 2023, an estimated 1,400 articles on COVID-19 and related matters have been published with participation by KI researchers.

At KI, eight groups were quickly formed in February and March 2020 to facilitate coordination and collaboration within the institute and to provide advice and make resources available to the community at large, including the Public Health Agency and the media and health services. After much work on this during the pandemic, a Centre for Health Crises was established to permanently ensure capacity to catalyze research, training, and action and to provide expertise and drive policy, all to contribute to a society better prepared for future national and international health crises.

3.3.3 *Vaccinations*

The Swedish strategy on vaccinations was characterized by a gradual, step-by-step introduction of the vaccines to priority groups, eventually offered to the whole population above 18. This was very much dependent on the speed with which the vaccines could be delivered by the manufacturers. It has been argued that Sweden, in comparison with other Nordic countries, was relatively quick in immunizing the elderly once the vaccines became available (Yarmol-Matusiak *et al.*, 2021).

All matters related to the administration of the vaccines were with the regions. In some instances, regions would choose slightly different strategies, which was quickly picked up in public debate as unfair and inequitable (SVT, 2020). All in all, such contentious issues faded away within a short time as vaccines increasingly became available.

The number of vaccinations given in total is shown in Figure 3.6. Vaccinations started at the very end of 2020 and increased rapidly up to the second quarter of 2021, after which the rate of vaccination leveled off. On March 14, 85% of the population above 12 had received at least one dose and 83.7% at least two doses (Folkhälsomyndigheten, 2023c).

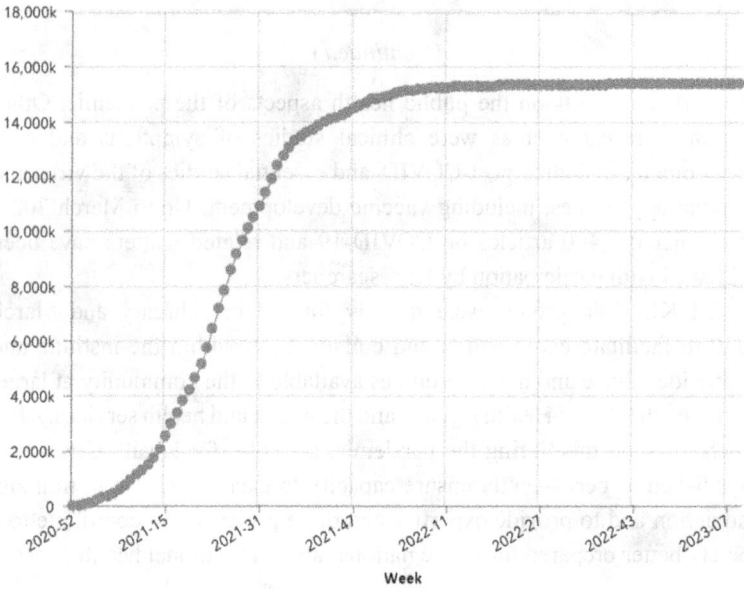

Figure 3.6. Cumulative number of vaccinations per week in thousands, Sweden. December 24, 2020–March 14, 2023 (Folkhälsomyndigheten, 2023b).

On February 25, 2021, the Public Health Agency lifted restrictions on elderly in nursing homes who had had two doses of vaccine. Two weeks after the second dose, these seniors were allowed to see symptom-free family members.

The Public Health Agency issued a series of recommendations on vaccinations to the population as vaccines became available, gradually expanding the eligible target groups. Priority was usually applied so that those in the highest need would get the vaccines first. All vaccinations were voluntary, but overall compliance was high. Some resistance to vaccination was seen but not to the point that it affected the vaccine coverage to any larger degree (Folkhälsomyndigheten, 2021b). Lindvall and Rönnerstrand found that the largest group of vaccine-hesitant individuals said they were reluctant to take the vaccine for the simple reason that they were young and felt they ran a low risk of developing serious illness from the COVID-19 virus (Lindvall & Rönnerstrand, 2022). Still, an anti-vax movement was also active in Sweden. On at least three occasions in 2021, demonstrations against the pandemic control measures and the COVID-19 vaccination were arranged in Stockholm with up to around a thousand participants, thereby violating the special pandemic law according to which public gatherings of more than 500 persons were prohibited (SVT, 2023). The most recent recommendations from the Public Health Agency on vaccinations against COVID-19 are given in Table 3.3.

Table 3.3. Recommendations from the Public Health Agency on vaccinations against COVID-19 as of March 23, 2023.

Target group	Recommendations	Comments
Persons >80 years and persons living in nursing homes (SÄBO)	Two doses with at least 6 months interval during the period March 1, 2023–February 29, 2024.	This is for those persons who have already received basic vaccination with three doses. Those who have not should be given these vaccinations first. Two doses + booster at earliest 4 months after the first.
Persons 65–79 years and persons in risk groups from 18–64 years	One dose during the period March 1, 2023–February 29, 2024, by preference before the autumn/winter 2023/24. One more dose will be available to be given after at least 6 months.	Recommended irrespective of earlier doses. Base vaccination recommended to this group: Two doses + booster at earliest 4 months after the first.
Persons 50–64 years	One dose, by preference before the autumn/winter 2023/24.	Recommendation irrespective of earlier doses. Vaccine to be given after an interval of at least 9 months since previous dose.
Persons 18–49 years	No recommendation on booster. However, people who live close to an elderly or a person in a risk group can get a dose.	The recommendation on base vaccination with three doses came to an end on March 1, 2023.
Persons with immunodeficiencies	A vaccination program specially developed by the FoHM for this group should be followed.	

The Swedish Agency for Health and Care Services Analysis (Vård-och omsorgsanalys) published a report in October 2022 on how well the Swedish regions had managed to reach those groups in society that were deemed to be of highest risk to be neglected in a general vaccination campaign with COVID-19 vaccinations. The study used interviews, a survey, and statistics in its work. The tool Tailoring Immunization Programmes (TIP) developed by WHO's Regional Office in Europe formed the basis for the assessment (Vård-och omsorgsanalys, 2022).

The report concluded that the work in the regions regarding reaching out with vaccinations could have been more evidence-based and targeted. After consultations with the regions, the Public Health Agency published a guideline, based on TIP, in July 2022 on how to reach people with vaccinations. Some regional staff expressed in interviews that they would have liked to have seen more of such guidance from the national level earlier. On the other hand, FoHM representatives expressed in their interviews that advice given by them was not always followed by the regions. Furthermore, regions and municipalities did not carry out surveys of their populations in the early phases of the pandemic to identify risk groups regarding vaccination coverage. The position was rather one of "expectation" until it became clear that vaccines would become available and, later, that there would be sufficient supplies to cover the larger part of the population in Sweden. In the review from the agency, it is said that already early in the pandemic, it was clear that COVID-19 hit significantly harder those born abroad as well as socio-economically vulnerable groups, and that it was known that those factors were also linked to lower coverage of vaccinations in general. The authors of the report suggested that the regions therefore could have prepared targeted vaccination efforts in these groups earlier in the pandemic than what they did.

A key recommendation in the review was that the government should clarify the division of responsibilities and roles between authorities and between the national and regional levels to create better conditions for future vaccination work. The same conclusion was drawn by the Corona Commission, a commission appointed by the government to review how the pandemic control was managed in Sweden (SOU, 2022:10). It criticized the government for not taking clear national leadership and larger responsibility in communicating with the public. It was also stated that the government was too dependent on assessments from the Public Health Agency.

With that said, a recent study concluded that Sweden was one of few countries that could return to its pre-pandemic life expectancy in 2021 after having experienced a decline in 2020. The study identified a rapid roll-out of vaccinations of those above 80 years or older as one of the possible reasons for this positive change in 2021 (Schöley *et al.*, 2022).

It can be concluded that Sweden acted swiftly to reach the high-risk group of elderly with vaccinations, while others that were also hit more than proportionally by the disease could have been identified and reached earlier.

3.3.4 *Consensus and critique*

The pandemic control measures that were enacted as laws were taken in broad political agreement within Parliament. Generally, the actions taken by the government and its agencies were supported by most of the parties in the political opposition and led to little criticism in Parliament. The party most critical was the Swedish Democrats, a populist and anti-immigrant party, that claimed that the government exceeded the temporary mandate given to it by the parliament (SFS, 2021:4) to act swiftly in the early phase of the pandemic (TT, 2022). Formal criticism was also given by entrepreneurs who were against a law that gave the government the legal right to close restaurants and other public places without supporting evidence to show that the measures taken were sufficiently effective in the control of the pandemic in relation to the significant costs to society linked to closures. Also, the gains from the restrictions on the constitutional rights of freedom of movement, and of conducting business freely, should be weighed against their costs to society (Krassén, 2022).

Criticism against the pandemic control strategies was also raised by some academics who felt that the approach taken was too lenient, that more active and legally binding control measures should be imposed, and that the government gave the Public Health Agency too extensive a mandate (King *et al.*, 2020; Hanson *et al.*, 2021; Lindström, 2020). Meanwhile, other researchers acted in support of the approaches taken or at least did not argue against them. This was not least true for those who appeared in public service media channels.

In the media, there was also a very active debate about the pandemic. On March 17, 2020, a count showed that articles on the coronavirus and outbreak had been shared about 7 million times on Swedish social media (Wikstrand, 2020). Leading editorials criticized the government for the absence of control measures like more active border controls and isolation of cases (Wolodarski, 2020). These critics were met by researchers who feared that scientific evidence was not given due respect in the debate (von Schreeb, 2020). In international media, Sweden was quickly put in bad light with *Time* magazine saying that "The Swedish COVID-19 response is a disaster. It shouldn't be a model for the rest of the world" (Björklund & Ewing, 2020), the *New York Times* warning that "Sweden has become the world's cautionary tale" (Goodman, 2020), and the *Guardian* calling the strategy "a deadly folly" (Cohen, 2020). Later, international media returned to the "Swedish experience" and gave more balanced reports on it (Pearson, 2023).

3.4 Impact of the Pandemic and the Control Measures

The impact of pandemic control in Sweden can be measured in many ways. The primary purpose of actions taken was to control the disease. However, considerations also had to be given to other effects of the pandemic and control measures, such as effect on other health issues, not least mental health, social life, and the economy. Much has been written about this in traditional and social media. The government-appointed Corona Commission (SOU, 2022:10) also went through the effects in great depth, mostly during 2021.

Many articles have already been published on the impact of the pandemic control measures on the containment of the virus and society at large. Public media also continues to take an interest in what measures were successful and which were not. The development of findings and positions calls for caution in drawing early conclusions on the pandemic and its effects. There is a continuous need to study the corona pandemic and its short- and long-term consequences on many variables. Not least is it too early to fully understand the consequences of post-COVID syndrome and, on a wider societal scale, the effects of lockdowns on learning and mental health, especially among the young.

3.4.1 *Mortality impact*

The effects on health were initially dramatic with high mortality, in relation to other OECD countries, in elderly and some other risk groups, like persons with immigrant background in socio-economically deprived areas. However, over time the mortality gradually stabilized and decreased as many other countries saw the mortality increase. Today, we find that Sweden did not fare much worse regarding overall COVID-19 mortality than many other countries.

In Sweden, much consideration was also given to healthcare that had to be postponed due to the pressure that COVID-19 put on health services. So far, there are no indications that overall mortality due to other reasons than COVID-19 has increased since the pandemic started. Overall mortality due to other reasons decreased slightly in 2020 which is in line with a declining mortality trend seen since 2001 (Folkhälsomyndigheten, 2021c).

It is somewhat complicated to categorize causes of death since only one cause can be documented per death. This means that in documented data those who have died from COVID-19 could not have died of other causes in 2020. However, we know that COVID-19-related deaths were concentrated in older ages, as is general mortality. As previously mentioned, nursing homes and special accommodations providing care for elderly with medical needs were particularly affected by the pandemic. Patients in these homes are already fragile. Around 20% of the clients in nursing homes in Sweden expire within 6 months of admission to these institutions. The average length of stay for all clients is around 24 months. Similarly, the seasonal influenza was mild in 2019 and therefore expected to be worse in 2020 than the previous year. However, since the flu season did not occur (as with other viruses, such as Respiratory Syncytial Virus (RSV)), there was no flu-related mortality. It can be assumed that some of those who died from COVID-19 would have passed away in 2020 due to other diseases.

At the beginning of the pandemic, much attention was brought to the high mortality rate in Sweden. More recently, there has been a debate

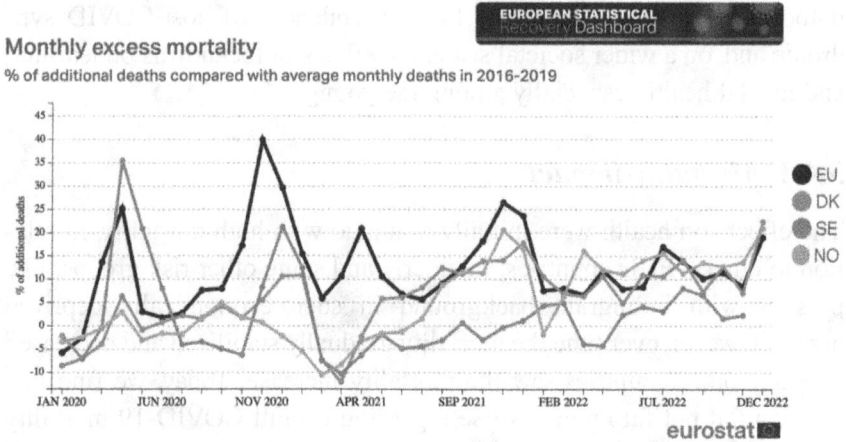

Figure 3.7. Monthly excess mortality in EU, Denmark, Sweden, and Norway (*Eurostat*, 2023).

around the fact that Sweden does not stand out in the EU in regard to excess mortality (Bergstedt, 2023), shown in Figure 3.7. On the contrary, Sweden has one of the *lowest* excess mortality rates in Europe.

3.4.2 *Life and mental health impact*

A report from FoHM on how public health was affected by the pandemic in 2020 in Sweden showed that people's lifestyles were affected in different ways and to a varying extent.

People were less physically active and increased unhealthy eating habits. This was especially the case for young people aged 16–29. However, there was no increase in the number of regular smokers, and people actually tended to reduce their intake of alcohol (Folkhälsomyndigheten, 2021a).

No dramatic changes were found in the first year of the pandemic on the mental health of the Swedish population. Mild emotions of distress and sleep problems increased during the autumn of 2020 but not severe psychological problems. The emergency operators reported having more calls linked to suicidal thoughts during the pandemic. Yet in 2020, there was no increase in suicide rates or in the number of people admitted to hospitals due to suicide attempts. The Public Health Agency reported growing symptoms of anxiety, worry, and depression among groups that were vulnerable before the pandemic, such as migrants, LGBTQI people, and children in families with mental health problems, addiction, or violence (Folkhälsomyndigheten, 2021a).

Among young people aged 16–29, the percentage with problems of anxiety, worry, or anxiety increased from 41% to 57% during the period 2015–2021. The rise in 2021 followed the same trend as in previous years and thus did not deviate from that trend during the pandemic. Analyses of the age group 16–19 showed similar results. In the group aged 16–29, in 2021, 30% stated that they had quite a lot or a lot of trouble with loneliness and isolation during the pandemic (Folkhälsomyndigheten, 2022). For children, the pandemic may have affected their daily life less as regular routines with school and social contacts continued.

Some persons who contract COVID-19 infection and disease will develop post-COVID syndrome. This is defined as a condition that occurs more than four weeks after a primary COVID-19 infection. As many as 62 different symptoms and conditions have been associated with post-COVID. Many of the conditions are serious and potentially life-threatening, such as pulmonary embolism and cerebrovascular disease. The prevalence of any post-COVID-19 condition symptom estimates vary widely, from 12.7% to 50.6% in community groups (European Centre for Disease Prevention and Control, 2022).

The incidence of post-COVID syndrome in Sweden has not been studied in a systematic way, but the condition has been so apparent that facilities for providing care to post-COVID patients were established in several regions. In August 2022, 12 regions out of 21 had such specialist centers. However, several of them have subsequently decided to close the centers and refer patients to primary care. Swedish media has given considerable publicity to post-COVID syndrome (European Centre for Disease Prevention and Control, 2022).

3.4.3 *Impact on the economy*

The Swedish economy was negatively affected by the pandemic and the subsequent lockdowns in Sweden and elsewhere. The Gross Domestic

Product (GDP) decreased by 2.4% in 2002. The GDP growth in 2019 was 2.0% and in 2021, 4.9%. Hence, there was a clear dip in the economy in 2020 followed by a considerable recovery in 2021. GDP per capita decreased from SEK 516,600 in 2019 to SEK 500,600 in 2020. However, in 2021, it was SEK 522,200 (*Ekonomifakta*, 2022b).

The number of persons in employment was 5,034,700 in February 2020 but then started to fall to reach its lowest in January 2021 with 4,853,800 in employment. After that, employment increased continuously and reached its highest ever in September 2022 with 5,224,490 in the work force. Furthermore, salaries in real terms increased by 1.6% in 2020 (*Ekonomifakta*, 2022a).

The rather remarkable development of the economy was facilitated by government interventions to support companies which experienced a dip in activities and demand. This allowed companies to keep much of their workforce during the short recession in the first half of 2020. All in all, the national government estimated in February 2021 that it had spent SEK 389 billion to keep up the economy during the COVID-19 pandemic. This corresponds to approximately 15% of the total national expenditures in a year. The support was made possible by a strong financial government balance at the beginning of 2020 (*Ekonomifakta*, 2022c).

3.5 Lessons Learned

The Swedish experience with the pandemic control had many interesting characteristics from which lessons can be learned. Some of them are as follows:

(1) A slow start in pandemic control can hit hard, but its repercussions can be balanced by more active action once the alert signals have become strong enough to mobilize the community at all levels. This may provide time to anchor decision-making in stakeholder groups and prepare the public for required control measures, factors that are likely to increase efficiency in implementation.

(2) A balance between actions to contain the spread of a virus causing an epidemic and the consequences on broader public health outcomes as well as on society at large from these actions should be sought.

(3) In a decentralized government system, significant decision-making power can be given to specialized expert agencies, such as the Public Health Agency in Sweden. The effort to base decision-making on evidence and accumulated knowledge is laudable but may also become a hindrance to effective decision-making at national government level.

(4) Legal frameworks and coordination of actors are setting the scene for pandemic control and are therefore essential to design and prepare for any system challenges that future pandemics may pose.

(5) Measures to contain an epidemic should be carefully reviewed and their potential gains should be weighed against their risks. Caution and discretion may at times be a defendable strategy given that quick action may miss its purpose and be met with resistance from the community.

(6) Academia can respond swiftly to the challenges posed by a pandemic and can make positive contributions to pandemic control.

Here we elaborate further on these and additional lessons learned during the pandemic.

The Swedish corona pandemic was characterized by a relatively slow start in public health actions once the pandemic reached Europe and Sweden. The first early cases were imported and isolated in hospitals. No community spread was documented from them. Within 5–6 weeks, when more cases occurred at great speed in Europe and cases were reported from different regions in Sweden, the government started to take action.

From early on, the Public Health Agency was given a prominent role in epidemic control. The agency acted as an advisor to the government throughout the pandemic and also took many actions within its jurisdiction. As the Public Health Agency originally was set up to integrate health promotion and prevention of both communicable and non-communicable diseases, it gave due attention to all aspects of the pandemic control, including effects on mental health and well-being from various actions to reduce the transmission of the virus, such as restricting movements in the community and closing public spaces. The government took the larger responsibility for the overall impact on society from potential and actual public health measures. For these reasons, the Swedish approach to the pandemic balanced the urgency to control the spread of the virus against the potential negative impact on society in general, and specifically in terms of mental health, especially from strict measures to reduce contact between people, restrict free movements, and isolate infected persons.

The Swedish approach, as illustrated earlier, received much attention in the early stages of the pandemic when many countries imposed very strong restrictions on people's right to move freely in the community. Among the more contentious elements in Sweden was that people continued to move around freely at their own will, while being advised to keep a distance from others, and that schools below the level of high school were kept open. Sweden was among the few countries that decided to keep schools open. Later research has suggested that school closing was not an essential intervention in the pandemic control package (Shapiro *et al.*, 2021). In some countries, such as Norway, there was criticism of the lack of consideration given to children's needs from leading authorities (Jakobsen, 2023). It remains an open question whether school closing should be applied in pandemic control in order to contain viral spread in the community. Also, much discussed nationally and internationally was that specific measures to protect people in homes for the elderly, nursing homes, were said not to be swift enough, especially in the early stages of the pandemic. This became particularly highlighted when Sweden showed considerably higher mortality from COVID-19 than most European countries, including the Nordic countries, during the first 6 months of the pandemic (European Centre for Disease Prevention and Control and the Joint Research Centre of the European Commission, 2023).

As the pandemic continued, Swedish mortality rates went down, and 34 months after the pandemic started, the country does not stand out as worse hit by the pandemic than many other countries. However, as described on page 55 Sweden was worse hit than its Scandinavian neighbors, countries that Sweden has much in common with.

Why did Sweden choose a somewhat different strategy than other countries, including the neighboring Scandinavian countries? This is a question that cannot be easily answered. Initially, it seemed that the difference was mainly due to slow reaction from the Swedish side when the first cases occurred. The other countries were quicker and more decisive at taking decisions to isolate cases and initiate testing as soon as testing became available (Yarmol-Matusiak *et al.*, 2021). It has been argued that one reason for the difference is that the governing system in Sweden is more decentralized with respect to the government expert agencies, while in Denmark and Norway, there is more direct rule by the political government of the administrative structures at national level (Askin & Bergström, 2022). The difference in governance allowed the national governments in Denmark and Norway to act swiftly when the pandemic threat became apparent, while the Swedish way was to rely more on the general directorates, such as the Public Health Agency, and the regions and municipalities.

Strang argues that there is a strong tradition in Sweden of thinking that a functioning economy is a prerequisite for people's well-being and health and that the economic aspects of the pandemic control measures were much more central in the Swedish discussion, and at a much earlier stage, than in the other Scandinavian countries (Strang, 2020). This would have made the government more cautious in locking down society and introducing strict border controls and travel regulations. Decision-making in Sweden sought to balance pros and cons in an overall assessment of the total effect on society from potential interventions to contain the pandemic.

Another possible reason for the difference in action taken in the Scandinavian countries is the proposed difference in trust in the state in these countries, insofar as Swedes in particular tend to follow advice from authorities and the national government (Raffetti *et al.*, 2022). Hence, there would be less need for mandatory rules in Sweden as compared to Norway and Denmark (Moodie, 2021).

It has been pointed out by Baum and colleagues that efforts to find systematic country or system patterns in the management and outcome of the pandemic have generally been less than rewarding. The authors argue that cross-country comparisons often overlook important differences, such as dynamic political, economic, and social structures and systems (Baum *et al.*, 2021). Other researchers have argued that the unscientific use of international comparisons of case and mortality data in public discourse, media reporting, and policymaking on intervention effectiveness should be subject to greater scrutiny (Thomson *et al.*, 2022).

What can be concluded from the "Scandinavian comparison" is that Sweden chose a somewhat different strategy to control the pandemic than Norway and Denmark and that Sweden ended up with a higher overall mortality from COVID-19 than these countries. The exact reasons for the differences in outcome need further exploration, including more in-depth studies of transmission patterns, reporting routines, and actual compliance with advice, rules, and regulations to control transmission in the population. Still, a full assessment of the pandemic experience in the countries should be comprehensive and include all effects on society. A study showed, for instance, that in Norway, 69% lived a more sedentary life during the pandemic versus 50% in Sweden, and 44% in Norway ate more versus 33% in Sweden. More people were depressed and sad in Norway than in Sweden (21% and 41% in Norway and 15% and 18% in Sweden, respectively) (Helsingen *et al.*, 2020). Furthermore, differences in the relative importance of foreign-born persons in the pandemic in the countries as well as any difference in the conditions for the elderly, in particular those with chronic diseases, should be studied.

Policies regarding disease control in Sweden are guided by the *Communicable Diseases Act*. It stipulates that containment measures must be proportionate and based on science and proven experience. In Sweden, there were few dramatic lockdowns and, to the extent possible, there was a policy to keep an open society with restrictions on factors, such as opening hours, number of customers allowed, and placement of clients in restaurants and bars. The authority of the public health actors in the communicable disease system remained and was not changed from the national level. The restrictions imposed at the national level were mainly focused on the public. For instance, private visits to nursing homes were prohibited under the "Pandemilagen" (SFS, 2021:4). Furthermore, significant energy was put into communication to the public on the importance of keeping a physical distance of two meters, handwashing, working from home, and, in particular, staying at home when signs of illness occurred.

The legal framework played a role in the Swedish pandemic control as Swedish politicians and officials are prevented by the constitution from restricting people's freedom of movement. As previously mentioned, temporary acts first had to be taken by the parliament before certain restrictions to contain the COVID-19 virus could be introduced by the government.

Interestingly, the dominant perspective on the pandemic and the Swedish pandemic control actions have changed from one of being much discussed and questioned to one in which there is now more overall relief and satisfaction with the way the pandemic was handled. For instance, a population-based survey in 2021 showed that the respondents rated the Public Health Agency higher than any other government agency (*Statskontoret*, 2022).

A reason for the positive assessment of the Swedish handling of the pandemic may well be that Sweden does not stand out anymore as an international "loser" in pandemic control, given the current mortality rates, compared to how it was portrayed at the beginning of the pandemic. Another reason for the assessment is that there have been many reports from other countries on the negative consequences for people from the drastic lockdowns imposed on them by their governments. Prolongation of restricting measures must be endured by the population. In many parts of the world, including countries close to Sweden, there were protests, some violent, as reactions to lockdowns and more so those that lasted for long. Sweden saw little of that, possibly because of the relative open pandemic control policy.

Many Swedes were pleased that they could continue to live a life that did not restrict their outdoor activities and allowed them to continue to interact in small numbers with relatives and friends. The restriction on visits to elderly relatives, especially in nursing homes, was a bad enough experience to make many Swedes feel gratitude that they were not subjected to complete lockdown and disruption of their daily lives.

The Swedish experience from the corona pandemic is much less discussed in Sweden today than in the years 2020–2021. It was not an issue in the election campaign in September 2022. After the elections, a new government was formed by the parties that were in opposition during the pandemic, but no political analysis has identified the management of the pandemic as a reason for why the previous government lost the election. In fact, the main party in the then-government, the Social Democrats, received increased support from the voters in the election.

The Director General of the Public Health Agency, who was appointed in 2022, has identified five areas that need to be strengthened in view of the experiences with the COVID-19 pandemic. They are (1) a revision of the *Communicable Disease Protection Act*, (2) a central body in each region for accelerating all necessary functions in case of need for rapid communicable disease control, (3) improved generation of, access to, and active use of health data, (4) strengthened capacity to store equipment and medical consumables required in an epidemic at regional and municipal levels; strengthen medical competence, in particular at the municipal level, and (5) scale-up efforts to reach quality care on equal terms for the entire population (Tegmark Wisell, 2023).

Several government commissions are now reviewing how the legal and administrative systems can be improved to ensure better preparedness for the next pandemic. The cross-sectoral interaction at the national level must be strengthened. Further, the roles and responsibilities of regions and municipalities in overlapping tasks must become clear and collaboration should be institutionalized. A call for strengthened intersectoral collaboration is also needed (Buse *et al.*, 2022). As pointed out by Kriegner and colleagues, public health interventions may be more effective if the strategies chosen are deployed so that they reinforce each other, value outcomes beyond health, and are tailored to maximize political priority for the intervention across sectors (Kriegner *et al.*, 2021). This approach should appeal to Swedish decision-makers as it fits well into the policy and legal framework for public health that has been described in this chapter.

Many lessons were learnt during the COVID-19 outbreak in Sweden. Operations must be carried out within existing structures, even in times of a pandemic crisis. Drastic measures must be supported by special legal action by the Parliament, something that may challenge the constitutional basis of the political and legal system. The extent to which such action can be taken may be restricted by cultural and constitutional traditions. The pandemic made it clear that the governance system at large must be prepared for any unforeseen large-scale emergency before, and not during, the emergency and that action must be carried out within the established system. The current post-pandemic development in Sweden suggests that focus will be on such preparation, rather than on any major reforms of the current system, including the system for public health protection. If major reforms of the governance system will come, they will do so for other reasons than the experience from the COVID-19 pandemic.

The Swedish case illustrates the challenge of when and how to evaluate public health interventions to draw stable and reliable conclusions from actions taken. It also serves as a case for comparing Sweden's experience with other countries' experiences to assess the impact of pandemic-driven complex, large-scale disruptions of society. Such actions have been linked to increased inequalities in access to resources and were deemed to diminish the rights to healthcare, education, and social protection (Tomson *et al.*, 2021). Such impact should be considered from the start of an epidemic to strike an appropriate balance between measures that are effective in containing an epidemic and those that are potentially harmful to society and people. Being prepared also means investing in people requiring stronger and more accountable health systems as well as fair and effective governance that engages multiple stakeholders.

The lessons learned in this study are supportive of the recommendations given by the Director General as described earlier. The review of these lessons is not exhaustive and the pandemic experience should be further studied in Sweden. Special attention should be drawn to the emergency preparedness in the regions to enhance the overall resilience of the Swedish health system to be better prepared for future pandemics and crises.

References

Anell, A., Glenngård, A. H., and Merkur, S. (2012). Sweden health system review. *Health systems in transition, 14*(5), 1–159.

Askin, J. and Bergström, T. (2022). Between lockdown and calm down. Comparing the COVID-19 responses of Norway and Sweden. *Local Government Studies, 48*(2), 291–311. DOI: 10.1080/03003930.2021.1964477.

Baum, F., Freeman, T., Musolino, C., Abramovitz, M., De Ceukelaire, W., Flavel, J., Friel, J., Guigliani, C., Howden-Chapman, P., Huong, N. T., London, L., McKee, M., Popay, J., Serag, H., and Villar E. (2021). Explaining COVID-19 performance: What factors might predict national responses? *The BMJ, 372*(91). DOI: 10.1136/bmj.n91.

Bergstedt, T. (February 25, 2023). *Sveriges överdödlighet en av de lägsta i Europa.* Stockholm: Svenska Dagbladet. https://www.svd.se/a/qWrrlO/sveriges-overdodlighet-ar-nast-lagst-i-norden.

Björklund, K. and Ewing, A. (October 14, 2020). The Swedish COVID-19 response is a disaster. It shouldn't be a model for the rest of the world. *Time.* https://time.com/5899432/sweden-coronovirus-disaster/.

Buse, K., Tomson, G., Kuruvilla, S., Mahmood, J., Alden, A., van der Meulen, M., Ottersen, O. P., and Haines, A. (2022). Tackling the politics of intersectoral action for the health of people and planet. *The BMJ, 376*, e068124. DOI: 10.1136/bmj-2021-068124.

Cohen, N. (May 23, 2020). Sweden's COVID-19 policy is a model for the right. It's also a deadly folly. *The Guardian.* https://www.theguardian.com/world/commentisfree/2020/may/23/sweden-COVID-19-policy-model-for-right-also-a-deadly-folly.

Coronavirus Resource Center (2023). Baltimore: Johns Hopkins University & Medicine. https://coronavirus.jhu.edu/region (Accessed on March 12, 2023).

Ekonomifakta (2022a). Arbetslöshet. https://www.ekonomifakta.se/Fakta/Arbetsmarknad/Arbetsloshet/Arbetsloshet/.

Ekonomifakta (2022b). BNP-Sverige. https://www.ekonomifakta.se/Fakta/Ekonomi/Tillvaxt/BNP---Sverige/.

Ekonomifakta (2022c). Stödåtgärder — coronakrisen. https://www.ekonomifakta.se/Fakta/Offentlig-ekonomi/Statsbudget/stodatgarder-coronakrisen/.

European Centre for Disease Prevention and Control and the Joint Research Centre of the European Commission (2023). Response measures database. https://covid-statistics.jrc.ec.europa.eu/RMeasures (Accessed on March 22, 2023).

European Centre for Disease Prevention and Control and the Joint Research Centre of the European Commission (February 26, 2023). Dashboard. https://covid-statistics.jrc.ec.europa.eu/Home/Dashboard.

European Centre for Disease Prevention and Control (October 27, 2022). *Prevalence of Post COVID-19 Condition Symptoms: A Systematic Review and Meta-analysis of Cohort Study Data Stratified by Recruitment Setting.* Stockholm: ECDC. https://www.ecdc.europa.eu/sites/default/files/documents/Prevalence-post-COVID-19-condition-symptoms.pdf.

Eurostat (2023). Excess mortality by month. https://ec.europa.eu/eurostat/databrowser/bookmark/2860d38c-740d-4bbc-89c7-2ab912afee05?lang=en (Accessed on March 20, 2023).

Folkhälsomyndigheten (2021a). Hur har folkhälsan påverkats av COVID-19-pandemin? — Samlad bedömning utifrån svensk empiri och internationell forskning under 2020. Stockholm. https://www.folkhalsomyndigheten.se/publikationer-och-material/publikationsarkiv/h/hur-har-folkhalsan-paverkats-av-COVID-19-pandemin/.

Folkhälsomyndigheten (2021b). Hög vaccinationsvilja mot COVID-19. Stockholm. https://www.folkhalsomyndigheten.se/contentassets/ba207c42c89c46f58bec596e3d2b67a5/vaccinationsvilja-COVID-19-mars-2021.pdf.

Folkhälsomyndigheten (2021c). Överdödlighet och dödlighet i COVID-19 i Sverige under 2020. Stockholm. https://www.folkhalsomyndigheten.se/publikationer-och-material/publikationsarkiv/oe/overdodlighet-och-dodlighet-i-COVID-19-i-sverige-under-2020/.

Folkhälsomyndigheten (2022). Unga och COVID-19-pandemin — ungas livsvillkor, levnadsvanor och hälsa. Stockholm. https://www.folkhalsomyndigheten.se/publikationer-och-material/publikationsarkiv/u/unga-och-COVID-19-pandemin/?

Folkhälsomyndigheten (2023a). När hände vad under pandemin. https://www.folkhalsomyndigheten.se/smittskydd-beredskap/utbrott/aktuella-utbrott/covid-19/nar-hande-vad-under-pandemin/ (Accessed on March 3, 2024).

Folkhälsomyndigheten (2023b). Folkhälsodata. Stockholm. https://www.folkhalsomyndigheten.se/fall-covid-19/ (Accessed on June 3, 2023).

Folkhälsomyndigheten (2023c). Vaccinationer mot COVID-19 i Sverige. Stockholm. https://www.folkhalsomyndigheten.se/faktablad/vaccination-covid-19/ (Accessed on March 22, 2023).

Fredriksson, M. and Hallberg, A. (2021). COVID-19 testing in Sweden during 2020-split responsibilities and multi-level challenges. *Frontiers in Public Health*, 9. DOI: 10.3389/fpubh.2021.754861.

Goodman, P. S. (December 15, 2020). Sweden has become the World's cautionary tale. *New York Times*. https://www.nytimes.com/2020/07/07/business/sweden-economy-coronavirus.html.

Hanson, C., Luedtke, S., Spicer, N., Stilhoff Sörensen, J., Mayhew, S., and Mounier-Jack, S. (2021). National health governance, science and the media: Drivers of COVID-19 responses in Germany, Sweden and the UK in 2020. *BMJ Global Health*, 6, e006691. DOI: 10.1136/bmjgh-2021-006691.

Helsingen, L., Refsum, E., Gjøstein, D., Løberg, M., Bretthauer, M., Kalager, M., …
    Clinical Effectiveness Research group (2020). The COVID-19 pandemic in
    Norway and Sweden — Threats, trust, and impact on daily life: A compara-
    tive survey. *BMC Public Health*, *20*(1), 1597. DOI: 10.1186/s12889-020-
    09615-3.
HSLF-FS (2017:40). (n.d.). Socialstyrelsens föreskrifter och allmänna råd om
    vårdgivares systematiska patientsäkerhetsarbete. https://www.socialstyrelsen.
    se/globalassets/sharepoint-dokument/artikelkatalog/foreskrifter-och-
    allmanna-rad/2017-5-24.pdf.
IVO (2017). Samverkan för multisjuka äldres välbefinnande — Nationell tillsyn
    inom hälso-och sjukvård. Stockholm: Inspektionen för vård och omsorg.
    https://www.ivo.se/aktuellt/publikationer/rapporter/samverkan-for-multisjuka-
    aldres-valbefinnande/.
IVO (2019). Vad har IVO sett 2018? Iakttagelser och slutsatser om vårdens och
    omsorgens brister för verksamhetsåret 2018. Stockholm: Inspektionen för
    vård och omsorg. https://www.ivo.se/aktuellt/nyheter/nyheter-2019/vad-har-
    ivo-sett-2018---risker-och-brister-i-vard-och-omsorg/.
Jakobsen, J. (March 17, 2023). *Tiltagsbyrden*. Copenhagen, Denmark:
    Weekendavisen.
King, C., Einhorn, L., Brusselaers, N., Carlsson, M., Einhorn, S., Elgh, F., Frisén,
    J., Gustafsson, Å., Hanson, S., Hanson, C., Hedner, T., Isaksson, O., Jansson,
    A., Lundkvist, Å., Lötvall, J., Lundback, B., Olsen, B., Söderberg-Nauclér, C.,
    Wahlin, A., Steineck, G., and Vahlne, A. (2020). COVID-19 — A very visible
    pandemic. *The Lancet*, *396*(10248), e15. DOI: 10.1016/S0140-6736(20)
    31672-X.
Krassén, P. (April 1, 2022). Pandemilagen — saknad av få, sörjd av ingen.
    Stockholm: Företagarna. https://www.foretagarna.se/nyheter/riks/2022/april/
    pandemilagen--saknad-av-fa-sorjd-av-ingen/.
Kriegner, S., Ottersen, T., Røttingen, J.-A., and Gopinathan, U. (2021). Promoting
    intersectoral collaboration through the evaluations of public health interven-
    tions: Insights from key informants in 6 European Countries. *International
    Journal of Health Policy and Management*, *10*(2), 67–76. DOI: 10.34172/
    ijhpm.2020.19.
Krisinformation (February 1, 2020a). Regeringen klassar coronavirus som sam-
    hällsfarlig sjukdom. https://www.krisinformation.se/nyheter/2020/februari/
    regeringen-klassar-corona-som-samhallsfarlig.
Krisinformation (February 26, 2020c). Nytt bekräftat fall av COVID-19 i
    Sverige. https://www.krisinformation.se/nyheter/2020/februari/nytt-bekraftat-
    fall-av-COVID-19-i-verige.

Krisinformation (January 31, 2020b). Första bekräftade fallet av coronavirus i Sverige. https://www.krisinformation.se/nyheter/2020/januari/forsta-bekraftade-fallet-av-coronavirus-i-sverige/.

Krisinformation (March 24, 2020d). Folkhälsomyndighetens råd om träning och idrott. https://www.krisinformation.se/nyheter/2020/mars/folkhalsomyndig hetens-rad-om-traning-och-idrott.

Läkartidningen (March 3, 2022). Regeringens förslag: Pandemilagen slopas-COVID-19 klassas om i april. Stockholm. https://lakartidningen.se/aktuellt/ nyheter/2022/03/regeringens-forslag-pandemilagen-slopas-COVID-19-klassas-om-i-april/.

Lindström, M. (2020). The COVID-19 pandemic and the Swedish strategy: Epidemiology and postmodernism. *SSM Popul Health*. DOI: 10.1016/j.ssmph.2020.100643.

Lindvall, J. and Rönnerstrand, B. (2022). Challenges for public-service delivery: the case of COVID-19 vaccine hesitancy. *Journal of European Public Policy*. DOI: 10.1080/13501763.2022.2123024.

Moodie, J. (July 2, 2021). Sweden's response to COVID-19 and the limits of individualism. https://www.coronatimes.net/sweden-response-covid-19-limits-individualism/.

Pearson, A. (2023). Lockdown was never on the agenda in Sweden. *The Daily Telegraph*, April 23. London: Daily Telegraph.

Prop. (2017/18:249). God och jämlik hälsa — en utvecklad folkhälsopolitik. https:// www.regeringen.se/rattsliga-dokument/proposition/2018/04/prop.-2017 18249.

Prop. (2021/22:137). Upphävande av COVID-19-lagen och lagen om tillfälliga smittskyddsåtgärder på serveringsställen. Retrieved on March 3, 2024 from https://www.regeringen.se/rattsliga-dokument/proposition/2022/03/prop.-202122137.

Raffetti, E., Mondino, E., and Di Baldassarre, G. (2022). COVID-19 vaccine hesitancy in Sweden and Italy: The role of trust in authorities. *Scandinavian Journal of Public Health*, 50(5), 803–809. DOI: 10.1177/14034948221099410.

Rechel, B., Maresso, A., Sagan, A., Hernández-Quevedo, C., Williams, G., Richardson, E., Jakubowski, E., and Nolte, E. (2018). *Organization and Financing of Public Health Services in Europe: Country Reports*. Copenhagen: European Observatory on Health Systems and Policies.

SCB Statistikdatabasen (2023). *Population by Country of Birth, Age and Sex. Year 2000 — 2022*. Örebro: Statistics Sweden.

SCB (2022). *Population Statistics*. Örebro: Statistics Sweden.

Schöley, J., Aburto, J. M., Kashnitsky, I., Kniffka, M., Zhang, L., Jaadla, H., Dowd, J. B., and Kashyap, R. (2022). Life expectancy changes since COVID-19. *Life Expectancy Changes Since COVID-19*, 6(12), 1649–1659. DOI: 10.1038/s41562-022-01450-3.

SFS (2001:453). The Social Services Act. Retrieved on March 3, 2024 from https://www.riksdagen.se/sv/dokument-lagar/dokument/svensk-forfattnings-samling/socialtjanstlag-2001453_sfs-2001-453.

SFS (2004:168). Smittskyddslagen. https://www.riksdagen.se/sv/dokument-lagar/dokument/svensk-forfattningssamling/smittskyddslag-2004168_sfs-2004-168.

SFS (2006:544). Lag om kommuners och regioners åtgärder inför och vid extraordinära händelser i fredstid och höjd beredskap. Retrieved on March 3, 2024 from https://www.riksdagen.se/sv/dokument-lagar/dokument/svensk-forfattningssamling/lag-2006544-om-kommuners-och-regioners_sfs-2006-544.

SFS (2008:962). The Act on Systems of Choice (LOV). Retrieved on March 3, 2024 from https://www.riksdagen.se/sv/dokument-lagar/dokument/svensk-forfattningssamling/lag-2008962-om-valfrihetssystem_sfs-2008-962.

SFS (2010:659). The act of patient safety in health care. Retrieved on March 3, 2024 from https://www.riksdagen.se/sv/dokument-lagar/dokument/svensk-forfattningssamling/patientsakerhetslag-2010659_sfs-2010-659.

SFS (2014:821). The Patient Act. Retrieved on March 3, 2024 from https://www.riksdagen.se/sv/dokument-lagar/dokument/svensk-forfattningssamling/patientlag-2014821_sfs-2014-821.

SFS (2017:30). Hälso-och sjukvårdslagen. Retrieved on March 3, 2024 from https://www.riksdagen.se/sv/dokument-lagar/dokument/svensk-for fattningssamling/halso--och-sjukvardslag_sfs-2017-30.

SFS (2017:612). Lagen om samverkan vid utskrivning från sluten hälso-och sjukvård (LUS). Retrieved on March 3, 2024 from https://www.riksdagen.se/sv/dokument-lagar/dokument/svensk-forfattningssamling/lag-2017612-om-samverkan-vid-utskrivning-fran_sfs-2017-612.

SFS (2021:4). Lag om särskilda begränsningar för att förhindra spridning av sjuk-domen COVID-19. Retrieved on March 3, 2024 from https://www.riksdagen.se/sv/dokument-lagar/dokument/svensk-forfattningssamling/lag-20214-om-sarskilda-begransningar-for-att_sfs-2021-4.

SFS (2022:524). Förordning om statliga myndigheters beredskap. https://www.riksdagen.se/sv/dokument-lagar/dokument/svensk-forfattningssamling/forordning-2022524-om-statliga-myndigheters_sfs-2022-524.

Shapiro, B., Rahamim-Cohen, D., Tasher, D., Geva, A., Azuri, J., and Ash, N. (2021). COVID-19 in children and the effect of schools reopening on potential transmission to household members. *Acta Paediatrica*, *110*(9), 2567–2573. DOI: 10.1111/apa.15962.

Socialstyrelsen (2021). Vård och omsorg om äldre. Lägesrapport 2021. Stockholm. https://www.socialstyrelsen.se/globalassets/sharepoint-dokument/artikelkata log/ovrigt/2021-3-7249.pdf.

Socialstyrelsen (2022a). Öppna jämförelser — Äldreomsorg. Stockholm. https://www.socialstyrelsen.se/statistik-och-data/oppna-jamforelser/social tjanst/aldreomsorg/.

Socialstyrelsen (2022b). Utrikesfödda och covid-19 — samsjuklighetens påverkan. Stockholm. https://www.socialstyrelsen.se/globalassets/sharepoint-dokument/ artikelkatalog/ovrigt/2022-1-7736.pdf.

SOU (2020:80). Äldreomsorgen under pandemin. https://www.regeringen.se/rattsliga-dokument/statens-offentliga-utredningar/2020/12/sou-202080/.

SOU (2021:89). Sverige under pandemin. https://www.regeringen.se/contentassets/e1c4a1033b9042fe96c0b2a3f453ff1d/sverige-under-pandemin-volym-1_webb-1.pdf.

SOU (2022:10). Sverige under pandemin. https://www.regeringen.se/rattsliga-dokument/statens-offentliga-utredningar/2022/02/sou-202210/.

Statskontoret (2022). Allmänhetens uppfattning om kvaliteten i de statliga verksamheterna. Stockholm. https://www.statskontoret.se/fokusomraden/ fakta-om-statsforvaltningen/allmanhetens-uppfattning-om-kvaliteten-i-de-statliga-verksamheterna/.

Strang, J. (April 6, 2020). Why do the Nordic countries react differently to the COVID-19 crisis? https://nordics.info/show/artikel/the-nordic-countries-react-differently-to-the-COVID-19-crisis/.

SVT (2023). *"Rörelsen"*. *Documentary*. Stockholm: Sveriges Television.

SVT (December 3, 2020). *Oklart hur svenska covid-vaccineringen ska gå till — bara en region har färdigskriven Plan*. Stockholm: Sveriges Television. https://www.svt.se/nyheter/inrikes/oklart-hur-svenska-vaccineringen-ska-ga-till-bara-en-region-har-fardigskriven-plan.

Tegmark Wisell, K. (May 12, 2023). *Så måste Sverige rusta inför nästa Pandemic*. Stockholm: Dagens Nyheter. https://www.dn.se/debatt/sa-maste-sverige-rusta-infor-nasta-pandemi/.

Thomson, S., Ip, E. C., and Lee, S. F. (2022). International comparisons of COVID-19 case and mortality data and the effectiveness of non-pharmaceutical interventions: A plea for reconsideration. *Journal of Biosocial Science*, *54*(5). DOI: 10.1017/S0021932021000547.

Tomson, G., Causevic, S., Ottersen, O., Swartling Peterson, S., Rashid, S., Wanyenze, R. K., and Yamin, E. (2021). Solidarity and universal preparedness for health after COVID-19. *The BMJ*, *372*, n59. DOI: 10.1136/bmj. n59.

Tidningarnas Telegrambyrå (TT) (January 12, 2022). SD begär granskning av regeringens beslut om restriktioner under pandemin. https://via.tt.se/pressmeddelande/sd-begar-granskning-av-regeringens-beslut-om-restriktioner-under-pandemin?publisherId=3236128&releaseId=3315524.

Vårdföretagarna (2019). Privat vårdfakta. Stockholm. https://www.vardforetagarna.se/privat-vardfakta-2019/.

Vård-och omsorgsanalys (2022). Riktade vaccinationsinsatser. Stockholm. https://www.vardanalys.se/rapporter/riktade-vaccinationsinsatser/.

von Schreeb, J. (March 15, 2020). Wolodarski undergräver svensk expertis. Svenska Dagbladet. https://www.svd.se/a/9vdW8l/johan-von-schreeb-wolodarski-bidrar-till-kunskapsforaktet.

Wikstrand, J. (March 19, 2020). Orosdebatten kring corona dominerar på sociala medier. *Retriever*. https://www.retrievergroup.com/sv/blogg/orosdebatten-kring-corona-dominerar-pa-sociala-medier.

Wolodarski, P. (March 12, 2020). Stäng ned Sverige för att skydda Sverige. *Dagens Nyheter*. https://www.dn.se/ledare/peter-wolodarski-stang-ned-sverige-for-att-skydda-sverige/.

Yarmol-Matusiak, E. A., Cipriano, L. E., and Stranges, S. (2021). A comparison of COVID-19 epidemiological indicators in Sweden, Norway, Denmark, and Finland. *Scandinavian journal of Public Health*, *49*(1), 69–78. https://doi.org/10.1177/1403494820980264.

https://doi.org/10.1142/9789811296307_0004

Chapter 4

Canada

Peter Berman and Candice Ruck

4.1 Introduction: Upstream Factors Shaping Authority and Decision-Making in a Public Health Crisis

Although Canada has a long, and not entirely glorious, history of government action to control threats of imported epidemic disease (Humphries, 2012), the impact of perceived failures to address the Sudden Acute Respiratory Syndrome (SARS) pandemic of 2003 awoke a renewed commitment to pandemic preparedness in Canada. As a result of the post-SARS reforms, the Global Health Security Index (Centre for Health Security, 2019) of 2019 ranked Canada number five globally in its readiness to handle a new pandemic threat. However, not uniquely among high-income countries (Goldschmidt, 2022), this did not prove to be an accurate prediction of Canada's real-world response to the COVID-19 pandemic.

Although Canada's collective performance in responding to the COVID-19 pandemic was considered moderately successful by the standards of global comparisons, within Canada large variations were observed in what was done, when it was done, and how well it was done, despite the guidance of national organizations that were established post-SARS to assure a more coherent national response. A study assessing the consistency of the pandemic response across Canada found that, of 24 public health interventions analyzed, only 57% were implemented by all provinces and territories (Cyr *et al.*, 2021). The authors also reported that there was a wide range in the timing of implementation for many of these interventions. Further, implementation was not found to be consistent with the number of positive cases, suggesting that other factors were also influencing decision-making (Cyr *et al.,* 2021). Policies that determined when and how restrictions were relaxed also tended to vary considerably between provinces. At the provincial level, a report by the Auditor General in Ontario identified a number of deficiencies in that province's response, including not being guided by scientific expertise and not being led by public health officials (Auditor General of Ontario, 2020).

Canadian provinces differ with respect to their demographics, density, and the structure and funding of their public health systems, which explains some of the diversity in pandemic response. However, we posit that much of the difference observed between provinces during COVID-19 can be more adequately explained by the influence of key upstream factors, namely Institutions, Politics, the Organization of Public Health Systems, and Governance (IPOG). In previous work, we have expanded on IPOG as a conceptual framework for analysis of the COVID-19 response in different jurisdictions and provided some definitions of the terms represented by IPOG (Brubacher *et al.,* 2022).

The **Institutional** context in Canada involves a federated system composed of the national government and 10 provincial governments. Additionally, there are three territories that do not have constitutional powers in their own right but rather exercise powers delegated by Parliament, although authority has been gradually devolving from the federal to the territorial level (Government of Canada, 2022). It is particularly noteworthy that the federal structure in Canada protects provincial autonomy from a wide range of specific types of action by the national government.

This represents one important dimension of many Canadians' perception of the "rules of the game" in terms of proper scope of action accorded to different levels of government. In situations where stronger collective action may be merited, such as when facing a rapidly moving infectious disease threat with significant unknowns, as was the case in the first half of 2020, this has posed a challenge for the country. Provinces also differ substantially in terms of values widely held about individual autonomy and collective action and social solidarity.

Understanding the influence of the Canadian **Political** context should involve considering the ideologies and policies of the various political parties and their elected or competing leaders across both the provincial and national scenes. In particular, it must be recognized that policies and strategies promoted by political parties in national elections and office are only partially aligned with the policies and strategies of the same parties at the provincial level. Similarly, the roles and authorities of legislators differ across provinces as does the degree to which political leadership is realized in the administrative organs of government.

The **Organizations** that encompass the public health services of Canada are for the most part subordinate structures situated within what may best be characterized as a medical care system since Canada's single-payer Medicare structure emphasizes guaranteed access to medically necessary treatments. At the provincial level, public health organizations within the medical care system are established under provincial laws and regulations and differ considerably across provinces in their legal authority, organization, and financing, especially in relation to deemed public health emergencies (Marchildon, 2008).

These variations in institutions, politics, and public health organizations intersect in the decision-making processes that shape the response to a public health emergency, such as the COVID-19 pandemic. Incorporating the role of **Governance** examines decision-making and implementation processes which are the locus of this intersection. For example, when assessing a particular key decision such as the decision to enable emergency powers in response to an emerging pandemic, it is necessary to consider what exchanges took place between political and public health organizational actors, how these exchanges were shaped by wider institutional factors, and how the decisions emerging from these processes reflected the influence of these different factors.

To provide insights into the importance of these upstream factors, we examine here the Canadian response to COVID-19 from the perspective of how Canadian institutions, politics, organization of public health systems, and governance processes contributed to specific national and provincial responses to COVID-19.

4.2 Structure of the Canadian Medical Care and Public Health Systems

Medical care in Canada is an amalgam of federal, provincial, and regional responsibility. Under the publicly funded medical care system, the federal government provides funding and, through the Canada Health Act established in 1984, sets out the criteria for medical care that must be available to all individuals (Urrutia *et al.*, 2021), organized around the five governing criteria of (1) Public Administration, (2) Comprehensiveness, (3) Universality, (4) Portability, and (5) Accessibility (Health Canada, 2015). These criteria must be adhered to in relation to all "medically necessary care" in order for provinces to receive the substantial "Canada health transfer" — an annual financial subvention.

The Canada Health Act establishes the baseline that all provinces must meet. Beyond this, provinces do not follow a singular model in the structuring of their medical care systems so there is considerable diversity between provincial systems. Within the organizational structure of each province's medical care system, key public health functions are embedded in different organizational structures with differing levels of authority, scope, and empowerment (see Figure 4.1).

4.2.1 *Public health changes prompted by SARS*

Many aspects of the Canadian response to COVID-19 were informed and shaped by the outbreak of SARS in 2003, during which Canada was the worst affected region outside Asia. Intergovernmental collaboration between federal and provincial governments was identified as a major factor in the failed response to SARS, and as such efforts have been made toward improvement. Yet in many aspects of pandemic response, intergovernmental collaboration remains voluntary, except for certain authorities given to the federal government, such as the management of international borders or the regulation of medical goods. Collaboration is facilitated by the Conference of Federal-Provincial-Territorial Ministers of Health, as

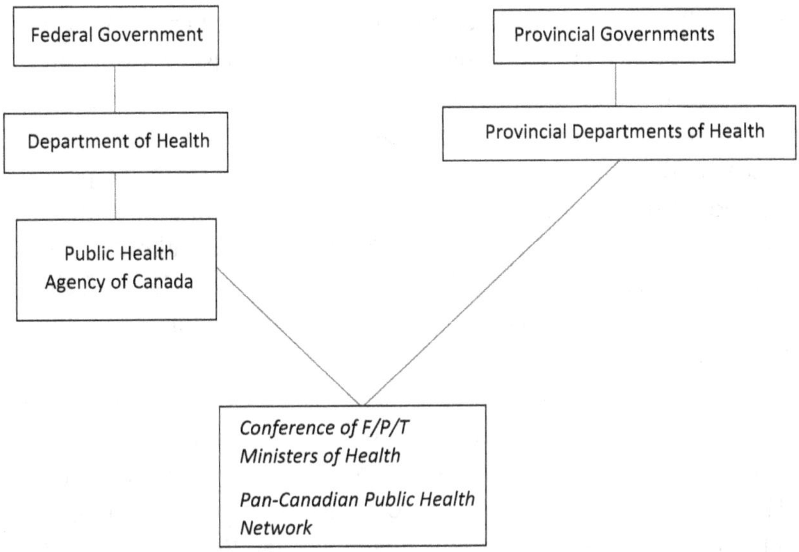

Figure 4.1. Public health governance in Canada.

well as by a similar mirror committee of the Deputy Ministers of Health (Marchildon, 2008; O'Reilly, 2001).

The aftermath of SARS also saw the development of the Pan-Canadian Public Health Network (PHN), which was created to further facilitate intergovernmental coordination and cooperation across jurisdictions. The PHN, which includes the lead health officer (Provincial Health Officer or PHO) from each of the provinces/territories as well as Canada's Chief Public Health Officer (CPHO), reports to the Conference of the Federal/Provincial/Territorial Deputy Ministers of Health. In response to a public health emergency, the PHN may establish a Special Advisory Committee (SAC) for the purpose of establishing a time-limited governance structure to lead a pan-Canadian response to the crisis. It is worth noting that within their respective provinces, the PHOs may hold different authorities which in some cases exceed those of the deputy ministers.

4.2.2 *Public Health Agency of Canada (PHAC)*

At the time that SARS emerged in 2003, Canada did not have a National Public Health Institute (NPHI). The Canadian response to SARS was beset by difficulties and failures, which were summed up in the *Learning from SARS* report produced by the National Advisory Committee on SARS and Public Health, chaired by Dr. David Naylor, and commissioned by the federal government (Naylor *et al.*, 2003). In the years that followed, approximately 80% of the recommendations made in that report were addressed (Webster, 2020), the most significant of which was the establishment of the PHAC. The operational structure and authority of PHAC has evolved since its inception, influenced by a range of IPOG factors. In turn, this has impacted how the agency has functioned in the response to COVID-19.

A Working Group was set up after the Naylor report was released to establish the structure of the future public health agency. Influenced by the findings of the *Learning from SARS* report, which envisioned that a future NPHI be granted considerable autonomy and be legislatively empowered to set priorities and steer the public health agenda, PHAC was established as a stand-alone agency that was partnered with, rather than subordinate to, Health Canada, the department of the federal government that serves as an umbrella agency under which numerous aspects of federal health policy are encompassed (Fafard & Forest, 2016). As part of the overall federal Health Portfolio, PHAC was to be reportable to the Minister of Health.

The Naylor report also recommended the establishment of the position of CPHO, a federal counterpart to the provincial-level PHOs. Such a role exists across numerous federations and is often designated as simultaneously being an advisor to the government and an independent watchdog for the public (MacAuley *et al.*, 2022). However, it has been suggested that encompassing both of these functions within a single role is untenable (Fafard *et al.*, 2018).

To imbue the CPHO role with both autonomy and authority, the report further recommended that the CPHO position should also be responsible for leading the new NPHI (Naylor *et al.*, 2003). Thus, when the PHAC was established by the then-Liberal government in 2004, the CPHO was designated at the rank of a Deputy Minister, and positioned as the deputy head of PHAC, with the Minister of Health as the head (Marchildon, 2008).

Under the Conservative government that took over in 2006, a shift began to emerge in the relationship between the federal government and PHAC. Critics claimed that the organization was skewed too heavily toward public health experts with few civil service managers, although the involvement of experts at the most senior levels was emphasized by the Working Group when the agency was established (Fafard & Forest, 2016). In 2010, the role of Executive Vice-President was appointed to effectively manage the operations side of the agency, unofficially splitting the public health and operational roles for the first time.

Following the retirement in 2013 of the first head of PHAC, Dr. David Butler-Jones, the role of CPHO was left vacant for 16 months amidst criticisms that the government was increasingly attempting to assert influence over what was supposed to be an apolitical appointment, making it difficult to attract suitable candidates (Robertson, 2014). The ideological clash between politics and public health came to a head in 2014, when the government formally separated the roles of CPHO and PHAC head by creating the position of President to lead PHAC. Under this new structure, the CPHO no longer had control over the PHAC budgets or staff and the role became more advisory than authoritative (Grant, 2014). This move was met with criticism among many in the public health community, who expressed concern that it would hamper the autonomy and authority of the agency, particularly as the position of President is not required to have a medical or scientific background. The Health Minister at the time countered these concerns by stating that the move was meant to free the CPHO from the administrative burden of leading the PHAC, supported by then-CPHO Dr. Gregory Taylor's testimony before a Senate committee supporting the creation of the position of President to lead the day-to-day running of the agency (Fafard & Forest, 2016).

Although the declared intent of these changes was to provide a more balanced structure to the agency, there have since been concerns that the balance has shifted too far to the other end of the spectrum. In the ensuing years since the agency was restructured, management roles at the PHAC have increasingly been filled by civil servants, regardless of medical or scientific training, prompting the departure of many senior-level experts (Robertson, 2020). The effect of these changes was to weaken the influence of experts in the operation of the agency. Not surprisingly, PHAC has been criticized for not having medical or scientific experts at the highest decision-making levels during the response to COVID-19 (Tumilty, 2021). However, it is also worth noting that the Working Group that originally established the structure of PHAC also explicitly rejected the notion that the CPHO be authorized to act autonomously during a public health emergency, where far-reaching actions would be required (Fafard & Forest, 2016).

4.3 Canada's Medical Care and Public Health Systems at the Outset of the Pandemic

Although the generally accepted view is that Canada's COVID-19 response has been moderately successful, in a country as large and diverse as Canada, a consolidated view obscures some of the more dire effects of the pandemic. Case counts and mortality varied widely between provinces. In the early phases of the pandemic, the Atlantic provinces compared favorably with the COVID-19 success story in New Zealand, while Quebec more closely resembled France (Poirier and Michelin, 2021). Further, the response throughout the first phase was not without blind spots. COVID-19 swept through long-term care (LTC) facilities seemingly at will, with LTC fatalities accounting for approximately 67% of COVID deaths in Canada up to February 15, 2021 (Betini *et al.*, 2021).

Some of this variation was simply due to chance; the higher rates of infection experienced by Quebec at the start of the pandemic were attributed in part to that province having an earlier spring break than other provinces, and thus a higher volume of returning travelers from other affected areas, such as Western Europe and Iran, before border restrictions were implemented (Allin *et al.*, 2022). However, there were also larger institutional and organizational factors that contributed to the variances in interprovincial response. These include Canada's federal structure, provincial variations in public health system organization, and how these were situated within the overall structure of medical care delivery. A closer consideration of these factors is necessary to fully reveal the upstream determinants of the observed variation in responses and outcomes.

4.3.1 *Initial response (Spring–Summer 2020)*

In accordance with the decentralized structure of the Canadian healthcare system, the responsibilities of the federal government in responding to COVID-19 were largely limited to implementing restrictions on travel and control of the borders, economic measures, and vaccine procurement. The implementation of non-pharmaceutical interventions as well as the policies determining the distribution of the vaccines were under provincial jurisdiction, with the federal government serving in an advisory role via the PHAC as well other advisory bodies such as the National Advisory Committee on Immunization (NACI).

The first COVID-19 case in Canada was confirmed on January 25, 2020. In January 2020, PHAC activated the Emergency Operations Centre and initiated the F/P/T Public Health Response Plan for Biological Events (Urrutia *et al.*, 2021). Actions taken at the governance level to facilitate intergovernmental and interagency coordination, an issue identified after the failed response to SARS, included the creation of a federal cabinet committee for the purpose of facilitating a whole-of-government response (Urrutia *et al.*, 2021) and activation of a SAC for COVID-19 (Piper *et al.*, 2022).

Beyond these measures, Canada took no substantive action at the federal level until after the WHO declared COVID-19 to be a pandemic on March 11, 2020. Calls for border restrictions were resisted in accordance with the guidance of the WHO and the IHR to which Canada is a signatory (Piper *et al.*, 2022). In Canada, as elsewhere, the imposition of travel restrictions was also complicated by a lack of clear scientific direction combined with competing economic interests. Particularly early in the pandemic, it remained unclear to what extent travel restrictions actually inhibited the spread of the virus. Despite this uncertainty, public support for travel restrictions was high, with only 19% supporting a total absence of restrictions on both international and interprovincial travel (Angus Reid Institute, 2020).

Following the WHO's declaration, a succession of measures were introduced that were aimed at reducing international travel and restricting the borders as well as addressing the economic burden of the burgeoning pandemic (Canadian Public Health Association, 2021). These included banning entry to foreign nationals and imposing a mandatory 14-day isolation on international arrivals (PHAC, 2020). Points of entry for international travelers was reduced to only four airports across the country. Constitutional rights prevented the federal government instituting a ban on Canadians traveling internationally; instead, an advisory against international travel was issued (Global Affairs Canada, 2020). Travel that was deemed essential was exempted from these policies, and categories of exempted travelers grew over time. With the exceptions of the Atlantic provinces, the territories, and the province of Quebec, domestic travel between provinces remained largely unrestricted at this stage, although both federal and provincial governments strongly recommended that people avoid non-essential travel of any kind (MacGregor, 2020).

The restrictions on international travel were also weakened by a lack of institutional capacity to monitor quarantines (Auditor General of Canada, 2021). Although the federal government has jurisdiction over air travel, and could therefore impose restrictions on incoming passengers, the provincial governments have civil jurisdiction over the land that the airports are on, and were thus largely responsible for the implementation of the regulations, including monitoring of quarantines. However, this frequently meant diverting resources that the provinces were devoting to other aspects of pandemic response. Further, provincial capacity was not equivalent across the board nor were the provinces equally affected from an economic standpoint by these travel restrictions. The federal travel measures and the manner in which they were enforced reveal the presence of political, economic, and institutional pressures on decision-making.

Concurrently with these actions, the provinces took responsibility for instituting a range of public health measures aimed at reducing the spread of the virus. These included restrictions on social gatherings, closures of schools and businesses, policies regarding the wearing of masks, testing, and case management. The provincial responses were broadly aligned due partly to pre-existing mechanisms for fostering intergovernmental coordination but were not entirely consistent in timing or stringency (Cassola *et al.*, 2021). Although all provinces had declared a state of emergency by the end of March 2020, there was considerable variation across provinces in the stringency of policies related to measures, such as testing and social distancing.

Although some of this disparity can also be traced to issues of capacity, as larger provinces tended to fare worse than smaller ones, the effect of pre-existing institutions was also a factor. British Columbia, which has a provincial Centre for Disease Control (BCCDC), had procedures and expertise that were more established than other provinces. By utilizing these capabilities to take a more aggressive approach early on, British Columbia became the exception to the trend of larger provinces having worse outcomes (Migone, 2020).

The different interpretations of the role of provincial Chief Medical Officers of Health (CMOH), titled in some provinces as the PHO to distinguish from regional-level CMOH positions, were also on display through the response to COVID-19. The position of CMOH is complex and multifaceted, encompassing advisory, managerial, and communications roles, particularly in the context of a pandemic. Similar to their federal counterpart, provincial CMOHs are expected both to act as a politically neutral scientific advisor to the government as well as to communicate government policy to the public, a duality that is not without friction (Fafard, 2018). Further, each province is distinct in how the role is structured both legislatively and within the larger public health system, and in how much emphasis is placed on each of these functions (Cassola *et al.*, 2022; Fafard, 2018).

The degree to which the response was centralized or decentralized also differed between provinces, reflecting the pre-existing institutional structures that were in place prior to the pandemic. Provinces such as British Columbia and Nova Scotia demonstrated a more centralized leadership strategy, with the CMOH as the main decision-makers while political leaders were engaged in less visible roles. It is worth noting that the provinces that employed this more centralized approach experienced lower rates of transmission and mortality in the early phases of the pandemic (Snowdon, 2021).

Initially, the emergency nature of the situation sparked considerable cooperation between the provincial and federal governments, all of whom were seemingly aligned on the potential seriousness of the burgeoning pandemic. This was not a foregone conclusion, as conflicts between the federal and provincial governments are part of the established pattern of intergovernmental relations in Canada and have less to do with political ideology than with division of authority. With some notable recent exceptions, successive federal governments have long adopted a strategy of not angering the provinces, a path that they also opted for in the early days of COVID-19 by, for example, not invoking the *Emergencies Act*.

As COVID-19 spread, the provinces largely expressed support for the policy decisions of the federal government (Migone, 2020). For their part, the federal government upheld provincial jurisdiction over healthcare and did not invoke the federal *Emergencies Act*, which would have temporarily given them increased dominion over the pandemic response. It is worth noting that the *Emergencies Act* had never been used since it was first tabled in 1987, indicative of the extent to which the federal government has historically avoided inflaming tensions with the provinces (Attaran, 2020).

In response to the emerging crisis that was COVID-19, the government briefly considered invoking the *act* during the early months of the pandemic. However, provincial leaders opposed ceding their jurisdiction over healthcare and argued that they could act more effectively if their autonomy was preserved (*The Globe and Mail*, 2020). The Council of the Federation, comprised of the provincial and territorial Premiers, informed the federal government that they considered it "neither necessary nor advisable to invoke the *Act* at this time" (Public Safety Canada, 2020). In the face of such opposition, the federal government assessed that any potential benefits of a more centralized response would be undermined by provincial resistance and the ensuing intergovernmental conflict (Cassola *et al.*, 2021).

Other options for a more centralized response exist within section 91 of the Constitution, which gives the federal government an option to pass legislation if the failure of one province would affect other provinces. However, it has not previously been established whether this power can be exerted without the consent of the provinces who, in rejecting the use of the *Emergencies Act*, had already tacitly rejected an increased federal presence (Canada, Parliament, Senate, Standing Senate Committee on Social Affairs, Science and Technology, 2010). Thus, both by design and default, the response Canadian institutions adopted to COVID-19 was cooperative rather than co-opted.

4.4 Responses During Subsequent Waves of Infection: Fall/Winter 2020–Fall 2021

The initial measures taken to "flatten the curve" in Canada yielded results, and from a peak near the end of April, cases fell throughout the month of

May 2020 (Our World in Data, 2022). In response, provinces began to relax their restrictions throughout the summer of 2020. As new variants of concern, including the highly transmissible Delta variant, began to circulate widely in late 2020, new measures were introduced at both federal and provincial levels to curb the spread of infection and avoid overwhelming the healthcare systems.

The ruling Liberal party called an election in the fall of 2021, just 2 years after being reduced from a majority to a minority government in the 2019 election. It was widely supposed that the timing was meant to take advantage of the generally favorable opinion the electorate had of the government's handling of the pandemic to restore the Liberals to a majority. However, the timing and cost of the election proved to be widely unpopular and became one of the major themes of the campaign. Polls showed that 69% of voters felt that the election should not have been called (Bricker, 2021). Voters expressed their displeasure at the polls, returning the Liberals to power with another minority government. In contrast, BC had called an election in October 2020 and the NDP party then in power was elevated from a minority to a majority government, largely influenced by public approval of how the provincial government had handled the pandemic response to that point. The difference in these respective outcomes reflects not only the different contexts (at the time of the provincial election, BC had the best pandemic response of the six large provinces) but also the decline in public support and positive perception of the pandemic response between the autumn of 2020 and 2021.

As the pandemic continued and the virus evolved, considerable heterogeneity developed between jurisdictions in the implementation of various interventions. Some of this was due to geographic and demographic variations, which saw the effect of the pandemic differentially distributed across jurisdictions. However, social, political, and institutional contexts also factored into the difference in responses.

Additionally, there were numerous competing interests beyond the scientific that necessarily influenced decision-making, including economic effects on businesses and households, the mental health impact of social distancing restrictions, and the institutional and political contexts in which policy decisions were made. These and other factors combined to produce increasingly distinct responses among the provinces throughout late 2020/early 2021 (Inverardi-Ferri & Brown, 2020). Further, policy responses seemed to be increasingly removed from the advice of experts, despite repeated assertions by governments at all levels that their policies were driven by science (Inverardi-Ferri & Brown, 2020; Yang & Allen, 2020; McEwan, 2020).

Communication was also key to establishing public trust and buy-in. The function and role of the CMOHs provide some insight into how communication strategies differ across the country. As previously mentioned, the provinces vary in how the role of the CMHO is structured with respect to their advisory, management, and communication functions (Fafard *et al.*, 2020). These differences were often reflected in the tone and content of the messaging relayed by the CMHO to the public. The extent to which the CMHO was the primary conveyor of information to the public was also influenced by these distinctions. In provinces such as BC, where the response had a more centralized structure, the CMHO was the primary spokesperson, with political figures taking a background role, while in provinces such as Alberta and Nova Scotia, the CMHO was more typically accompanied by an elected official (Fafard *et al.*, 2020). These different approaches fed into public perceptions of transparency, autonomy, and the role of experts in decision-making.

As the pandemic entered its second year, public confidence was also undermined by numerous instances in which government figures either denied responsibility for surges in case numbers or avoided being questioned by the public altogether (Inverardi-Ferri & Brown, 2022; Yang & Allen, 2020). Together, the lack of transparency, real or perceived, as to how the evidence actually informed decisions (Piper *et al.*, 2022) combined with a lack of accountability, growing disparities between provincial policies and the frequency with which policies changed all contributed to increasing skepticism among the public.

4.4.1 *Federal travel restrictions*

Starting in early 2021, a series of new travel measures was introduced. These included requirements that international travelers show a negative PCR test within 72 hours of traveling, as well as testing upon arrival. Air travelers were additionally required to quarantine for 3 days at a government-designated hotel (PHAC, 2021), a restriction that was not imposed on those crossing the border by land. Again, essential travelers were exempted from these restrictions.

Compared to previous restrictions, the implementation of these new measures was met with much more resistance. Some of this was driven by skepticism over government claims that the measures were based on scientific evidence. The extent to which data drove policies was not always transparent. The 3-day quarantine imposed on air travelers, an attempt to find a middle ground between tougher restrictions and the strict 14-day quarantine imposed by countries such as Australia, was criticized for lacking scientific legitimacy and for allowing travelers a loophole at land crossings. Researchers reviewing the available data found that there was insufficient evidence to support these policy decisions (Lee & Nicol, 2021). Much of the resistance was based on concerns that the new rules didn't go far enough to be sufficiently effective, with the vast majority of Canadians supporting restrictions on international travel (Canseco, 2020). As debates over the new restrictions intensified, the political cohesion that had marked the earlier phase of the pandemic disintegrated.

4.4.2 *Provincial travel restrictions*

The gradual erosion of social solidarity and cohesion was also visible at the provincial level. Up to this point, restrictions on travel between provinces had varied throughout most of 2020 with most provinces opting to advise against non-essential travel but not going as far as enforceable restrictions. The exception was the four Atlantic provinces, which jointly formed the so-called "Atlantic Bubble." This agreement allowed unrestricted travel between those four provinces but restricted the entry of residents from other Canadian provinces. The three territories also displayed regional unity, acting with similar timing and stringency (Cameron-Blake *et al.*, 2021). Although the Atlantic and Territorial regions no doubt benefitted from their relative geographic isolation, the unity of their responses undoubtedly contributed to their success in controlling COVID-19, with the Atlantic provinces recording the lowest case numbers throughout the first year of the pandemic (VOCM, 2020).

Despite the potential benefits, there were questions regarding the constitutionality of these restrictions under Section 6 of the Charter, which guarantees Canadians freedom of movement between provinces. This was cited by some provinces as justification for why they did not pursue similar measures. The Canadian Civil Liberties Association filed a charter challenge against the restrictions in Newfoundland. The Supreme Court there upheld the restrictions and ruled that they were allowed under Section 1 of the Charter, which permits justifiable exemptions to the charter (Cooke, 2020).

As the Delta wave drove infection numbers and stretched healthcare capacities, provinces such as British Columbia that had previously relied on recommendations rather than restrictions finally began to restrict both interprovincial as well as intraprovincial travel (BC Public Safety and Solicitor General, 2021). Public pressure also played a role in these decisions, as public support was high for both interprovincial (82%) and interprovincial (75%) travel restrictions by December 2020 (Canseco, 2020). The timing and extent of the new restrictions varied from province to province. Apart from the Atlantic and Territorial regions, there was little coordination, cooperation, or communication between provinces on limiting the interprovincial movement of people (Cameron-Blake *et al.*, 2021). These disparities between provinces in the type, timing, and stringency of travel restrictions, not to mention in the scientific evidence upon which they were supposedly based, fueled increasing levels of anger and frustration among the public.

4.4.3 Vaccinations: Procurement, distribution, and mandates

Canadians showed strong support for COVID-19 vaccination (Statistics Canada, 2021), with approximately 84% of the country having received at least two doses of vaccine as of October 2022 (Holder, 2022). There is some regional variation in public enthusiasm for the vaccine, as reflected in differing rates of vaccination across the country. Newfoundland has the highest rate at >91%, while the remote territory of Nunavut has 73% fully vaccinated (Little, 2022).

The vaccination campaign was not without some early difficulties. Vaccine procurement, licensing, and production are the responsibility of the federal government, and lack of vaccine production facilities within Canada meant that domestic production was not available. Canada initially signed procurement deals with seven manufacturers in both the US and Europe and had committed to agreements to procure enough doses to vaccinate 400% of the population (Cameron-Blake *et al.*, 2021). Despite this, the initial rollout was beset by delays. Due to export bans in the US, the first doses from those suppliers were not shipped until mid-March 2021. There were early criticisms that Canada was not receiving doses as quickly as other countries (Ling, 2021).

Delays caused by federal procurement difficulties were also exacerbated by the fact that there did not appear to be adequate preparedness plans to support mass vaccination campaigns at either federal or provincial levels (Snowdon *et al.*, 2021). Vaccine distribution and administration strategies were determined at the provincial/territorial level. Effectively, this meant that there was no central distribution policy, although the federal government provided advice through a variety of federal agencies and committees, including Health Canada, PHAC, the Council of Chief Medical Officers of Health, and the expert advisory NACI. In the early stages, this decentralization imposed an additional delay in administering doses (Marchildon, 2021). The provinces leveled heavy criticism at the federal government, but this was at least partly intended to deflect criticism away from their own inadequacies in implementing effective distribution strategies.

The vaccine distribution process has also been criticized for a lack of transparency (Ling, 2021). As an independent advisory committee, NACI is committed to transparency in their process (Ismail *et al.*, 2021); however, as NACI is only empowered to advise, the vaccination policies developed by each province were not always consistent with their recommendations. Due to an early shortage of doses, BC opted to extend the interval between doses beyond that recommended by the manufacturers and the federal government to ensure that more first doses could be administered (Tauh *et al.*, 2021). At the time, there was scant scientific evidence to support this capacity-driven policy, although upon further review it was subsequently adopted by NACI as the recommended dosing strategy (NACI, 2021).

In the fall of 2021 as cases again began to rise, the provinces began to implement policies restricting access to specific venues based on vaccination status (Han & Breton, 2022). These policies and their implementation varied by province, but most instituted some form of "vaccine passport" (Durrani, 2021). Vaccine-related controversies began to escalate in response, not only among those opposed to vaccination but also among those confused about the inconsistency between provinces as well as the businesses that bore the brunt of enforcing these policies.

4.5 Early 2022

Public unrest reached new highs in the early months of 2022, sparked by an announcement in late 2021, shortly after the election, that from January 15 truckers would be required to adhere to vaccine mandates and mandatory quarantine when crossing the border (*Reuters*, 2022). As an essential service, trucking had previously been exempt from COVID-related border restrictions. This exemption, motivated by a desire to minimize disruption to the supply chain, was not without controversy, as essential service providers had comprised the vast majority of border crossings following federal restrictions on non-essential travel.

In response to the new restrictions, convoys consisting mostly of trucks made their way to Ottawa in late January 2022, where large protests were staged. Although initially peaceful, the protests devolved into an occupation-style movement that became highly disruptive while also sparking protests in cities across the country. As the protest devolved into disorderly and illegal conduct, protesters blocked a number of border crossings between Canada and the US, including the Ambassador Bridge in Windsor Ontario, (*Reuters*, 2022). On February 15, the federal government invoked the *Emergencies Act* to deal with the protests, a move that enabled the government to impose bans on public assembly in certain regions of Ottawa and gave banks the power to freeze the accounts of individuals linked to the protests (*BBC News*, 2022). It is notable that this was the first time during the course of the pandemic that the

Emergencies Act was used, having previously been rejected by the provinces in the initial phase of the COVID-19 response.

From their origins as a reaction to vaccine mandates, the protests evolved to include all COVID-19 restrictions, despite many of these being under provincial, rather than federal, control. They also become a megaphone for anti-government sentiment and a rallying cry for the far-right, not only in Canada and the United States but also around the world (Scott, 2022). Hacked records of the crowdsourcing site GiveSendGo revealed that nearly half of the donations to fund these protests originated in the US (Cardoso, 2022). The leader of the Opposition Conservative Party was removed as the head of his party. While this was largely the result both of his failure to win the recent election and his reversal of opposition to federal carbon tax and assault weapons policies, a reluctance to voice support for the movement was also seen to be a contributing factor. Notably, a member of the Conservative Party that vocally supported the protests became the next elected leader of the party.

The extent to which the so-called "freedom convoy" arose as a response to frustrations around the cross-border vaccine mandate is debatable. While the restrictions imposed on truckers acted as the spark, the anger that fueled these protests pre-dated the new restrictions and even the pandemic. Anger still simmered from what many perceived as an ill-timed and pointless election in the fall of 2021. Provinces were becoming less cohesive in the imposition of restrictions and poor communication combined with a perceived lack of transparency, particularly regarding the imposition of vaccine mandates, exacerbated these disparities and drove confusion and frustration among the public (Fafard *et al.*, 2020). Combined with pandemic fatigue and economic hardships, this set the stage for increased resistance and defiance.

Anti-government sentiment, much of which pre-dated the pandemic, also fueled the protests (Cardoso, 2022). The convoy, which originated in Western Canada, also tapped into long-standing feelings of alienation between the western provinces and the federal government. Organizers of the movement had previously been involved with the yellow vest movement of 2018/2019 that protested against the impact of federal carbon tax policies (Crawford, 2022). This sense of alienation among the western provinces is also driven by longstanding feelings of disconnect resulting from political, institutional, economic, and cultural influence being concentrated in the two most populous provinces of Ontario and Quebec.

4.6 How Could Understanding IPOG Factors Improve Canada's Future Crisis Response?

Overall, our case study research and observations support the observation that the interactions among institutions, politics, and the organization of public health systems, as evidenced and expressed through decision-making processes (our "governance"), are important explanatory factors under-pinning a wide diversity of responses in Canada to the COVID-19 pandemic. The following are some suggestions of how greater attention to these "upstream" determinants could strengthen preparedness and response to future public health crises.

At the level of "institutions," the evolution of the pandemic exposed profound differences in values and expectations for the role of the state in the lives of Canadians. During the first wave of the pandemic, the advice of health experts was given primacy reflecting a general sense of social solidarity in response to an urgent crisis of unknown severity. However, as the pandemic extended in time, there was growing dissatisfaction with the imposition of restrictions on individuals' freedoms, reflecting a different set of institutional norms, those questioning the legitimacy of government interference in people's lives, even when justified by the common good. This also became entwined with many Canadians' distrust of federal authority. The leanings of Canadian law and governance institutions toward provincial autonomy justified resistance to increasing federal powers.

These experiences suggest that both health and other leaders need to consider a wider framing than just health outcomes to sustain popular support for control measures. And more generally it is challenging to sustain a solely health-focused emergency posture for longer periods when needing to balance health threats with other social consequences.

We observed in several places and at several times the strong influence of political actors on the substance and timing of emergency response decision-making. The timing of several provincial elections and the national election suggested politicians sought to take advantage of their perception that the public perceived their leadership positively. Some of these elections were associated with delays or modifications in short-term decision-making in response to the changing pandemic which may have had negative health consequences.

There were significant differences across Canada's provinces in leadership roles taken by elected figures relative to those given to scientists and public health experts. At the federal level, the role and authorities observed in PHAC and various advisory councils could be seen as unduly weakened by authority imposed by political actors over the recommendations initially adopted to establish these agencies.

In several instances, we felt that pandemic responses could be improved through decision-making processes that better integrate both federal and provincial agencies in making decisions. The mixed experiences in vaccine procurement, distribution, and roll-out across the provinces were good examples of where greater integration might have improved trust and compliance.

Overall, this would suggest that enabling legislation for public health authorities should provide clearer roles and functions in such crises that are protected from modification during a crisis. Also, public health leaders may need to be better prepared for public leadership roles often filled by politicians, including communication skills relating to both traditional and new media.

The organization of public health services and systems is another important dimension associated with the diversity of responses in Canada. The structure and placement of public health services in Canada's provinces are determined by laws and regulations in each province. The main role of provincial health ministries is financing and provision of medical services. Public health functions are embedded in these systems in a variety of ways with implications for their voice in decision-making and their capacity to execute decisions at population and community levels. Federal-level organizations have specific authorities over things that affect provinces' ability to act, such as procurement and regulation of vaccines and medicines and control over international borders. But they have limited abilities beyond advice to influence provincial actors. Overall, further analysis and evaluation of how difference in organizational structure and function influenced decision-making and implementation is needed, with guidance provided to how provinces might improve their legislation and structures to be more effective. One might consider whether some public health functions might be better served by having distinct vertical organizations rather than being embedded in organizations mainly charged with clinical services.

4.7 Conclusion

COVID-19 exposed weaknesses within the structure of the 2020s Canadian public health system, as SARS did 20 years ago. Responses to the crisis were not dependent upon technical capacity alone but were influenced by institutional, political, and organizational factors which resulted in significant differences in decisions taken and implemented despite many common features of social, economic, and informational context. Our studies suggest that improving understanding of the role these factors played in the pandemic response is essential to better prepare for future responses to the public health crises that will certainly recur in the coming years and decades.

References

Allin, S., Campbell, S., Jamieson, M., Miller, F., Roerig, M., and Sproule, J. (2022). *Sustainability and Resilience in the Canadian Health Care System*. London: LSE consulting.

Angus Reid Institute (2020). From sea to locked down sea: Most want US border to stay closed, reluctant to welcome interprovincial visitors. https://angus-reid.org/covid19-canada-usa-border/ (Accessed on November 17, 2022).

Attaran, A. (2020). The failing federation: Why Canada is ineffective at COVID-19. *Journal of National Security and Policy*, *11*, 229–246.

Auditor General of Canada (2021). The public health agency of Canada falls short on the enforcement of border control measures. 2021 Reports 12 to 15 of the Auditor General of Canada. *oag-bvg.gc.ca* (Accessed on October 26, 2022).

Auditor General of Ontario (2020). Auditor general special report news release: Ontario's COVID-19 response faced systemic issues and delays.

News Release: COVID-19 Preparedness and Management Special Report (auditor.on.ca) (Accessed on February 2, 2023).

BBC News (2022). Canada protests: Police push back demonstrators in Ottawa. https://www.bbc.com/news/world-us-canada-60420469 (Accessed on November 12, 2022).

BC Public Safety and Solicitor General (2021). Province introduces travel restrictions to curb spread of COVID-19. https://news.gov.bc.ca/releases/2021PSSG0029-000758 (Accessed on November 18, 2022).

Betini, R., Milicic, S., and Lawand, C. (2021). The impact of the COVID-19 pandemic in long-term care in Canada, *Healthcare Quarterly, 24*, 13–15.

Bricker, D. (2021). *Conservatives Could Benefit from Ballot-Box Bonus on e-Day, but COVID Concerns, Apathy Make Election Outcomes Uncertain.* Toronto: Ipsos. https://www.ipsos.com/en-ca/news-polls/conservatives-could-benefit-from-ballot-box-bonus-on-e-day (Accessed on November 6, 2022).

Brubacher, L. J., Hasan, Md. Z., Sriram, V., Keidar, S., Wu, A., Cheng, M., Lovato, C. Y., UBC Working Group on Health Systems' Response to COVID-19 and Berman, P. (2022). Investigating the influence of institutions, politics, organizations, and governance on the COVID-19 response in British Columbia, Canada: A jurisdictional case study protocol. *Health Research Policy and Systems,* 20.

Cameron-Blake, E., Breton, C., Sim, P., Tatlow, H., Hale, T., Wood, A., Smith, J., Sawatsky, J., Parsons, Z., and Tyson, K. (2021). *Variation in the Canadian Provincial and Territorial Responses to COVID-19.* Oxford: Blavatnik School of Government. *ox.ac.uk* (Accessed on October 26, 2022).

Canada, Parliament, Senate, Standing Senate Committee on Social Affairs, Science and Technology (2010). Canada's response to the 2009 H1N1 influenza pandemic, committee report 15. http://sencanada.ca/Content/SEN/Committee/403/soci/rep/rep15dec10-e.pdf (Accessed on November 6, 2022).

Canadian Public Health Association (2021). Review of Canada's initial response to the COVID-19 pandemic. https://www.cpha.ca/review-canadas-initial-response-covid-19-pandemic (Accessed on November 3, 2022).

Canseco, M. (2020). Canadians endorse travel restrictions during COVID-19 pandemic. https://researchco.ca/2020/12/01/canada-covid19-2/ (Accessed on November 16, 2022).

Cardoso, T. (2022). *Data Leak Reveals Canadians, Americans Donated Millions to Fund Trucker Convoy Protests.* Toronto: *The Globe and Mail.* https://

www.theglobeandmail.com/canada/article-data-leak-reveals-canadians-americans-donated-millions-to-fund-convoy/ (Accessed on November 16, 2022).

Cassola, A., Fafard, P., MacAuley, M., and Palkovits, M. (2021). *The Politics and Policy of Canada's COVID-19 Response, in Coronavirus Politics: The Comparative Politics and Policy of COVID-19*. USA: University of Michigan Press, pp. 459–476.

Cassola, A., Fafard, P., Nagi, R., and Hoffman, S. J. (2022). Tensions and opportunities in the roles of senior public health officials in Canada: A qualitative study. *Health Policy, 126*, 988–995.

Centre for Health Security (2019). *Global Health Security Index: Building Collective Action and Accountability*. USA: Johns Hopkins Bloomberg School of Public Health.

Cooke, R. (2020). *N.L. Travel Ban Upheld in Provincial Supreme Court Ruling*. Toronto: CBC. https://www.cbc.ca/news/canada/newfoundland-labrador/nl-travel-ban-supreme-court-decision-1.5727549 (Accessed on December 8, 2022).

Crawford, B. (2022). *Who is Tamara Lich — The 'Spark that Lit the Fire'*. Ottawa: Ottawa Citizen (Accessed on November 16, 2022).

Cyr, A., Mondal, P., and Hansen, G. (2021). An Inconsistent Canadian Provincial and Territorial response during the early COVID-19 pandemic. *Frontiers in Public Health, 9*, 708903.

Durrani, T. (2021). *Across Canada, Vaccine Passports are a Patchwork. Here's What That Looks Like*. Toronto: *BNN Bloomberg*. https://www.bnnbloomberg.ca/across-canada-vaccine-passports-are-a-patchwork-here-s-what-that-looks-like-1.1647710 (Accessed on November 12, 2022).

Fafard, P. and Forest, P.-G. (2016). The loss of that which never was: Evaluating changes to the senior management of the Public Health Agency of Canada. *Canadian Public Administration, 59*, 448–466.

Fafard, P., McNena, B., Suszek, A., and Hoffman, S. J. (2018). Contested roles of Canada's Chief Medical Officers of Health. *Canadian Journal of Public Health, 109*, 585–589.

Fafard, P., Wilson, L. A., Cassola, A., and Hoffman, S. J. (2020). Communication about COVID-19 from Canadian provincial chief medical officers of health: A qualitative study. *CMAJ Open, 8*, E560–E567.

Global Affairs Canada (2020). Government of Canada advises Canadians to avoid non-essential travel abroad. Canada.ca (Accessed on October 21, 2022).

Goldschmidt, P. G. (2022). The Global Health Security Index: Another look. *Front. Epidemiology, 2*.

Government of Canada (2022). Interdepartmental affairs: Provinces and territories. *Canada.ca* (Accessed on January 30, 2023).

Grant, K. (2014). Ottawa to limit power of Canada's top doctor. *The Globe and Mail.* https://www.theglobeandmail.com/news/politics/ottawa-to-limit-power-of-canadas-top-doctor-the-chief-public-health-officer/article21550260/ (Accessed on November/December 3, 2022).

Han, J. Y. and Breton, C. (2022). *Provincial Paths Diverge on Vaccine Mandates and Passports.* Montreal: Policy Options.

Health Canada (2015). *Canada Health Act: Annual Report.* Ottawa: Health Canada. 2015-cha-lcs-ar-ra-eng.pdf (canada.ca) (Accessed on December 18, 2022).

Holder, J. (2022). *Tracking Coronavirus Vaccinations Around the World.* New York: *New York Times.* https://www.nytimes.com/interactive/2021/world/covid-vaccinations-tracker.html (Accessed on December 13, 2022).

Humphries, M. O. (2012). *The Last Plague Spanish Influenza and the Politics of Public Health in Canada.* Canada: University of Toronto Press.

Inverardi-Ferri, C. and Brown, T. (2020). Territories, politics and governance of the COVID-19 pandemic. *Territory, Politics, Governance, 10,* 751–758.

Ismail, S. J., Langley, J. M., Harris, T. M., Warshawsky, B. F., Desai, S., and FarhangMehr, M. (2021). Canada's National Advisory Committee on Immunization (NACI): Evidence-based decision-making on vaccines and immunization. *Vaccine, 28,* A58–63.

Lee, K. and Nicol, A. (2021). *Why Canada Doesn't Know How Many COVID-19 Cases are Linked to Travel.* Toronto: The Conversation. https://theconversation.com/why-canada-doesnt-know-how-many-covid-19-cases-are-linked-to-travel-154321 (Accessed on November 16, 2022).

Ling, J. (2021). *Where did Canada's Vaccine Effort Actually Go Wrong?* Toronto: Macleans. https://www.macleans.ca/news/canada/where-did-canadas-vaccine-effort-actually-go-wrong/ (Accessed on December 13, 2022).

Little, N. (2022). COVID-19 vaccination tracker. https://covid19tracker.ca/vaccinationtracker.html (Accessed on December 13, 2022).

MacAulay, M., Macintyre, A. K., Yashadhana, A., Cassola, A., Harris, P., Woodward, C., Smith, K., de Leeuw, E., Palkovits, M., Hoffman, S. J., and Fafard, P. (2022). Under the spotlight: Understanding the role of the Chief Medical Officer in a pandemic. *Journal of Epidemiology and Community Health, 76,* 100–104.

MacGregor, S. (2020). *Canada's Provinces Introduce New Coronavirus Travel Regulations to Limit Domestic Travel.* New Jersey: *Forbes.* https://www.

forbes.com/sites/sandramacgregor/2020/04/03/canadas-provinces-introduce-new-coronavirus-travel-regulations-to-limit-domestic-travel/?sh=3bb6ea 4c15c2 (Accessed on October 22, 2022).

Marchildon, G. P. (2008). Canada, health system of. *International Encyclopedia of Public Health,* 381–391.

Marchildon, G. P. (2021). The rollout of the COVID-19 vaccination: What can Canada learn from Israel? *Israel Journal of Health Policy Research*, 10.

McEwan, T. (2020). Alberta medical experts call for mandatory COVID-19 restrictions based on hospitalization numbers. CBC. https://www.cbc.ca/news/canada/edmonton/alberta-hospitalization-health-measures-1.5770314 (Accessed on November 3, 2022).

Migone, A. R. (2020). Trust, but customize: Federalism's impact on the Canadian COVID-19 response, *Policy and Society*, *39*, 382–402.

National Advisory Committee on Immunizations (NACI) (2021). *Extended Dose Intervals for COVID-19 Vaccines to Optimize Early Vaccine Rollout and Population Protection in Canada in the Context of Limited Vaccine Supply.* Ottawa: Health Canada. https://www.canada.ca/en/public-health/services/immunization/national-advisory-committee-on-immunization-naci/extended-dose-intervals-covid-19-vaccines-early-rollout-population-protection.html (Accessed on November 4, 2022).

Naylor, D., Basrur, S., Bergeron, M. G., Brunham, R. C., Butler-Jones, D., Dafoe, G., Ferguson-Pare, M., Lussing, F., McGeer, A., Neufeld, K. R., and Plummer, F. (2003). Learning from SARS: Renewal of public health in Canada, Health Canada. https://www.canada.ca/en/public-health/services/reports-publications/learning-sars-renewal-public-health-canada.html (Accessed on December 12, 2022).

O'Reilly, P. (2001). The federal/provincial/territorial health conference system. In D. Adams (ed.), *Federalism, Democracy and Health Policy in Canada* (pp. 107–129). Montreal and Kingston: McGill-Queen's University Press.

Our World in Data (2022). Canada: Coronavirus pandemic country profile. https://ourworldindata.org/coronavirus/country/canada (Accessed on December 3, 2022).

Piper, J., Gomis, B., and Lee, K. (2022). Guided by science and evidence? The politics of border management in Canada's response to the COVID-19 pandemic. *Frontiers in Political Science*, 4, 834223.

Poirier, J. and Michelin, J. (2021). Facing the coronavirus pandemic in the Canadian federation. In N. Steytler (ed.), *Comparative Federalism and COVID-19* (pp. 200–219). New York: Routledge.

Public Health Agency of Canada (PHAC) (2020). Government of Canada updates mandatory requirements for travelers entering Canada. *Canada.ca* (Accessed on October 21, 2022).

Public Health Agency of Canada (PHAC) (2021). Additional testing and more stringent requirements for travel to Canada. https://www.canada.ca/en/public-health/news/2021/02/additional-testing-and-more-stringent-quarantine-requirements-for-travel-to-canada.html (Accessed on November 16, 2022).

Public Safety Canada (2020). Emergency management act and emergencies act. https://www.publicsafety.gc.ca/cnt/trnsprnc/brfng-mtrls/prlmntry-bndrs/20200730/017/index-en.aspx (Accessed on November 12, 2022).

Reuters (2022). Key events in Canada's trucker protests against COVID curbs. *Reuters* (Accessed on November 4, 2022).

Robertson, D. (2014). Federal government hasn't filled top doctor's job, 15 months later, Ottawa Citizen. https://ottawacitizen.com/news/politics/federal-government-hasnt-filled-top-doctors-job-15-months-later (Accessed on December 3, 2022).

Robertson, G. (2020). We are not prepared': The flaws inside public health that hurt Canada's readiness for COVID-19. *The Globe and Mail*. https://www.theglobeandmail.com/canada/article-we-are-not-prepared-the-flaws-inside-public-health-that-hurt-canadas/ (Accessed on November 27, 2022).

Scott, M. (2022). *Ottawa Truckers' Convoy Galvanizes Far-right Worldwide*. Virginia: Politico. https://www.politico.com/news/2022/02/06/ottawa-truckers-convoy-galvanizes-far-right-worldwide-00006080 (Accessed on November 4, 2022).

Snowdon, A. W. (2021). An evidence-based strategy to scale vaccination in Canada. *Healthcare Quarterly*, *24*, 28–35.

Statistics Canada (2021). COVID-19 vaccine willingness among Canada's population groups. https://www150.statcan.gc.ca/n1/pub/45-28-0001/2021001/article/00011-eng.htm (Accessed on November 12, 2022).

Tauh, T., Mozel, M., Meyler, P., and Lee, S. M. (2021). What is the evidence for extending the SARS-CoV-2 (COVID-19) vaccine dosing schedule? *BC Medical Journal*, *63*, 67–70.

The Globe and Mail (2020). Premiers don't want emergencies act used during COVID-19 pandemic. *The Globe and Mail* (Accessed on November 12, 2022).

Tumilty, R. (2021). Why wasn't public health prepared? Parties agree on need for post-pandemic review. *National Post*. https://nationalpost.com/news/politics/why-wasnt-public-health-prepared-parties-agree-on-need-for-post-pandemic-review (Accessed on November 28, 2022).

Urrutia, D., Manetti, E., Williamson, M., and Lequy, E. (2021). Overview of Canada's answer to the COVID-19 pandemic's first wave (January–April 2020). *International Journal of Environmental Research and Public Health, 18*, 7131.

VOCM (2020). COVID cases in Atlantic Canada remain low as cases grow across Canada. *VOCM, St. John's.* https://vocm.com/2020/12/23/covid-cases-in-atlantic-bubble-remain-low-as-cases-grow-across-canada/ (Accessed on November 16, 2022).

Webster, P. (2020). Canada and COVID-19: Learning from SARS, *Lancet, 395*, 936–937.

Yang, J. and Allen, K. (2020). *Ontario Rejected It's Own Public Health Agency's Advice When It Launched Its Colour-coded Plan for COVID-19 Restrictions.* Toronto: Toronto Star. https://www.thestar.com/news/gta/2020/11/11/ontario-rejected-its-own-public-health-agencys-advice-when-it-launched-its-colour-coded-plan-for-covid-19-restrictions.html (Accessed on November 3, 2022).

Chapter 5

Australia

Evelyne de Leeuw, Glen Ramos, and Patrick Harris

5.1 Introduction

The Commonwealth of Australia is a federated nation comprised of six states (Tasmania, Victoria, South Australia, New South Wales, Queensland, and Western Australia) and two self-governing territories (the Northern Territory and the Australian Capital Territory, largely equivalent to the agglomeration of Canberra and its connected — technically independent but not self-governing — Jervis Bay Territory which provides Commonwealth access to the Pacific Ocean). In addition to these "mainland" entities, there are seven external dependent territories (Ashmore and Cartier Islands, Christmas Island, the Cocos (Keeling) Islands, Coral Sea Islands, Heard Island and McDonald Islands, Norfolk Island, and the Australian Antarctic Territory) (Geoscience Australia, 2023) (Figure 5.1). As a result of cartographic projection distortions, there is a belief that Australia is a relatively small island toward the bottom of our planet. It is, however, Earth's sixth-largest country at 7,692,024 km².

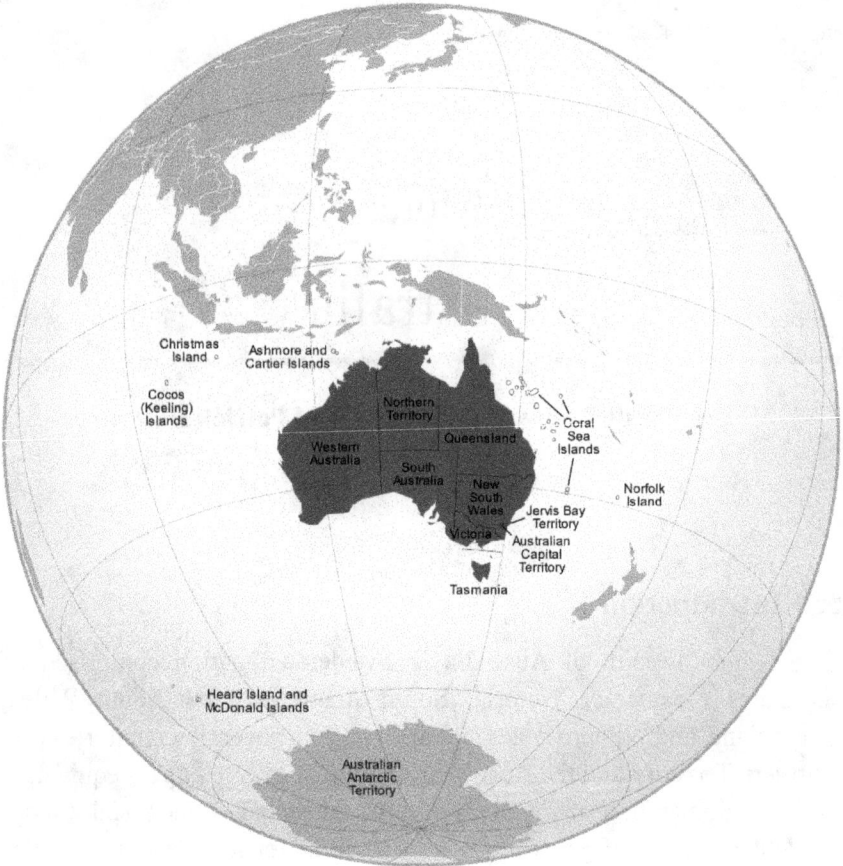

Figure 5.1.   Australia and its territories.

Note: From Lasunncty — Own work, CC BY-SA 4.0, https://commons.wikimedia.org/w/index.php?curid=49837804.

Australia has three tiers of government — federal (also known as the Commonwealth or Australian government), state and territory, and local — utilizing a mixed system comprising elements of representative liberal democracy, constitutional monarchy, and a federation of states (Parliamentary Education Office, 2022) which operate under the Westminster system at the federal, state, and territory levels (NSW Public Service Commission (NPSC), 2023). The Australian Constitution (there is no Bill of Rights) delineates the roles and responsibilities between the federal and state governments. Importantly, it also outlines the separation of powers between the three branches of government (Legislature — makes the laws; Executive — implements the laws; and Judiciary — interprets and upholds the laws) (NPSC, 2023).

States also have their own constitutions which, among other things, allow them to incorporate and legalize local governments. Across states and territories, these "Local Government Areas" differ vastly in size, population density and other demographic parameters, and natural environments and opportunities. The Australian Bureau of Statistics currently counts 566 of such "gazetted local government boundaries as defined by each state and territory" (Australian Bureau of Statistics, 2023).

This complexity and overlap can lead to governance and financial oddities. For Australia, specifically in health policy, the responsibility of primary care finance and regulation falls under federal authority, but primary care facilities are considered small business enterprises. General practitioners are rarely public sector employees. Their clinical work is subsidized (through patient rebates) on the basis of strictly priced engagements detailed in the Medicare Benefits Schedule (MBS) which lists the medical services subsidized by the Australian Government (Department of Health and Aged Care (DHAC), 2023b). There is general agreement that the current levels of subsidy are wholly insufficient to maintain an effective primary care system (Faux *et al.*, 2022; Langmaid, 2022) and that this necessarily has profound impacts on levels of equity and poverty in Australian society (Butler *et al.*, 2023). The other federal health scheme of note is the Pharmaceutical Benefits Scheme (PBS) which subsidizes — or, for example, in the case of approved essential vaccinations, provides for free — a very large collection of pharmaceuticals to Australian citizens and residents (DHAC, 2023c). The out-of-pocket pharmaceutical costs to these groups are considered modest (Lofgren, 2009), although still relatively significant if one is on or under the poverty line or in need of much medication.

On the other hand, tertiary care public hospitals are typically a state and territory responsibility and budgeted at that level. In the public sector at state level, staff in public hospitals are paid by the state government. However, these public hospitals are co-funded by the federal government and also receive funds from private health insurance and private patients (Hewett, 2022). There is a broad social and political consensus that Australia delivers universal health coverage, but in fact, the inequities and distributive injustices in the current system challenge this rhetoric (Fisher *et al.*, 2022).

Funding mechanisms between primary, secondary, and tertiary care are different and disjointed. This means coordination and continuity of care are a perennial Australian challenge. It also allows for clinicians and health services to perversely exploit the state–federal and public–private chasms. It is quite possible to be discharged in the morning from a public hospital by a surgeon and then be referred to their private consulting rooms (sometimes even in the same building) for profit-driven follow-up treatment in the afternoon. Conversely, a visit to the private rooms of a specialist can lead to a referral to "free" publicly funded diagnostics or radiology (via bulk-billed Medicare subsidy). The level of care, atmosphere, and quality of staffing and services may be radically different between the crowded public facilities and the well-appointed private ones.

To this complexity must be added the fact that — again because of its largely unresolved colonial past — Australia is generally classified as a liberal welfare state (in the classic Esping-Andersen typology), together with the United Kingdom and the United States. This dictates the primacy of entrepreneurship and market-driven healthcare delivery, although, nominally, Australians believe they can avail themselves of universal health coverage through its Medicare reimbursement system (Tikkanen *et al.*, 2020).

5.2 Trifle, Custard, and COVID-19

According to the Commonwealth Fund, Australia's formal responsibilities for the delivery of health and healthcare are organized in the following structure:

> **The federal government** provides funding and indirect support for inpatient and outpatient care through the Medicare Benefits Scheme (MBS) and for outpatient prescription medicine through the PBS. The federal government is also responsible for regulating private health insurance, pharmaceuticals, and therapeutic goods; however, it has a limited role in direct service delivery.
>
> **States** own and manage service delivery for public hospitals, ambulances, public dental care, community health (primary and preventive care), and mental health care. They contribute their own funding in addition to that

provided by federal government. States are also responsible for regulating private hospitals, the location of pharmacies, and the healthcare workforce.

Local governments play a role in the delivery of community health and preventive health programs, such as immunizations and the regulation of food standards (Tikkanen *et al.*, 2020, para. 6–8).

Much can be said about Australian health inequities and their relation to disease care delivery. Of particular note, there is a persistent failure of Australian governments at every tier to "Close the Gap" in relation to the unfair and avoidable health chasms between the First Nations' populations and other Australians (Bond and Singh, 2020; Pholi *et al.*, 2009). The track record in health promotion, disease prevention, and what is generally called — in a rhetorical perversity — "preventative health" is of greater interest. A new federal "National Preventive Health Strategy 2021–2030" (Department of Health (DoH), 2021) claims to present a systems-based approach to betterment of health, but who or what will be the delivery agent of, for instance, the "equity lens" on health remains unclear (is prevention implementation actually about creating health or preventing disease?). Institutionally, it is hard to determine how good "preventatatative" (not a typo) intentions will be evidence-based, developed, implemented and financed, coordinated, and monitored for quality, effectiveness, efficiencies, and equity.

While quarantine is the only specific public health activity the Australian Constitution grants exclusively to the Commonwealth over the states, there are a number of other areas from which many other aspects of public health can be (and are) administered. The Commonwealth's powers in relation to external affairs, corporations, taxation, and financial arrangements can shape and wield laws and powers which directly and indirectly, conditional on funding, could tie the states to specific public health policies (Reynolds, 1995). And while historically (prior to federation) and, continuing to this present day, public health functions have been seen as a primary domain of the states, the ability to exercise these constitutional powers together with accumulating High Court interpretations of these powers enables the federal government to exert broader and more centralized public health legislation (Baker *et al.*, 2022).

However, we observe the lack of central coordination (both locally, at state and territory level, and federally) for public health and health promotion. The nation does not have a central public health agency and only very recently — as of May 2023 — allocated funds for the establishment of a center for disease control, such as the US-based Centers for Disease Control and Prevention (CDC), the European Centre for Disease Prevention and Control (ECDC), Public Health Agency of Canada (PHAC), or the province-based Institut National de Santé Publique du Québec (INSPQ). In fact, the Australian Labor Party won the 2022 federal election committing to such a national center (its title being Australian Centre for Disease Control), the purpose being "to improve Australia's response and preparedness for public health emergencies" (DHAC, 2023a), although the architecture of this new institution at the time of writing remains unclear.

What we do have, though, is an absolute smorgasbord of committees, departments, and regulatory bodies that at the federal level, in relation to COVID-19, include, for example, (not exhaustive):

- Commonwealth Department of Health,
- Health Emergency Management Branch,
- Office of Health Protection,
- Australian Health Minister's Advisory Council (AHMAC),
- Numerous other Australian Government non-health Departments and agencies,
- Australian Health Protection Principal Committee (AHPPC),
- Communicable Diseases Network Australia (CDNA),
- Public Health Laboratory Network (PHLN),
- Australian Technical Advisory Group on Immunisation (ATAGI),
- National Immunisation Committee (NIC),
- Therapeutic Goods Administration (TGA),
- Advisory Committee on the Safety of Vaccines (ASCOV),
- National Health and Medical Research Council (NHMRC),
- Infection Prevention and Control Expert Group (IPCEG).

Beyond these functions, the federal government has taken on a variety of other public health roles and activities that include regulatory frameworks, nuclear safety, HIV programs, cancer screening, national health programs (e.g. diabetes and mental health), food standards, workplace safety, health and medical research funding, and aboriginal health (Baum, 2015). This leaves the states and territories to undertake the heavy lifting of epidemiological surveillance (identification, intervention, and monitoring of public health issues), policy development and statutory responsibility for communicable diseases, environmental health, emergency responses, prevention and early detection programs for cancer, maternal and child health, dental screening, and health promotion (Baum, 2015). Additionally, the states regulate local government public health functions that include food safety monitoring, environmental hazards, land use planning, and community services (Baum, 2015). In this way, the responsibilities for public health are thereby opaquely shared among the three tiers of government.

The one significant organizational change in relation to public health governance, significantly inspired by the pandemic, was the establishment of the National Cabinet on 13 March 2020 replacing the former Council of Australian Governments (COAG). Its first priority "…was to respond to the urgent health and economic impacts of the COVID-19 pandemic" (Department of the Prime Minister and Cabinet, 2023).

The Australian public health infrastructure can thus be characterized as a *trifle-covered-in-custard*. The foundation consists of a delightful diversity of fruits, cakes, jellies, and condiments. The custard topping appears solid and allows for light pressing with a finger or spoon but pressing hard or sharp onto a custard surface is potentially lethal (Waitukaitis and Jaeger, 2012). Running on custard is possible, but standing still leads to sinking. In other words, when the elements of the public health system of Australia's jurisdictions came under hard and sharp pressure during the pandemic, the response was panicked and haphazard (de Leeuw *et al.*, 2022). The fact that during the first year of COVID-19 the nation performed relatively well in comparison with other jurisdictions around the world has been deemed a triumph of the Australian people, not of the Australian government (Duckett, 2022).

In the remainder of this chapter, we first outline the ways in which the Australian governments and associated institutions may have anticipated a respiratory pandemic, such as the COVID-19 event. We then account for the existing architecture of the Australian public health system and pandemic response patterns. We end with a political appraisal of the antipodean response thus far.

5.3 Preparedness

Australia was not totally unprepared for a pandemic. Following historical precedent (McCracken and Curson, 2003), global guidance outlining the parameters of an appropriate response in the region of the Asia-Pacific (World Health Organization (WHO) Regional Office for the Western Pacific, 2017), consistent high scores across the International Health Regulations' Capacities on managing public health risks (WHO, 2023), a detailed "Emergency Response Plan for Communicable Disease Incidents of National Significance" (Communicable Diseases Network Australia, 2016), and scholarly warnings (Kamradt-Scott, 2018), in late 2019 the Commonwealth Department of Health issued an "Australian Health Management Plan for Pandemic Influenza" (AHMPPI) (DoH, 2019). Astutely and timely, literally days before the eruption of the COVID-19 emergency, the AHMPPI observed the following:

> Pandemics are unpredictable. When the next pandemic will occur, how rapidly it will emerge and how severe the illness will be are all unknown. What we do know is that even when the clinical severity of the disease is low, such as experienced in 2009, a pandemic can cause significant morbidity and mortality. It can overwhelm our health systems and in more severe scenarios, cause significant disruption to our economy and to society (DoH, 2019, p. 13).

To situate this formally adopted policy, the authors ascertained the following:

> This plan will sit under the Emergency Response Plan for Communicable Disease Incidents of National Significance (CDPLAN), one of the four plans under the Australian National Health Emergency Response Arrangements. It also supports the Emergency Response Plan for Communicable Disease Incidents of National Significance: National Arrangements (National CD Plan) (DoH, 2019, p. 16).

It then continues to outline where it fits among the federation:

The AHMPPI acknowledges that the primary responsibility for managing the impact of a severe outbreak of influenza, or a pandemic, lies with the state and territory governments and that each jurisdiction will have its own plans and protocols. Therefore the majority of operational detail will be found in these plans (DoH, 2019, p. 16).

The various elements and dimensions of AHMPPI are represented in Table 5.1.

Three months after this roadmap was presented, the pandemic in fact happened. A coronavirus jumped species, either in a market in Wuhan or as a gain-of-function experiment in a virological lab in the same town, and rapidly continued its mutation journey across the world: COVID-19 and its variants were born. In its wake, health bureaucrats must have quickly realized that even "the best laid schemes o' Mice an' Men, Gang aft agley" (Burns, 1785).

The 230-page AHMPPI specifies a series of steps and recommendations that are driven by an assessment of a manageable infectious respiratory disease, from mild to severe. But the interventions that have become part of the common global repertoire during the pandemic seem underemphasized in the document. Quarantine, for instance, is mentioned a few dozen times, but only in illustrative manners, and "lockdown" does not feature at all. Mass masking outside health service delivery systems (which have their own protocols separate from AHMPPI) is not mentioned at all in the policy. An assumption of calm and reason in the response to a threat pervades the policy but also, perhaps, a naïve sense of "governability" of the system.

The face-masking question is an interesting one. During the Spanish flu pandemic of the early 20th century, it had become clear, and often mandated, that reducing aerosol circulation prevented the transmission of disease (Harris *et al.*, 2022). Even then there were "mask slackers" (Navarro, 2020). After nearly a year of doubt and debate, by 2021 it was clear that the primary route of COVID-19 transmission was aerosols (airborne) and much less fomite (surfaces) (CDC, 2021). Better ventilation,

Table 5.1.   Dimensions and elements of the AHMPPI.

Preparedness No novel strain detected (or emerging strain under initial investigation)		• Establish pre-agreed arrangements by developing and maintaining plans; • research pandemic specific influenza management strategies; • ensure resources are available and ready for rapid response; • monitor the emergence of diseases with pandemic potential, and investigating outbreaks if they occur.
Response	Standby Sustained community person to person transmission overseas	• Prepare to commence enhanced arrangements; • identify and characterize the nature of the disease (commenced in Preparedness); and • communicate to raise awareness and confirm governance arrangements.
	Action Cases detected in Australia	Action is divided into two groups of activities: Initial (when information about the disease is scarce) • prepare and support health system needs; • manage initial cases; • identify and characterize the nature of the disease within the Australian context; • provide information to support best practice health care and to empower the community and responders to manage their own risk of exposure; and • support effective governance. Targeted (when enough is known about the disease to tailor measures to specific needs.) • support and maintain quality care; • ensure a proportionate response; • communicate to engage, empower and build confidence in the community; and • provide a coordinated and consistent approach.
	Standdown The public health threat can be managed within normal arrangements and monitoring for change is in place	• Support and maintain quality care; • cease activities that are no longer needed, and transitioning activities to seasonal or interim arrangements; • monitor for a second wave of the outbreak; • monitor for the development of antiviral resistance; • communicate to support the return from pandemic to normal business services; and • evaluate systems and revise plans and procedures.

Source: Key activities in each stage of the AHMPPI. Department of Health, 2019, *Australian Health Management Plan for Pandemic Influenza*, p. 15. (https://www.health.gov.au/sites/default/files/documents/2022/05/australian-health-management-plan-for-pandemic-influenza-ahmppi.pdf). Copyright 2019 Commonwealth of Australia.

introduction of high efficiency particulate air (HEPA) filters, social distancing, and mask-wearing were the keystones of the non-pharmaceutical intervention package. Oddly, none of these feature as recommended frontline tools in the AHMPPI (which ironically was designed to address transmission of a potentially airborne respiratory virus!).

The plan critically also contains a series of recommended interventions labeled "Menu of Actions" to manage a respiratory pandemic. These are summarized in Table 5.2.

The developers and health bureaucrats that put together AHMPPI were also aware of the particularities of actually implementing the measures: there is a "Guide to Implementation" buried in the "Support Documents" (DoH, 2019, pp. 164–169). The (third) worst-case scenario is described as follows:

> Widespread severe illness will cause concern and challenge the capacity of the health sector. Areas such as primary care, acute care, pharmacies, nurse practitioners and aged care facilities will be fully-stretched to support essential care requirements. Heavy prioritisation will be essential within hospitals in order to maintain essential services and mortuary services will be under pressure. The demand for specialist equipment and personnel is likely to challenge capacity. Staff absenteeism will compound these difficulties. Pressure on health services will be more intense, rise more quickly and peak earlier as the transmissibility of the disease increases. Secondary care services, such as blood services will be challenged to maintain capacities and the community focus will be on maintaining essential services. Pandemic emergency legislation may be needed to support pandemic specific activities. The level of impact may be similar to the 1918 Spanish flu (DoH, 2019 p. 164).

What follows in the plan, as implementation suggestions, is a series of almost clinically determined stacked boxes. Larger social disruption, and its management, is not considered in spite of lessons that might (or should) have been learned from earlier pandemics with a Spanish flu-type impact. It seems that this reference to the 1918–1919 pandemic is more a rhetorical incantation than a real call to full-scale preparedness. As podcaster Michael Adams has observed, and contrary to popular wisdom, history teaches us

Table 5.2.   A menu of actions in pandemic response.

Measure	Effectiveness assessment	Apply?
Infection Control Measures		
Communication strategies hand hygiene and cough/sneeze etiquette	Minor to moderate	Recommended
Personal Protective Equipment in healthcare	Moderate	Based on risk assessment
Mask wearing by symptomatic individuals	No evidence	May be considered by individuals
Border Measures		
Communication		
Pandemic specific inflight announcements	Little direct evidence	Recommended
Communication materials high risk	Minor effect	Recommended
Travel advice	Minor	Recommended
Information for border staff	No direct evidence	Strongly recommended
Identification		
Entry screening — negative pratique	Minor	Recommended only when asymptomatic carriage is unlikely. Not recommended once community transmission is established
Entry screening — passenger locator documents	For detection of case: minor For awareness raising: no evidence	Recommended only when asymptomatic carriage is unlikely. Not recommended once community transmission is established.
Entry screening — thermal scanners	Minor	Not recommended
Entry screening — border nurses	Depends on the effectiveness of identification measures, which is likely to be low	Not recommended
Entry screening — passengers on cruise ships	Minor	Not recommended (unless there is evidence of clinical severity)
Entry screening — voluntary isolation	Minor	May be considered

Table 5.2. (*Continued*)

Measure	Effectiveness assessment	Apply?
Entry screening — voluntary quarantine	Minor	Not recommended
Exit screening	Minor	Not recommended
Internal travel restrictions	Minor to none	Not recommended
Social Distancing Measures		
Proactive school closure	Moderate	Not generally recommended
Reactive school closure	Variable to minor	Not recommended
Workplace closure	Moderate	Not generally recommended
Working from home	Minor	May be considered
Cancellation of mass gatherings	Some evidence	Not generally recommended
Voluntary isolation	Minor	Recommended
Voluntary quarantine	Moderate	Recommended in the Initial Action stage, and consider in the Targeted Action stage,
Contact tracing	Minor	Important part of initial enhanced surveillance activities
Pharmaceutical Measures	Minor	Antivirals for treatment of cases
	Dependent on severity and timeliness of delivery	Antivirals for post-exposure prophylaxis for contacts
	Moderate, initially, but generally protective against death.	Antivirals for post-exposure prophylaxis for contacts in at-risk groups
	Minor	Antivirals for post-exposure prophylaxis for contact healthcare workers
	Moderate	Candidate pandemic vaccine
	Moderate	Customized pandemic vaccine
	Moderate	Seasonal influenza vaccine

Source: Adapted from Department of Health, 2019, AHMPPI, pp. 115–162. (https://www.health.gov.au/sites/default/files/documents/2022/05/australian-health-management-plan-for-pandemic-influenza-ahmppi.pdf). Copyright 2019 Commonwealth of Australia.

nothing (Adams, 2022). Admittedly, the vast volumes of scholarly work inspired by, and unleashed on, the pandemic may prove us wrong, though. The "paperdemic" (Yang *et al.*, 2023) may still change complacency.

Similarly, the federal bureaucrats recognized that good communication of the plan, its management, and consequences would be pivotal to successful implementation and general responses of authorities at all levels and of the population. Another flowchart was developed (Figure 5.2) outlining, in a cascading avalanche of acronyms, who was to be guided by what and whom at what level.

The federal government was aware, as Tables 5.1, 5.2, and Figures 5.2, 5.3 show, of the complex governance and accountability arrangements a federated nation-state has to put in place for a coordinated and strong response. Laudably, the intent of the management plan was to have a Whole-of-Government approach (see also de Leeuw (2022), but a flowchart is much easier designed than implemented, as real-world events a few months later demonstrated. Also, an examination of other pandemic preparedness plans across the various Australian constituencies (in the Australian Disaster Resilience Hub (Australian Institute for Disaster Resilience, n.d.)) shows divergent levels of awareness and coordination between them. The reliance then, on the states' operational capacity for public health emergency management as proposed in the AHMPPI, was perhaps overly optimistic, if not mislaid.

5.4 COVID-19 Hits the Turbofan

The story of COVID-19 has been told innumerable times now — and in Australian lore, March 15, 2020 was the day that turbofan (and jet) powered aircraft stopped disgorging potentially COVID-19-carrying humans freely on the shores of the sunburnt country. Incoming travelers were to be subject to mandatory a 14-day quarantine, whether symptomatic or tested positive for COVID-19 or not.

5.4.1 *Quarantine*

Quarantine stations as had been used a century earlier were closed (Longhurst, 2018), and their use (or use of other facilities for that

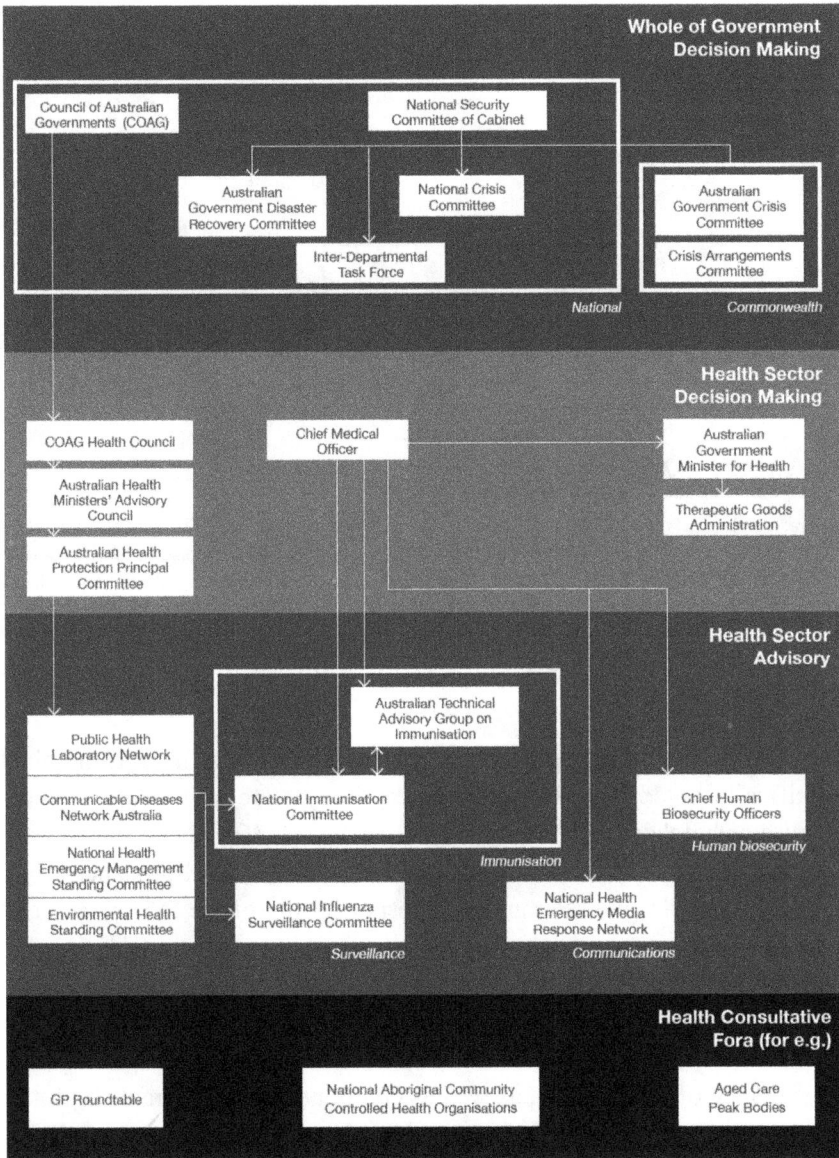

Figure 5.2.   Whole-of-government response: The ideal.

Source: Whole of government, health sector, health advisory, and consultative committees involved in decision-making for an influenza pandemic in Department of Health, 2019, AHMPPI, p. 34. (https://www.health.gov.au/sites/default/files/documents/2022/05/australian-health-management-plan-for-pandemic-influenza-ahmppi.pdf). Copyright 2019 Commonwealth of Australia.

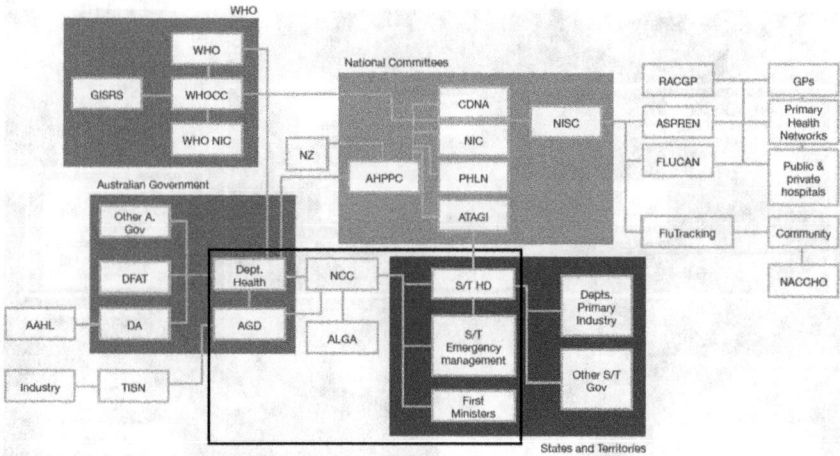

Figure 5.3.   Pandemic communication: The ideal.

Source: Pandemic Preparedness and Response Communication Channels. Department of Health, 2019, AHMPPI, p. 65. (https://www.health.gov.au/sites/default/files/documents/2022/05/australian-health-management-plan-for-pandemic-influenza-ahmppi.pdf). Copyright 2019 Commonwealth of Australia. This figure was in the original documentation (both Word and PDF versions) available for download. It was removed from the Word version in 2019 and the PDF version in 2023. It is uncertain if these channels were considered in Australia's response to COVID-19.

purpose) was not anticipated in the preparedness plans. In fact, the plan specifically noted that "No quarantine premises are currently available, and use of hotels is problematic" (DoH, 2019, p. 140). States and territories had to improvise and were offered very little, if any, guidance from any authority (despite seemingly the responsibility of the federal government, according to the Australian constitution). In an improvised strategy, incoming air passengers across Australia were collected at airports and transported to hotels and hotel-like serviced apartments (Haire *et al.*, 2022) — all converted to makeshift quarantine stations. Monitoring and surveillance of this process, as well as compliance with quarantine protocol, were put in the hands of impromptu developed institutions, often a mix between public (police) officers and private (security) personnel. Training, briefing, and debriefing of these officials were assessed as of variable quality, leading to dramatic incidents.

For instance, lack of job security and the generally precarious nature of the labor market in Australia mean that increasing number of people are part of the gig economy, having to work two or more jobs to stay above the poverty line. For hastily recruited private security staff, this often meant a second job as a food deliverer (in popular demand during lockdowns), a third job as an Uber driver, and a fourth job as handyman in an aged care institution. Paired with inconsistent public health guidance for infection control (to the extent that, reportedly, security guards in Melbourne quarantine hotels engaged in sexual exchanges with quarantined guests), the lackluster development and operation of the quarantine system may have created more, rather than less, spread of the pandemic (Thiessen, 2020). Initially, only one place in Australia could be used for "proper" quarantine: a former housing estate for mining employees in the Northern Territory (Trewin *et al.*, 2022). Following the — relative — success of this facility and a review of hotel quarantine (Halton *et al.*, 2021), the Commonwealth commissioned the building of more of such facilities, benignly called "Centres of National Resilience" (Department of Finance, 2021). The first came online at the very moment restrictions had been lifted and quarantine was no longer considered necessary.

The chaotic development of quarantine processes at international airports was also caused by a realization that there was a conundrum of accountability and governance in a federated nation between national border control and the actual place where people and goods enter the country: locally. Although quarantine (and border control and defense) is nationally framed, local street-level bureaucrats are to implement the operational dimensions of the policy. Nowhere more dramatically was the inconsistency and impotence of governance demonstrated than at Circular Quay (in Sydney), NSW, with the arrival of the cruise ship the Ruby Princess (Ito *et al.*, 2020). In spite of what many believed were clear protocols, over 900 COVID-19-positive passengers were freely released (against Public Health Orders) into the community (Walker, 2020), causing a significant spike in infections across Australia and indeed, the world. Contrastingly, two weeks later, the MS Artania cruise ship docked in Freemantle, WA, with 58 positive and suspected COVID-19 cases, the better management of which led to no infections spreading to the Western Australia community (Codreanu *et al.*, 2021).

As COVID-19 arrived on Australian shores and international borders were closed, the states and territories also embarked upon border closures between themselves. With their own constitutional independence, the states enacted a variety of public health emergency laws that included closing or restricting borders and access to those with permits (McCann *et al.*, 2022). Non-residents traveling to other states (without exemptions, which were very hard to come by) were generally required to self-isolate for 14 days.

From March 19–24, 2020, Tasmania, Northern Territory, South Australia, Western Australia, and Queensland announced a variety of border closures. The Queensland/New South Wales border had last closed to contain the Spanish flu over 100 years ago (Palaszczuk, 2020). Queensland Premier Palaszczuk was quite adamant at the time, stating, "Let me make it very clear, Queenslanders should stay in Queensland, people in New South Wales should stay in New South Wales and people in Victoria should stay in Victoria" (Ludlow, 2020). Western Australia remained closed for 697 days and was the last to reopen, with its premier claiming them to be "… an island within an island" (Hondros, 2020). It was a rapid, haphazard, and far from cohesive approach that the states undertook in a fervor of political and state parochialism in an effort to be seen to be acting in some meaningful and measurable manner on the pandemic.

Among the obvious challenges that these border restrictions placed on commerce, travel, social, financial, emotional, and medical needs, some communities were harder hit. A number of heated flashpoints erupted, particularly in border towns which, in some instances, were literally split down the middle, isolating families and preventing access to employment or schooling. Tweed Heads–Coolangatta, on the New South Wales/Queensland border, became a regular lightning rod for those protesting anything COVID-19 related, from border closures to vaccine mandates. Additionally, a number of states concurrently applied further internal border closures along local government areas during lockdown periods, with NSW contentiously restricting the access and movement of people living in (already socio-economically disadvantaged) western Sydney and not those in the (predominantly very affluent) east and northern suburbs to the same degree.

5.4.2 *Public health expertise and legitimacy*

Cool-headed biosecurity experts have repeatedly scratched their heads as to why nearly two centuries of accumulated public health evidence on infectious disease control could not be mobilized into policy interventions. Our earlier description of the Australian pandemic preparedness shows part of the cause underlying this concern. The public health community is often too beholden to a "clinical gaze" which dictates a focus on particular pathogens, clinical characteristics of disease, and a preference for quantifications of aetiologies. In Table 5.2, "evidence" almost exclusively is biomedical, not social science evidence. Biostatistical and epidemiological data, while absolutely critical and necessary to pandemic management, appear to drive the policy framework. Societal context, local conditions, mass behavioral sentiment, social practices, emotion, and livelihoods are absent from the gauging of evidence and feasibility of interventions.

This was no better reinforced than through the daily media briefings provided by the various state premiers, health ministers, and chief medical office (CMO) or chief health officers (CHO) where barrages of numbers and statistics (on cases, deaths, and hospitalizations) were provided in the attempt to demonstrate understanding and the appearance of management and, to a certain extent, control of the pandemic. In the existing public health structures, it is certainly much easier to capture this epidemiological data than to measure emotional, psychological, and social well-being of those impacted by the policies. The catch-all phrase wheeled out at every opportunity by politicians and bureaucrats to demonstrate authority was "we're following the medical advice." A major point of public contention that arose, however, was that, given the same medical advice, why were there such varying degrees of differences between policies on border restrictions and non-pharmaceutical interventions (NPIs).

And yet, this is precisely the anticipated role of public health leadership, in both senses: the public's health and public sector health leadership. There is no one organizational or statutory definition of this role: in Australia, the legalities of public health leadership vary significantly across states, territories, the Commonwealth, and in some case, localities. The Queensland CMO has the legal potential to declare draconian social and policy measures and in effect, shut down the state. In Victoria, however, the CHO is a senior leader within the Department of Health but otherwise merely an advisor of the Premier and political executive. The CMO at the federal level has arguably the least formal power of all — their influence mainly came through chairing the national committee of state and territory CMOs and CHOs.

These CMOs and CHOs are all under significant pressure, between the rock of evidence and the hard place of politics neither the Scylla of fact nor the Charybdis of belief are coherent and predictable. In spite of the best intentions of the preparedness plan, the scientific advice supporting actions to address COVID-19 was uncontained, chaotic, incoherent, and unpredictable. The neoliberal lack of a national institute coordinating (or dominating?) the public health response created opportunities for the emergence of new centers of trust and excellence, competition for confidence of politics and population, and ammunition for conspiracists (Bruns et al., 2020). Interestingly, for many Australians, the most trustworthy assessment of the COVID-19 state of play did not come from public authorities but from physician-journalist Norman Swan's "Coronacast" (Nee & Santana, 2022).

Admittedly, the CMOs and CHOs did not necessarily wield their authoritative power as well as they might have. Research into the role of the CMOs during the early COVID-19 period has revealed as much. The reality of the CHO/CMO role is one that juggles an evidence-based authoritative persona with behind-the-scenes political acumen to influence political masters (MacAuley et al., 2022). That juggling has been well described in the political science literature (Cairney et al., 2016). Evidence, that body of work explains, is but one of a great number of issues to battle out (or wield) in the political arena. The battle is most important, not the evidence. For instance, the right-leaning, neoliberal coalition in power at the federal level as the pandemic arrived had very little interest in public health measures that would negatively impact the economy. The CHOs, therefore, designed an elaborate strategy to force the hand of the federal health minister and — as it turns out, very much under the power of the Prime Minister — to accept these measures, including lockdowns.

CHOs at the same time became beholden to the difficult realities of what previous UK Prime Minister Harold McMillan famously explained as "Events" outside their control. Quarantine, for instance, was historically the preserve of federal legislation. During COVID-19 however, quarantine decisions were directed to the states. Governance of quarantine was not generally under the power or experience of the CHOs and routinely became the source of infections (Davey, 2020). This risk manifested across the country. Following success in suppressing infections through strict public health orders across 2020 and 2021, a third wave of COVID-19 hit the population because of a single infected driver taking passengers from the airport into quarantine (Franks, 2021). That single infection necessitated another round of measures, stretching the patience of the public and political support for continued interventions.

In a retrospective analysis, three CHOs addressed the 2022 Australian Population Conference. Rather than facilitate a generation of "political nous" (Harris *et al.*, 2021) however, the presenting CHOs surprised the public health community not with deep insight into the social and political dimensions of the course of the pandemic but rather with colloquial observations that Asia has a different tradition in the use of face masks, of which Australians might well learn something (Dow, 2022).

5.4.3 *Vaccines*

As outlined in the introduction, Australia is a large country; and yet, it is situated on the periphery of the more populated continents. With our neighbor antipodeans "across the ditch" (in Aotearoa/New Zealand), this may have initially presented the insular opportunity to close international borders and contain the pandemic. But this peripheral spatial position also means a distance to centers of power in terms of geopolitics and commercial wherewithal. With a relatively small population and a "backyard" of sparsely populated Pacific Islands, Australia is not necessarily in an advantageous position for high-end manufacturing. For instance, the automobile industry has withdrawn from the nation (Beer, 2018), despite the fact that a successful innovative mobility sector (in electro-voltaic or hydrogen futures) has been supported by past governments.

A similar pattern can be observed for pharmaceuticals' development and innovation. Australia is not the home of any major global pharma player, with the possible exception of CSL (formerly known as Commonwealth Serum Laboratory, privatized in 1994). The country does not have a sovereign pharmaceutical production capability and relies on imports from Europe and North America and, increasingly, India. In spite of rhetoric to the contrary, Australia does not "punch above its weight" (de Leeuw *et al.*, 2022). In the corridors of power in Canberra, someone must have been aware of this reality — and when Pfizer and AstraZeneca announced they might have a viable vaccine, the country started ordering doses excessively. In total, the federal government ordered 280.8 million vaccine doses, but because of a lack of effective international geopolitical engagement missed out on the timely delivery of many of these. In what appeared a coming tsunami of vaccines, Australia in fact experienced shortages, compromised supply lines, and failures in distribution and prioritization (for instance, into aged care facilities and First Nations communities). On top of this, the more than a quarter billion doses did not benefit the UN-led and global solidarity-inspired COVID-19 Vaccines Global Access (COVAX) mechanism as well as they might or should have (Gleeson *et al.*, 2022).

Criticism of the bungling of vaccine ordering and early distribution shortages was dismissed by the Prime Minister in his now (in)famous comment — "It's not a race" — about the speed of the vaccine rollout (dubbed by many a "stroll out") (Taylor, 2022). The lackadaisical speed left much to be desired, and a number of states expedited the process through the establishment of their own pop-up clinics and vaccination hubs (Cormack *et al.*, 2021). In fact, the vaccine delivery schedule was falling behind so much that the Australian Defence Force was called in to assist in its delivery (Reuters, 2021). In the best of Australian traditions, an inquiry was announced, led by Jane Halton (the consultant who, at one point in her career, was responsible for the very vaccine procurement policy she now assessed) (Halton, 2022). Its recommendations were as follows:

Recommendation 1: Public health campaigns designed to encourage sustained booster uptake for those that will benefit should be developed and delivered during 2023 and 2024 to improve coverage.

Recommendation 2: A clear, updated, policy framework including objectives for the management of COVID-19 should be developed to inform decision-making, purchasing, clinical decision-making, and resource allocation. A statement of risk appetite should form a part of this framework.

Recommendation 3: Advisory structures should be streamlined, and advice should be integrated to enable decision-makers to undertake their role. The role of decision-makers and advisors should be clarified. Reasons for decisions should be evidenced including indicating where they are based on judgment. Care should be taken to prevent confusion at the clinical level about who is eligible to receive vaccines/treatments and recommendations for use including in respect of target populations.

Recommendation 4: Procurement decisions should be made in the context of agreed policy objectives, risk appetite (the acceptability of failure to supply), knowledge/predictions in respect of the evolution of the virus, and supply constraints, including knowledge of market behavior.

Recommendation 5: Vaccine distribution arrangements should be reviewed in order to test value for money and reduce wastage while ensuring timely access.

Recommendation 6: New mechanisms to manage stock held by the NMS for use in an ongoing pandemic or epidemic should be developed as a matter of urgency to enable greater transparency about and access to stock held.

Recommendation 7: The Department of Health and Aged Care should work with sponsors to ensure that adequate supplies of therapeutics are available to meet reasonably anticipated demand for the next 2 years. Mechanisms such as guarantees for minimum supply should be explored to ensure availability and access.

Recommendation 8: Steps should be taken, consistent with an agreed policy and risk appetite, to ensure adequate supplies of vaccines and treatments are available across 2023 and 2024 including in the event of spikes in demand. This should include additional Moderna vaccines in 2023 and, as a minimum and based on an assessment of "COVID-19 stability," doses necessary to meet baseline demand in 2024.

Apart from number 6, these recommendations appear to be basic and fundamental. That they had to be spelt out in a review of this nature demonstrates the poor foresight, lack of planning, and policy impotence which was in place at the beginning and during the pandemic in relation to vaccines.

5.5 Conclusion

Like the surface of the custard-covered trifle, international observers would have had the impression that Australia's management of the COVID-19 pandemic was equally smooth and stable. Yet, underneath this surface façade, and in the face of innumerable pandemic management plans, was a wholesale debacle of panic, confusion, and politicking.

It is difficult to determine what meaningful lessons have been learnt from the Australian experience. There have certainly been innumerable failures and consequently a lot to learn. Have the recommendations of the vaccine review been implemented? Will the National Cabinet continue to take a lead role in a future pandemic or will the soon-to-be-established Australian Centre for Disease Control (ACDC) take ownership (perhaps unlikely, given early announcements that it will initially be situated within the federal Department of Health)? Have the social aspects of public health been considered in future planning and management?

The challenge perhaps for Australia is in incorporating into future pandemic preparedness and management the lessons of the various failures that took place. In doing so, being able to navigate the neoliberal institutions and loud anti-science voices and broadening beyond the purely clinical and data-driven approaches will be challenging. These two aspects are essentially embedded within the fragmented public health structures.

When provided with the resources, the Australian community demonstrated a capacity and solidarity of action that served to overcome the shortfalls of the government's planning (or lack thereof). It was the "public" in public health that actually carried the COVID-19 pandemic response.

References

Adams, M. (July 28, 2022). 'Sydney Breathes Again!' The folly of declaring victory too soon in a pandemic [Conference Session]. Healthy Cities: How to make Sydney healthier and happier after the COVID-19? Sydney. https://medsydney.org/how-do-we-make-sydney-healthier-and-happier-after-covid-19/.

Australian Bureau of Statistics (2023). Local government areas. *Commonwealth of Australia.* https://www.abs.gov.au/statistics/standards/australian-statistical-geography-standard-asgs-edition-3/jul2021-jun2026/non-abs-structures/local-government-areas (Accessed on February 18, 2023).

Australian Institute for Disaster Resilience (n.d.). Australian disaster resilience knowledge hub: Pandemic plans. https://knowledge.aidr.org.au/resources/pandemic-plans/.

Baker, E., Daniel, L., Beer, A., Bentley, R., Rowley, S., Baddeley, M., London, K., Stone, W., Nygaard, C., Hulse, K., and Lockwood, A. (2022). An Australian rental housing conditions research infrastructure. *Scientific Data*, *9*(1), 33. https://doi.org/10.1038/s41597-022-01136-5.

Baum, F. (2015). *The New Public Health* (4th edn.). South Melbourne, Victoria, Australia: Oxford University Press.

Beer, A. (2018). The closure of the Australian car manufacturing industry: Redundancy, policy and community impacts. *Australian Geographer*, *49*(3), 419–438. https://doi.org/10.1080/00049182.2017.1402452.

Bond, C. J. and Singh, D. (2020). More than a refresh required for closing the gap of Indigenous health inequality. *Medical Journal of Australia*, *212*(5), 198–199.e191. https://doi.org/10.5694/mja2.50498.

Bruns, A., Harrington, S., and Hurcombe, E. (2020). 'Corona? 5G? or both?': The dynamics of COVID-19/5G conspiracy theories on Facebook. *Media International Australia*, *177*(1), 12–29. https://doi.org/10.1177/1329878x20946113.

Burns, R. (1785). To a mouse, on turning her up in her nest with the plough. Reprinted in W. E. Henley and T. F. Henderson (Eds.), *The Poetry of Robert Burns* (Vol. 1, pp. 152–154).

Butler, D. C., Larkins, S., and Korda, R. J. (2023). Association of individual-socioeconomic variation in quality-of-primary care with area-level service organisation: A multilevel analysis using linked data. *Journal of Evaluation in Clinical Practice*. https://doi.org/10.1111/jep.13834.

Cairney, P., Oliver, K., and Wellstead, A. (2016). To bridge the divide between evidence and policy: Reduce ambiguity as much as uncertainty. *Public Administration Review*, 76(3), 399–402. https://doi.org/10.1111/puar.12555.

Centers for Disease Control and Prevention (2021). Scientific brief: SARS-CoV-2 transmission. *US Department of Health and Human Services*. https://www.cdc.gov/coronavirus/2019-ncov/science/science-briefs/sars-cov-2-transmission.html.

Codreanu, T. A., Ngeh, S., Trewin, A., and Armstrong, P. K. (2021). Successful control of an onboard COVID-19 outbreak using the cruise ship as a quarantine facility, Western Australia, Australia. *Emerg Infect Dis*, *27*(5), 1279–1287. https://doi.org/10.3201/eid2705.204142.

Communicable Diseases Network Australia (2016). Emergency response plan for communicable disease incidents of national significance. *Department of*

Health. https://www.health.gov.au/sites/default/files/documents/2022/07/emergency-response-plan-for-communicable-diseases-of-national-significance-cd-plan.pdf.

Cormack, L., Carroll, L., and Ward, M. (July 31, 2021). Churches, mosques, community centres to become pop-up vax clinics in hotspots. *The Sydney Morning Herald*. https://www.smh.com.au/politics/nsw/churches-mosques-community-centres-to-become-pop-up-vax-clinics-in-hotspots-20210730-p58eis.html.

Davey, M. (July 18, 2020). 'A wicked enemy': Why Australia's second wave of coronavirus will be tougher to fight. *The Guardian*. https://www.theguardian.com/australia-news/2020/jul/18/a-wicked-enemy-why-australias-second-wave-of-coronavirus-will-be-tougher-to-fight.

de Leeuw, E. (2022). Intersectorality and health: A glossary. *Journal of Epidemiology and Community Health*, *76*(2), 206. https://doi.org/10.1136/jech-2021-217647.

de Leeuw, E., McCracken, K., Harris, P., and Yashadhana, A. (2022). Underpromise and overdeliver: The failure of political rhetoric in managing COVID-19 in Australia. In R. Akhtar (Ed.), *Coronavirus (COVID-19) Outbreaks, Vaccination, Politics and Society: The Continuing Challenge* (pp. 17–31). Springer International Publishing. https://doi.org/10.1007/978-3-031-09432-3_2.

Department of Finance (2021). Centres for national resilience. *Commonwealth of Australia*. https://www.finance.gov.au/government/property-and-construction/centres-national-resilience.

Department of Health (2019). Australian health management plan for pandemic influenza. *Commonwealth of Australia*. https://www.health.gov.au/sites/default/files/documents/2022/05/australian-health-management-plan-for-pandemic-influenza-ahmppi.pdf.

Department of Health (2021). National preventive health strategy 2021–2030. *Commonwealth of Australia*. https://www.health.gov.au/sites/default/files/documents/2021/12/national-preventive-health-strategy-2021-2030_1.pdf.

Department of Health and Aged Care (2023a). Australian Centre for Disease Control. *Commonwealth of Australia*. https://www.health.gov.au/our-work/Australian-CDC.

Department of Health and Aged Care (2023b). MBS online — Medicare benefits schedule. *Commonwealth of Australia*. http://www.mbsonline.gov.au/internet/mbsonline/publishing.nsf/Content/Home.

Department of Health and Aged Care (2023c). Pharmaceutical benefits scheme. *Commonwealth of Australia*. https://www.pbs.gov.au/pbs/home.

Department of the Prime Minister and Cabinet (2023). About. *Commonwealth of Australia*. https://federation.gov.au/about.

Dow, A. (September 22, 2022). Sutton argues Asia can teach us about mask protocols. *The Age*. https://www.theage.com.au/national/sutton-argues-asia-can-teach-us-about-mask-protocols-20220922-p5bk4l.html.

Duckett, S. (2022). Public health management of the COVID-19 pandemic in Australia: The role of the Morrison government. *International Journal of Environmental Research and Public Health, 19*(16). https://doi.org/10.3390/ijerph191610400.

Faux, M., Adams, J., Dahiya, S., and Wardle, J. (2022). Wading through molasses: A qualitative examination of the experiences, perceptions, attitudes, and knowledge of Australian medical practitioners regarding medical billing. *PloS one, 17*(1), e0262211. https://doi.org/10.1371/journal.pone.0262211.

Fisher, M., Freeman, T., Mackean, T., Friel, S., and Baum, F. (2022). Universal health coverage for non-communicable diseases and health equity: Lessons from Australian primary healthcare. *International Journal of Health Policy and Management, 11*(5), 690–700. https://doi.org/10.34172/ijhpm.2020.232.

Franks, R. (June 21, 2021). Health expert blames quarantine arrangements for Sydney's latest covid outbreak on sunday project. news.com.au. https://www.news.com.au/national/nsw-act/news/health-expert-blames-quarantine-arrangements-at-sydney-airport-for-latest-covid-outbreak/news-story/0df7bcc94bf94cb34517e571d2c89b09.

Geoscience Australia (2023). Remote offshore territories. *Commonwealth of Australia*. https://www.ga.gov.au/scientific-topics/national-location-information/dimensions/remote-offshore-territories.

Gleeson, D., Tenni, B., and Townsend, B. (2022). Four actions Australia should take to advance equitable global access to COVID-19 vaccines. *Australian and New Zealand Journal of Public Health, 46*(4), 423–425. https://doi.org/10.1111/1753-6405.13268.

Haire, B., Gilbert, G. L., Kaldor, J. M., Hendrickx, D., Dawson, A., and Williams, J. H. (2022). Experiences of risk in Australian hotel quarantine: A qualitative study. *BMC Public Health, 22*(1), 953. https://doi.org/10.1186/s12889-022-13339-x.

Halton, J. (2022). Review of COVID-19 vaccine and treatment purchasing and procurement — Summary and recommendations. *Commonwealth of Australia*. https://www.health.gov.au/sites/default/files/2023-02/review-of-covid-19-vaccine-and-treatment-purchasing-and-procurement-summary-and-recommendations.pdf.

Halton, J., Head, G., Collignon, P., and Wilson, A. (2021). National review of quarantine. *Department of the Prime Minister and Cabinet.* https://www.pmc.gov.au/sites/default/files/resource/download/national-review-of-quarantine.pdf.

Harris, P., Harris-Roxas, B., Prior, J., Morrison, N., McIntyre, E., Frawley, J., Adams, J., Bevan, W., Haigh, F., Freeman, E., Hua, M., Pry, J., Mazumdar, S., Cave, B., Viliani, F., and Kwan, B. (2022). Respiratory pandemics, urban planning and design: A multidisciplinary rapid review of the literature. *Cities, 127,* 103767. https://doi.org/10.1016/j.cities.2022.103767.

Harris, P., Yashadana, A., and de Leeuw, E. (September 17, 2021). Chief health officers are in the spotlight like never before. Here's what goes on behind the scenes. *The Conversation.* https://theconversation.com/chief-health-officers-are-in-the-spotlight-like-never-before-heres-what-goes-on-behind-the-scenes-166828.

Hewett, R. (2022). *Public Hospital Funding: An Overview.* Parliament of Australia. https://www.aph.gov.au/About_Parliament/Parliamentary_Departments/Parliamentary_Library/FlagPost/2022/July/Hospital-funding.

Hondros, N. (April 2, 2020). 'An island within an island': WA to close its border with the east. *WA Today.* https://www.watoday.com.au/national/western-australia/an-island-within-an-island-wa-to-close-its-border-with-the-east-20200402-p54gl6.html.

Ito, H., Hanaoka, S., and Kawasaki, T. (2020). The cruise industry and the COVID-19 outbreak. *Transportation Research Interdisciplinary Perspectives, 5,* 100136. https://doi.org/10.1016/j.trip.2020.100136.

Kamradt-Scott, A. (2018). Securing Indo-Pacific health security: Australia's approach to regional health security. *Australian Journal of International Affairs, 72*(6), 500–519. https://doi.org/10.1080/10357718.2018.1534942.

Langmaid, A. (September 26, 2022). Doctor warns failures in outdated Medicare bulk-billing system risk tipping health system over edge. *ABC News.* https://www.abc.net.au/news/2022-09-26/gp-mariam-tokhi-warns-medicare-failures-leave-vulnerable-at-risk/101447950.

Lofgren, H. (2009). Generic medicines in Australia: Business dynamics and recent policy reform. *Southern Med Review, 2.* https://doi.org/10.2139/ssrn.1471687.

Longhurst, P. (2018). Contagious objects: Artefacts of disease transmission and control at North Head Quarantine Station, Australia. *World Archaeology, 50*(3), 512–529. https://doi.org/10.1080/00438243.2018.1494624.

Ludlow, M. (March 24, 2020). Qld puts roadblocks on the NSW border. *The Australian Financial Review.* https://www.afr.com/politics/qld-puts-road-blocks-on-the-nsw-border-20200324-p54dby.

MacAulay, M., Macintyre, A. K., Yashadhana, A., Cassola, A., Harris, P., Woodward, C., Smith, K., de Leeuw, E., Palkovits, M., Hoffman, S. J., and Fafard, P. (2022). Under the spotlight: Understanding the role of the Chief Medical Officer in a pandemic. *Journal of Epidemiology and Community Health*, *76*(1), 100–104. http://dx.doi.org/10.1136/jech-2021-216850.

McCann, L., Thompson, S. C., Rolf, F., and Podubinski, T. (2022). Police, permits and politics: Navigating life on Australia's state borders during the COVID-19 pandemic. *Australian Journal of Rural Health*, *30*(3), 363–372. https://doi.org/10.1111/ajr.12845.

McCracken, K. and Curson, P. (2003). Flu downunder: A demographic and geographic analysis of the 1919 epidemic in Sydney, Australia. In J. S. Oxford, T. Ranger, D. Killingray, & H. Phillips (Eds.), *The Spanish Influenza Pandemic of 1918–1919: New Perspectives* (pp. 110–131). Routledge, Taylor and Francis Group. https://doi.org/10.4324/9780203468371.

Navarro, J. A. (July 13, 2020). Mask resistance during a pandemic isn't new — In 1918 many Americans were 'slackers'. *The Conversation*. https://theconversation.com/mask-resistance-during-a-pandemic-isnt-new-in-1918-many-americans-were-slackers-141687.

Nee, R. C. and Santana, A. D. (2022). Podcasting the pandemic: Exploring storytelling formats and shifting journalistic norms in news podcasts related to the coronavirus. *Journalism Practice*, *16*(8), 1559–1577. https://doi.org/10.1080/17512786.2021.1882874.

NSW Public Service Commission (2023). Westminster system. *NSW Government*. https://sef.psc.nsw.gov.au/understanding-the-sector/westminster-system.

Palaszczuk, A. (2020). Border control slows virus spread. *Queensland Government*. https://statements.qld.gov.au/statements/89585.

Parliamentary Education Office (2022). Australian system of government. *Commonwealth of Australia*. https://peo.gov.au/understand-our-parliament/how-parliament-works/system-of-government/australian-system-of-government/.

Pholi, K., New, H., Area, E., Service, H., Black, D., Retired, C., and Richards. (2009). Is 'close the gap' a useful approach to improving the health and well-being of indigenous Australians? *Australian Review of Public Affairs*, *2*, 1–14. https://www.nintione.com.au/?p=3921.

Reuters (2021). Australia armed forces called in to support COVID-19 immunization drive. https://www.reuters.com/article/us-health-coronavirus-australia-idUSKCN2AV01I.

Reynolds, C. (1995). Public health and the Australian Constitution. *Australian Journal of Public Health*, *19*(3), 243–249. https://doi.org/10.1111/j.1753-6405.1995.tb00438.x.

Taylor, N. (February 22, 2022). 'It's not a race': Morrison palms COVID responsibility to the states. *Independent Australia*. https://independentaustralia.net/politics/politics-display/its-not-a-race-the-last-straw-for-morrison-and-the-coalition,16023.

Thiessen, T. (2020). Australia: New coronavirus lockdown Melbourne Amid Sex, Lies, Quarantine Hotel Scandal. *Forbes*. https://www.forbes.com/sites/tamarathiessen/2020/07/07/australia-coronavirus-melbourne-lockdown-hotel-sex-scandal/?sh=65e9d88a131d.

Tikkanen, R., Osborn, R., Mossialos, E., Djordjevic, A., and Wharton, G. (2020). International health care system profiles: Australia. *The Commonwealth Fund*. https://www.commonwealthfund.org/international-health-policy-center/countries/australia.

Trewin, A., Curtis, S. J., McDermott, K., Were, K., and Walsh, N. (2022). Avoiding catastrophe in a high-risk environment: AUSMAT at Howard Springs. *Global Biosecurity*. https://doi.org/10.31646/gbio.162.

Waitukaitis, S. R. and Jaeger, H. M. (2012). Impact-activated solidification of dense suspensions via dynamic jamming fronts. *Nature, 487*(7406), 205–209. https://doi.org/10.1038/nature11187.

Walker, B. (2020). Report of the special commission of inquiry into the Ruby Princess. *State of NSW*. https://www.nsw.gov.au/sites/default/files/2023-07/Report-of-the-Special-Commission-of-Inquiry-into-the-Ruby-Princess.pdf.

WHO Regional Office for the Western Pacific (2017). Asia Pacific strategy for emerging diseases and public health emergencies (APSED III): Advancing implementation of the International Health Regulations (2005): Working together towards health security. *World Health Organization*. http://iris.wpro.who.int/handle/10665.1/13654.

World Health Organization (2023). Electronic state parties self-assessment annual reporting tool. https://www.who.int/publications/i/item/9789290618171.

Yang, Y., Zhao, N., Ma, T., Yuan, Z., and Deng, C. (2023). 'Paperdemic' during the COVID-19 pandemic. *European Journal of Internal Medicine, 108*, 111–113. https://www.ejinme.com/article/S0953-6205(22)00352-1/fulltext.

Chapter 6

France

Thibaud Deruelle

6.1 Introduction

France was severely affected by the COVID-19 pandemic, with 36 million recorded cases and more than 160,000 deaths between 2020 and 2022 (Santé Publique France Website, 2022). When the pandemic first hit the European continent, in January 2020, the French executive scrambled to come to terms with the scope of the crisis (Wheaton, 2020), as did many of its neighbors (Clemens & Brand, 2020; Pacces & Weimer, 2020; Renda & Castro, 2020). Data were scarce, and the virus unknown. The French government, as well as other European decision-makers and experts, was inclined to a normalcy bias, the heuristic that leads people to minimize threat warnings. This bias would only entirely dissipate once Italian authorities started to enforce localized lockdowns, at the end of February 2020 (European Centre for Disease Prevention and Control (ECDC), 2020). It took the months of January and February 2020 for the French government to seize the breadth of the crisis to come and for public health experts to successfully play their role of fire alarm (McCubbins

& Schwartz, 1984). From then on, France confronted a series of challenges: lack of personal protective equipment, hospital capacity, crisis management challenges (including the French executive approach to evidence-based policy), and ultimately growing public mistrust. These difficulties were alarming as, 20 years prior, the French healthcare system had been hailed by the World Health Organization (WHO) as the best in the world in terms of quality and provision (WHO, 2000).

The responsibility lies in the hands of the French executive. Because it operates within a centralized political system, as shown in Figure 6.1, the French executive has control over all levers available in managing the health crisis (Freeman, 2000). The French public health system is characterized by centralized structures of policymaking (Hornung, 2022a). At the level of the Ministry of Health, this includes the General Directorate of Health (French acronym, DGS) and the General Directorate of Health Care Services (French acronym, DGOS) which are responsible for ensuring monitoring, forecasting, regulation, and health security missions (Tabuteau, 2016). Experts are particularly institutionalized in the French public health arena (Rozenblum, 2021b), with three scientific agencies: the High Authority for Health (French acronym, HAS) for medicines, the

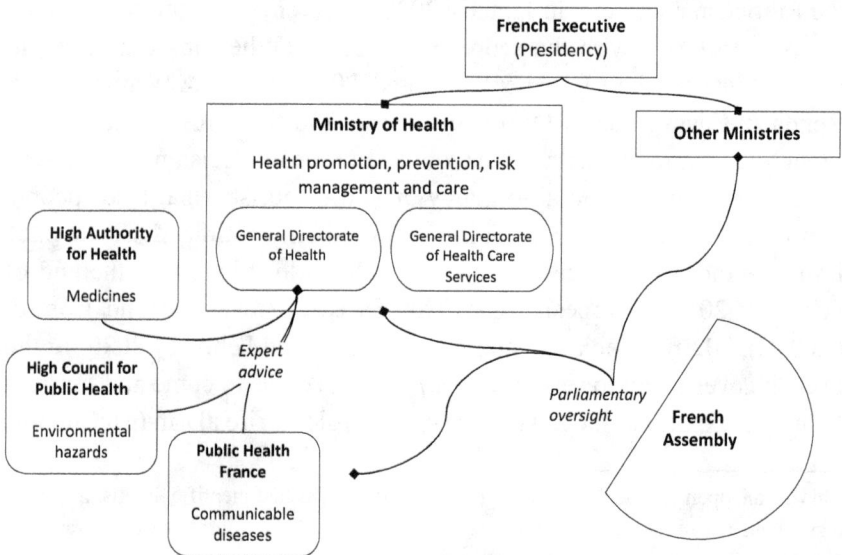

Figure 6.1.   Public health governance in France.

High Council for Public Health (French acronym, HCSP) for environmental hazard, and the Public Health France (Santé Publique France, SPF) for communicable diseases and which can all inform decision-making and crisis management. This governance system was nevertheless completely subverted amid the crisis.

The COVID-19 pandemic has created premium conditions in France to learn from the crisis (Deverell, 2009; Lee *et al.*, 2020; Stern, 1997; Vagionaki & Trein, 2019). But, despite a context that should be propitious to reforming health, the scope of reforms is limited. Two reforms were initiated in 2020: new investments in healthcare and a revamped strategy for preparedness, based on increased coordination with its neighbors, but, beyond fast-paced reforms amid crisis, there is no defined strategy to further reform public health and healthcare. Moreover, despite the temporary reconfiguration of crisis management institutions amid crisis, there is an apparent lack of self-reflection on the matter, with no institutional reform on the agenda.

This chapter discusses the limited successes as well as the hindrances to reforming the French health system in the (post-)COVID era. It analyses reforms kicked off by the French government since the beginning of the pandemic as well as the context of public health and healthcare pre-COVID-19. Strategic choices made in the 2010s and reforms made in the early days of the crisis shed an illuminating light on the lack of enthusiasm for engaging in in-depth reforms. Section 6.2 paints the context of public health reforms in France prior to COVID-19 through two key points: the recent reform of public hospitals and strategic choices made in terms of preparedness. Section 6.3 discusses fast-paced reforms kicked off in 2020 regarding the financing of healthcare and procurement of medical devices. Section 6.4 shifts the focus to the reconfiguration of the crisis management system and its effect on trust and evidence-based policymaking.

6.2 The Challenges of a Depleted Health System

From the early days of the pandemic, fundamental criticisms were made regarding the French government's lack of readiness for the crisis, especially with regard to protective personal equipment (PPE) and testing supplies as well as insufficient intensive care beds (Hassenteufel, 2020; Davet & Lhomme, 2020). The lack of capacity of the French response system, both in terms of preparedness and the provision of healthcare, was the result of health policies which had focused on cutting costs. But this late "New Public Management" turn occurs through different processes depending on whether we examine public health or healthcare. Regarding the lack of hospital beds, it can be traced back to the 2009 territorial reform of healthcare. Turning to preparedness, there are complex learning processes at play in which lessons learned from the 2009 H1N1 pandemic have — ironically — led to a depletion of PPE and testing supply.

6.2.1 *Healthcare access and the territorial reforms of healthcare pre-COVID-19*

Between 2000 and 2020, the number of hospital beds had decreased by 25%, with some regions showing a staggering 50% decrease (Ministère des solidarités et de la santé, 2022). On the eve of the COVID-19 pandemic, the number of intensive care beds was only 1 per 100,000 inhabitants. For comparison, on the same date, there were 35 per 100,000 in Germany (Naumann *et al.*, 2020).

When COVID-19 hit, Regional Health Agencies (French acronym, ARS) became easy scapegoats, especially for local civil servants having to deal with citizens' frustration regarding the lack of healthcare access. The ARS, created in 2009, carry out prevention and health planning missions at the regional level. They played a critical role during the COVID-19 crisis (Rozenblum, 2021b). In effect, ARS were in charge of reorganizing beds, canceling non-emergency medical interventions, supplying health personnel with PPE (by controlling the purchase of masks by local authorities), and organizing patient transportation (Hassenteufel, 2020). Local and regional authorities have no competences in health, therefore ARSs reported directly to the national health ministry.

The territorial reform that created ARS aimed at increasing access to healthcare and reducing disparities between French regions (see the 2009 law (*LOI N° 2009-879*) "On hospital reform, regarding patients, health and territories," also called "Hospital, patients, health, territories"). Territorial reforms are an important leitmotiv of French public policymaking. They usually aim to reduce inequalities between different portions of the French territory. Despite a long tradition of French centralization, the governance of healthcare provision was historically characterized by localist and centrifugal dynamics (Pasquier, 2016; Reiter & Kuhlmann, 2016). The 2009 reform tied hospital directors to regional agencies, which *prima facie* would mean a reinforcement of the regional governance level. But, in effect, the creation of ARS amounted to a process of centralization. The regional agencies were given little room to maneuver and were mandated to implement policy goals defined at national level in the DGOS (Hornung, 2022b). Budget-wise, the reform tied ARS to the Interministerial Committee for the Performance and Modernization of Hospital Care (Pierru, 2020) meant to create a leaner and less expensive management of healthcare, at the implementation level, i.e. across the French territory (Duchesne, 2018). Overall, the 2009 territorial reform, despite creating *regional* agencies, was actually an effort in centralizing the governance of healthcare, by reducing the discretion of ARS whether at policy or budgetary level, as illustrated in Figure 6.2.

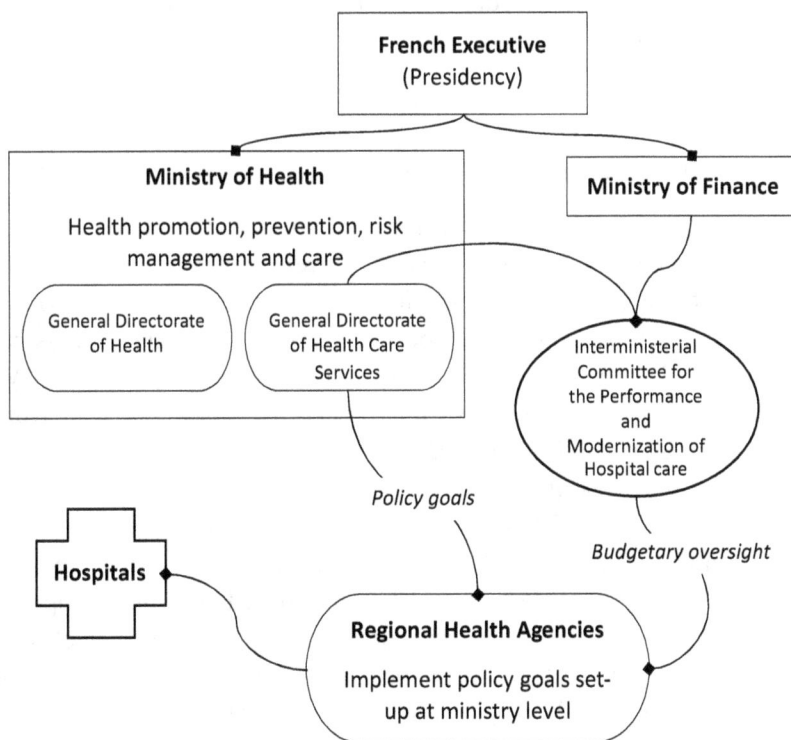

Figure 6.2.   Centralization of hospital care in France prior to the COVID-19 pandemic.

Once ARS were up and running, budgetary constraints as well as centralized objectives defined by Paris had a profound effect on access to healthcare. A big emphasis was put on hospitalization from home as well as the medicalization of retirement homes (acronym in French, EPHAD). ARS were particularly focused on profit margins to evaluate hospitals. This led to the drastic drop in number of hospital beds presented earlier. If the responsibility ultimately lies with the central state, it is worth noting that ARS are administrations that were always dedicated to imprint a New Public Management approach to healthcare management. Overall, while the territorial reform led to institutional change, it was mostly the vehicle of a budgetary-centered approach to healthcare which had a detrimental effect on access to life-saving care at the beginning of the pandemic. Ultimately, it inflicted an unmanageable burden on hospital services and patients. Budgetary constraints are thus a key element to understand the depletion of access to intensive care. Such constraints also play a role in the depletion of strategic stocks for preparedness.

6.2.2 Lessons in preparedness from the 2009 H1N1 crisis

In terms of preparedness, and across the European continent, lessons learned from the 2009 H1N1 pandemic were forgotten too soon, as the Director of the European Centre for Disease Prevention and Control Andrea Ammon mentioned in a podcast interview: "we have always had done lessons learned after the 2009 influenza pandemic, after Ebola. We have done really thorough 'Lessons Learned' exercises, but we haven't learned the lessons" (Gottlieb, 2021). Indeed, on the eve of the crisis, the French strategic stock of PPE and test kits was particularly low among EU member states (Bayer, 2020; Guarascio, 2020; Michalopoulos, 2020).

In contrast, prior to the 2009 H1N1 pandemic, the French executive was invested in enhancing preparedness. In 2007, France had adopted a protection mechanism for large-scale pandemics in the implementation of the law on the preparation of the health system for large-scale health threats ("loi relative à la préparation du système de santé à des menaces sanitaires de grande ampleur") and had created the office for the preparation and response to health emergencies (French acronym,

EPRUS), during the 2005 H5N1 influenza epidemic (Rozenblum, 2021b). Between 2005 and 2006, EPRUS created a strategic stock of 616 million masks.

The stock of masks did not end up being necessary to face the 2009 H1N1 pandemic. The H1N1 flu had a more moderate effect on mortality than initially feared (Nicoll & McKee, 2010) and the response of the French executive to the 2009 H1N1 pandemic appeared excessive at the time (Davet & Lhomme, 2020). Indeed, the then-Health Minister Roselyne Bachelot had promoted the generalized vaccination of the population and €195 million for masks, although H1N1 flu directly caused only 342 deaths. Ultimately, this explains why, after a few years, and in stark contrast with the lead-up to the H1N1 influenza outbreak, "lesson-learning" gave way to a form of relaxation *vis-à-vis* preparedness. Crucially, the budget of EPRUS was divided by 10 between 2007 and 2015 (Hassenteufel, 2020) and only an additional 98 million masks were purchased between 2015 and 2016. Public health literature underlines the emergence of the financial and budgetary crisis in Europe a few months after the outbreak as a determinant in understanding the shift in priorities (Brusaferro & Tricarico, 2017; Crosier *et al.*, 2015; Droogers *et al.*, 2019; Ekdahl, 2016).

However, a more important turn occurred in 2016 with the election of Emmanuel Macron as the President of the French Republic. At that date, there were 714 million masks in the strategic stock, however, in March 2020, only 117 million of them were left. Between 2016 and 2020 strategic decisions led to stock depletion (Davet & Lhomme, 2020). Here again, as in the case of ARS, there is an institutional reform leading to the creation of Public Health France (acronym in French, SPF) with the 2016 fusion of the National Institute for Public Health Surveillance, the National Institute for Health Prevention and Education, and EPRUS. The new organization, SPF, had a limited budget and was unable to fulfill its mission inherited from EPRUS to maintain a strategic stock of masks (Assembléee Nationale, 2020) without an intervention of the Ministry of Health to provide for extra financial resources.

The question of strategic stocks was, most likely, disregarded by the Ministry of Health, and specifically the DGS. Not only was there no new purchase from 2016 onward, but aging stocks were discarded

(Rozenblum, 2021b). Most of the 616 million masks purchased in 2005–2006 were destroyed between 2016 and 2020. When COVID-19 hit, only 117 million masks remained. Attributing blame remains difficult to this day. A recent Senate inquiry points out that the SPF was in charge of the masks and their destruction (Assembléee Nationale, 2020; Milon, 2020) and should have done more to alert on stock depletion. However, at the ministry level, an oversight could hardly be possible: masks were destroyed because they were deemed to have expired after an audit requested by the DGS.

Ultimately, the question of depleted strategic stocks appears to be the result of budget rationalizing. Low on the list of priorities, strategic stocks easily became depleted. This situation, coupled with the lack of bed availability, shook the French healthcare system.

6.3 Fast-paced Reforms' Intracrisis

When the COVID-19 pandemic hit, France was ill-prepared. The first year of the pandemic in France was thus characterized by important insufficiencies which led to two fast-paced reforms. First, the lack of intensive care beds led to a financial reform of the healthcare system. Second, on the problem of strategic stocks, after a strategy of avoidance, the French government turned to coordinated solutions with its European partners, thus reforming its own approach to procurement.

6.3.1 *Financial reform of healthcare*

The first wave of COVID-19 infections inflicted an important stress on the French hospital system. At its peak, more than 3,500 new patients would be admitted every day (Santé publique France Website, 2022). With the enormous risk that the hospital system could be overwhelmed, French patients were flown to Germany to avoid a saturation of hospital beds (Tidey, 2020). In the summer 2020, as the first wave ended, the Ministry held consultations known as *Ségur de la Santé*[1] with the goal of

---

[1] The origin of the name "Ségur" is the address of the Ministry of Health, *Avenue de Ségur* in Paris. This custom in naming large consultations takes its origin in another consultation,

reforming the financing of healthcare institutions. The consultation convened medical professional organizations which focused the attention on careers and remuneration. The consultation also included territory-specific feedback (Stromboni, 2022). The conclusions of the consultation were presented by the Ministry of Health on July 20, 2020, with the announcement that €19 billion will be spent over the next 5 years to improve the working conditions of doctors and nurses in French public hospitals and nursing homes.

This includes the financing of 4,000 beds "on demand" with an envelope of €50 million from winter 2020 to 2021 as well as €6 billion investments in medicalized homes for the elderly (acronym in French, EHPAD), one of the most affected population categories. Beyond the urgent access to intensive healthcare and hospital beds, a crucial question was salary increases for hospital personnel. Unions and the executive ultimately agreed on a base increase of €180 net per month for all non-doctor hospital staff in the public and private non-profit sectors (nurses, orderlies, technicians, stretcher-bearers, etc.). The agreement also provided for an increase of €160 for private sector personnel. Finally, unions of hospital practitioners (i.e. medical doctors) signed an agreement which provided for an envelope of €450 million to be distributed. Self-employed physicians who experienced a significant loss of income because of reduced activity during the lockdown also received financial aid (Gandre & Or, 2020).

But beyond a budgetary bump, stakeholders argued that the reform did not address the core issues (Stromboni, 2022), such as understaffed hospitals, that were causing poor working conditions for healthcare workers and patients. In the same vein, the issue of access to healthcare — to which the 2009 territorial reform was supposed to be the answer — was specifically addressed here by developing teleconsultations, rather than increasing a direct access to healthcare facilities through infrastructure development.

Finally, as described in Figure 6.3, stakeholders unsuccessfully advocated for "decentralizing" the French healthcare system, as ARS still

---

the 1968 "*Grenelle*" consultation organized by the Ministry of Labour situated *Rue de Grenelle*.

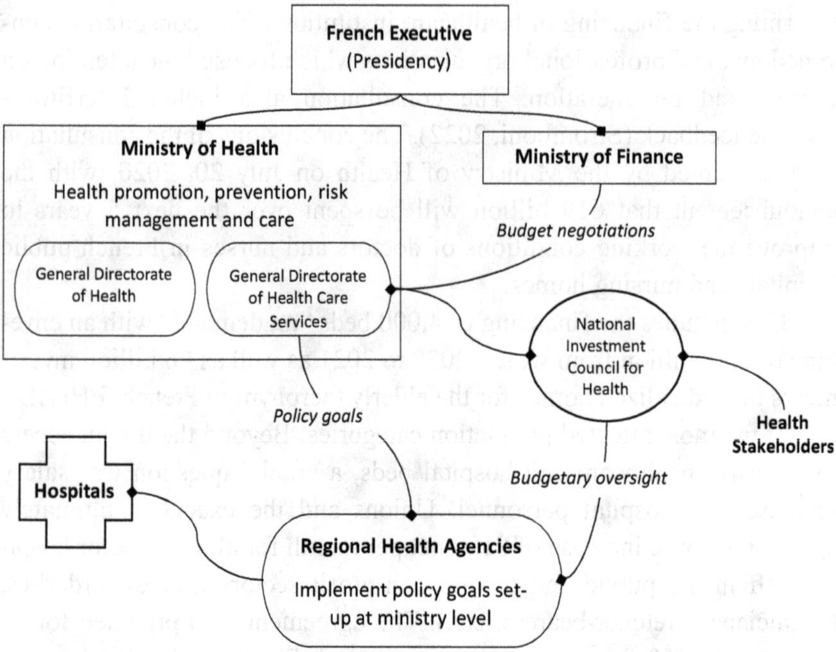

Figure 6.3.   Centralization of hospital care in France post *Ségur*.

implement centralized policy goals (Greer *et al.*, 2022). However, the reform created a National Investment Council for Health, made up of stakeholders and without the Ministry of Finance, replacing the Interministerial Committee for the Performance and Modernization of Hospital, which seemed to indicate that the focus had shifted away from budget rationalizing. Therefore, it will be necessary to reassess in the future if ARS are still the vehicle for a New Management approach to healthcare.

6.3.2 Coping with insufficient preparedness: Between avoidance and reforms

The use of masks was widely accepted as an efficient measure to reduce viral transmission of the COVID-19 virus, among other respiratory pathogens (Asscher, 2020). In the early weeks of the pandemic in France, this was nevertheless subject to debate. There was initially no mask mandate, and on April 9, 2020, the spokesperson for the French government even declared masks to be unhelpful in reducing infections (Fauvelle, 2020). This was in stark contrast with reports from the experience of Asian countries at the time which provided evidence of the benefits of implementing mask mandates. This communication was perceived as a clear strategy of avoidance to be held accountable regarding the depleted stock of PPE, especially because the executive's communication strategy changed as masks became increasingly more available (Hassenteufel, 2020). Ultimately, along with social distancing, masks became the heart of the prevention strategy. From May 2020 onward, i.e. at the end of first the lockdown, masks became mandatory in closed public places (workplaces, schools and universities, shops, etc.). This was followed on July 20, 2020 by a mask mandate for open public places, in a move that could be described as an overcompensation of the initial approach of the French government.

In the same vein, access to test kits was scarce, causing a consequent underdetection of cases (Pullano *et al.*, 2021). In a similar fashion to the mask issue, systematized territorialized screening was only implemented at the end of summer 2020 (Albouy-Llaty *et al.*, 2021). This testing strategy was nevertheless particularly criticized (Hassenteufel, 2020): laboratories were saturated, and results were delayed. Moreover, most of the tests were done at the hospital, adding to the pressure hospitals were experiencing at the time with intensive care. This partially explains why the triptych "testing, tracing and isolation" was never properly implemented in France (Greer *et al.*, 2022).

Since then, two parliamentary inquiry commissions (in the National Assembly and in the Senate, respectively) have pointed out the responsibility of the executive for the lack of preparedness, specifically the lack of strategic stocks of masks (Assembléee Nationale, 2020; Milon, 2020), as well as test kits. And blame attribution is not over: former Prime Minister Edouard Philippe was heard by Court of Justice of the Republic on charges of "manslaughter" and of "endangering the lives of others" on October 10, 2022 (Paun, 2020), and future rulings will be crucial in attributing blame. Unsurprisingly, the public health and health policy literature as well as news media (Davet & Lhomme, 2020; Fauvelle, 2020) have focused on holding the executive branch accountable for the lack of sincerity in attempting to mitigate the effects of a blatant lack of preparedness. Yet, it is worth analyzing the strategy to which the French executive resorted to cope with the situation. Indeed, the French case is not isolated, and many countries, including those on the European continent, were struggling with similar issues with purchasing masks in the early days of the crisis.

From early in the pandemic, EU member states were particularly interdependent in the face of the virus, due to freedom of movement. While EU treaties only allow for coordination of response measures, they had nevertheless allowed for the development of a mechanism for procurement of medical devices in the aftermath of the 2009 H1N1 crisis (Deruelle & Engeli, 2021). The mechanism had been overlooked in the years prior to the pandemic but became a key instrument in the arsenal against the pandemic particularly for France and its depleted stocks. EU member states activated the mechanism of joint procurement of medical equipment on February 28, 2020 for PPE and on March 17, 2020 for ventilators (European Commission, 2020). European coordination for procurement thus became a lifeline for France in the early months of the pandemic.

Coordination with other EU member states prevailed when the question of purchasing vaccines was raised. French representatives, among a few others, expressed their support for a coordinated vaccination plan and their interest in the joint procurement of COVID-19 vaccines. But it was not the only way through which France attempted to coordinate with its neighbors as, with Germany, Italy, and the Netherlands, they had reached a deal with AstraZeneca on the supply of up to 400 million doses of its vaccine. Taking place outside the EU framework (Deutsch, 2021a), the negotiations did not include some smaller member states which would have benefited the most from joint procurement. Ultimately, a form of "solidarity" (Deruelle & Greer, 2022) prevailed and, overall, from August 2020 until January 2021 the Commission signed so-called "advance purchase agreements" with six different companies, for a total of 2.3 billion doses. The first deal signed was with AstraZeneca in August for 400 million doses, largely converting the agreement initially sealed by Germany, France, Italy, and the Netherlands (Sánchez Nicolás & Zalan, 2021).

Moreover, early on in the crisis, the French executive was committed to developing a coordinated approach to procurement. On May 18, 2020, France and Germany jointly proposed setting up an EU "Health Task Force" (Ministère de l'Europe et des Affaires étrangères, 2020). This proposal ultimately took the form of the Health European Response Authority (HERA) (Deruelle & Cairó, 2021). The role of HERA, created on September 16, 2021, is to assist member states in purchasing medical equipment jointly, assist in the deployment of medicines and vaccines, as well as the development of new medicines and medical equipment by covering the whole value chain from conception to R&D and distribution. For instance, it launched the €75 million VACCELERATE project, a COVID-19 clinical research network involving scientific institutions from 16 EU member states including French partners.

Ultimately, the French executive's strategy *vis-à-vis* coordination with its neighbors proved successful in correcting its lack of preparedness. It led to a reconfiguration of the French response and crisis management system and, specifically, the institutionalization of a robust way to access medical devices via the joint purchasing mechanism. But European coordination is not the only force at play in this reconfiguration: the crisis has also given way to a reinforcement of the role of the executive, in which its ambiguous relationship with scientific advice plays a key role.

6.4 Reconfiguration of the Crisis Management System

Amid the crisis, the French executive initiated a fast-paced reconfiguration of the crisis management institutional system. Special measures for the management of the pandemic have given way to a reinforcement of the role of the executive (Presidency and Ministry of Health). This institutional reconfiguration was not permanent, but it bears some effect on the credibility of scientific advice and ultimately future reforms.

6.4.1 *The reinforcement of the executive in crisis management*

In France, the national executive often trumps all. As discussed in Section 6.1, the executive has a great deal of control in territorial terms, i.e. centralization, but this also holds true in institutional terms. As such the role of the executive in France is often analyzed with reference to the weakness and sidelining of other institutions, such as the French Parliament regarding presidentialization. The COVID-19 crisis created a context propitious to concentrating crisis management powers in the hands of the executive (Bergeron & Borraz, 2020; Pedrot, 2020). Ultimately, this institutional reconfiguration of the crisis management system has led to the sidelining of expert's agencies.

The concentration of powers within the hands of the executive is a formal process. The adoption of a Health Emergency Law on March 23, 2020 gave the executive broad powers, including the possibility of adopting many measures by decree, i.e. without parliamentary oversight. Despite legal limits on its length and possibility for extension, the state of emergency lasted from March 24, 2020 to November 10, 2021. The French executive was very creative in its strategy to maintain the state of emergency, using decrees to ensure continuity. The state of emergency was initially declared on March 24, 2020 for 2 months and then renewed up to July 9, 2020. This was followed by a "transition" period which ended on October 17, 2020 — only for a new state of emergency to be declared on the same day. It then was extended twice. The executive was able to take decrees and avoid parliamentary oversight, a matter particularly criticized in both chambers.

This amounted to a concentration of power in the hands of the President. During the state of emergency, decisions were taken by the "Defence Council," convened and chaired by the French President and composed of the Prime Minister and Ministers selected by the President. Decisions were made public by President Macron himself, especially regarding the details of the introduction of lockdowns or their lifting. It was as if the French President had taken the concept of health "security" quite literally, in stark contrast with the pre-COVID period. This approach has clear advantages: it legitimizes public health as high politics (Rozenblum, 2021a) and its inherent verticality allows for a reactive response. But it may also be perceived as arbitrary by the population. COVID-19 altered living conditions in a substantial manner, as a total of three "lockdowns" were declared over the years 2020–2021. It is worth noting that the enforcement of the lockdowns was particularly severe and

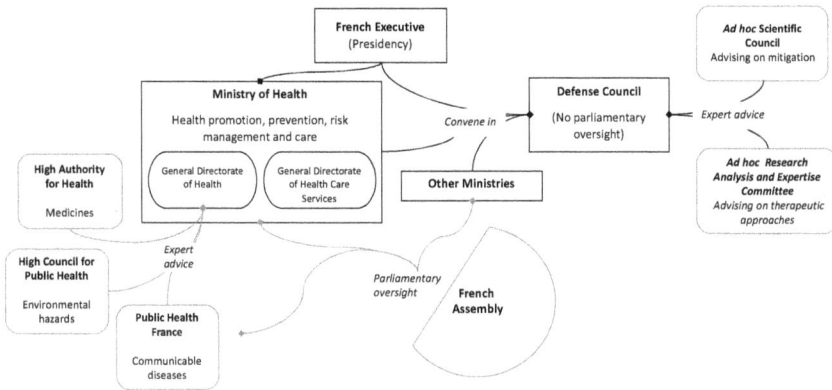

Figure 6.4. Public health governance in France under the Health Emergency Law.

required having to fill, date, and sign forms each time one would step out in the public space. Police repression was particularly brutal in some portions of the territory, as denounced by human rights NGOs (Willsher, 2020).

As described in Figure 6.4, this reconfiguration of the crisis management system also altered the role of scientific advice in decision-making: the President and its Security Council sidelined institutionalized scientific bodies to the benefit of *ad hoc* advisory committees. The first was the Scientific Council advising on strategic decision-making set up on March 12, 2020, and the second was the Research Analysis and Expertise Committee advising on innovative, scientific, technological, and therapeutic approaches and set up on March 24, 2020 (Assemblée Nationale, 2020). The creation of the *ad hoc* committees may seem superfluous in a system described as one of the densest public health networks in Europe. But in the context of French politics, it shows commitment to solving the crisis, especially since scientific bodies and agencies usually have a low profile in France.

The creation of the *ad hoc* committees with a direct line to the Security Council led to the marginalization of the High Council of Public Health (HCSP), Public Health France (SPF), and the HAS (Gergeron & Borraz, 2020; Pedrot, 2020). This marginalization was clear as SPF and the HCSP were invited by the Scientific Council to attend meetings as "permanent observers," without actually participating (Delfraissy, 2020). On top of that, there was a proper epistemic divide with the new *ad hoc* council being mostly made of medical doctors, while institutionalized scientific bodies were hosting public health experts (Rozenblum, 2021a). Throughout the pandemic, the snub was most evident for SPF. Its core missions are to prepare and respond to health threats, alerts, and crises by developing and implementing strategies to contain health crises (Article L.1413-1 of the Code of Public Health). SPF had already absorbed at least part of the blame for the lack of strategic stocks. Ultimately, it was relegated to risk assessment and surveillance and was sidelined from risk management.

But even on the matter of risk assessment and surveillance, the systemic understaffing of SPF made it difficult to produce reliable data, especially finer data, which is crucial information for Regional Public Health Agencies (Greer *et al.*, 2022). On top of that, SPF data had been discredited by the French executive, with the Prime Minister pointing out the "shallowness" of data reports (Hecketsweiler & de Royer, 2020).

Ultimately, this institutional "distortion" was only temporary: it ended with the withdrawal of the Health Emergency Law on July 31, 2022. However, it has reinforced centrifugal forces that concentrate powers in the hands of the executive with profound effects on the credibility of health agencies. Moreover, as the executive concentrates crisis management prerogatives in its hands, it also concentrates blame from both medical professionals and public opinion. This presents new challenges to reforming the health system.

6.4.2 *The legacy of the crisis on trust*

Because of early problems with masks and scientific advice, the French executive was the focus of the majority of the blame. According to the CEVIPOF's European opinion survey from May 2020, 62% of French respondents said they were dissatisfied with the government's action (Sciences Po CEVIPO, 2018). SPF shared some of the blame on strategy stocks (Assemblée Nationale, 2020) but many were dissatisfied with the severity of lockdowns. This was unsurprising as the pre-COVID context was already characterized by a growing discontent, with the yellow vest ("gilets jaunes") movement from autumn 2018 to spring 2019 and the strikes against pension reform from December 2019 to February 2020, ending days before the first lockdown.

Later on in the pandemic, an important point of defiance was the introduction of "health passes" in June 2021, which means only individuals who either had a proof of full vaccination, a negative virological test, or a certificate of recovery could access closed public spaces: cafes, restaurants, hospitals (except emergencies), retirement homes, airplanes, trains and buses for long-distance travel, and so on. The health pass has been criticized by a number of politicians, notably from La France Insoumise (far left) and the Rassemblement National (far right), who denounced a significant reduction in public freedoms and a vaccine mandate in disguise (Willsher, 2021). This was exacerbated over the question of mandatory vaccination for healthcare workers and caregivers — paradoxically, this measure came at a time of great tension in hospital services due to the lack of healthcare personnel. Nevertheless, this measure most likely supported and incited vaccination. An analysis by the Economic Analysis Council estimates that the introduction of the pass resulted in 13% more people being vaccinated, which would have prevented about 4,000 additional deaths (Conseil d'Analyse Economique *et al.*, 2022).

It seems likely that the ambiguous use of evidence-based policymaking and scientific advice contributed to eroding trust in the executive (Coste *et al.*, 2020). The French executive's communication regarding the stock of masks showed that it was not shy from adopting a head-in-the-sand approach when scientific advice was inconvenient. In a similar vein, the institutional reconfiguration of the crisis management system has led to the sidelining of public health experts in institutionalized bodies, in favor of medical doctors in *ad hoc* groups, which allowed for the executive to cherrypick between different advice. For instance, despite a negative opinion of SPF on maintaining the date of the 2020 local elections, the Security Council publicly invoked the *ad hoc* committees' decisions to justify their controversial decisions to maintain elections "on site." This demonstrates that the French executive has exploited the divide between *ad hoc* and institutionalized experts. Ultimately, the French executive engaged in a compartmentalization of risk assessment and risk management: while SPF had the data, other forms of scientific credibility were invoked to assert choices in terms of management. This strategy offers a great deal of freedom for the French executive from scientific advice — and data — in making choices regarding crisis management, but it contributes to maintaining a high level of ambiguity and ultimately undermining scientific advice.

6.5 Conclusion: A Not-So-Disruptive Pandemic?

The COVID-19 crisis was a profoundly disruptive event which affected French people. Yet its effect on health reforms remains limited. Two fast-paced reforms initiated in the early months of the crisis must nevertheless be noted: the financial reform of healthcare as well as the reform of procurement by way of European coordination. These reforms were a direct consequence of the lack of preparedness to face serious health threats (Jugl, 2022) and ultimately, a form of learning from the crisis. But while the pandemic has delivered lessons, some may have yet to be learned, as exemplified by the lack of reform of the crisis management system despite its overhaul amid crisis. Overall, the pandemic appears to have been less disruptive than one could expect.

The financial reform of healthcare, prepared on a time crunch, was both a social reform for hospital personnel and a reform of investment in healthcare; it has yet to be fully implemented, with many fearing budget cuts. The reform of procurement, a joint effort with France's European partners, has already changed the way preparedness is done at national level. This reform does not revolutionize crisis management but rather partially mutualizes the issue of procurement: the EU's action is still limited to coordination, albeit supported by much more sophisticated institutions than pre-pandemic (see Greer, this volume). However, a substantial leap would require a treaty change, and EU member states have shown little interest in proposals on the matter, such as the one formulated by the Conference on the Future of Europe (Deruelle & Engeli, 2021; Deruelle & Greer, 2022; Deruelle, 2021).

Future health reforms seem unlikely in the short or medium term. For instance, despite the fact that there was a complete overhaul of scientific bodies, there is an apparent lack of self-reflection on the matter. Moreover, other issues have taken front stage. On the internal front, the executive agenda is set on the reform of the pension system rather than of the health system, a reform that the French President has been preparing since 2017. On the external front, inflation and the crisis in Ukraine have steered attention away from health reforms. Beyond reforms of crisis management itself, the challenge ahead will be to avoid letting lessons learned about public health to be cannibalized by economic or defense affairs.

Ultimately, the legacy of the crisis is beyond reforms, in the practice of concentrating authority in the hands of the French executive. The pandemic confirmed the rationale for centralization of hospital care, albeit alleviated by the imperative of "modernization." It also led to a centralization of crisis management prerogatives in the hands of the executive, sideling not only the French Assembly but also institutionalized public health experts. Beyond the effects on trust documented in this chapter, the question remains to what extent such a lengthy centralized management in times of crisis may foreshadow the post-COVID era.

References

Albouy-Llaty, M., Martin, C., Benamouzig, D., Bothorel, E., Munier, G., Simonin, C., Guéant, J.-L., and Rusch, E. (2021). Positioning digital tracing applications in the management of the COVID-19 pandemic in France. *Journal of Medical Internet Research, 23*(10), e27301. https://doi.org/10.2196/27301.

Assemblée Nationale (June 3, 2020). Rapport d'information sur l'impact, la gestion et les conséquences dans toutes ses dimensions de l'épidémie de Coronavirus-COVID-19.

Bayer, L. (2020). EU response to corona crisis 'poor,' says senior Greek official. *POLITICO*, April 1. https://www.politico.eu/article/eu-response-to-coronavirus-crisis-poor-says-senior-greek-official/.

Bergeron, H. and Borraz, O. (March 31, 2020). *COVID-19: Impréparation et crise de l'Etat*. AOC. https://aoc.media/analyse/2020/03/30/covid-19-impreparation-et-crise-de-letat/.

Brusaferro, S. and Tricarico, P. (2017). How to include public health practice and practitioners in a European network. *European Journal of Public Health, 27*(suppl_4), 56–59. https://doi.org/10.1093/eurpub/ckx156.

Clemens, T. and Brand, H. (2020). Will COVID-19 lead to a major change of the EU public health mandate? A renewed approach to EU's role is needed. *European Journal of Public Health*. https://doi.org/10.1093/eurpub/ckaa103.

Conseil d'Analyse Economique (CAE), Martin, P., Pisani-Ferry, J., and Ragot, X. (July, 2022). Note du CAE n°57. "Une stratégie économique face à la crise".

Coste, J., Bizouarn, P., and Leplège, A. (2020). L'épistémologie troublée de la première vague de recherche sur la COVID-19. *Revue d'Épidémiologie et de Santé Publique, 68*(5), 269–271. https://doi.org/10.1016/j.respe.2020.09.001.

Crosier, A., McVey, D., and French, J. (2015). 'By failing to prepare you are preparing to fail': Lessons from the 2009 H1N1 'Swine Flu' pandemic. *European Journal of Public Health, 25*(1), 135–139. https://doi.org/10.1093/eurpub/cku131.

Davet, G. and Lhomme, P. (2020). 2017–2020: Comment la France a continué à détruire son stock de masques après le début de l'épidémie. *Le* Monde.fr, May 7. https://www.lemonde.fr/sante/article/2020/05/07/la-france-et-les-epidemies-2017-2020-l-heure-des-comptes_6038973_1651302.html.

Delfraissy, J.-F. (June 18, 2020). Président du Conseil scientifique COVID-19. Audition devant la Mission d'information parlementaire. Assemblée Nationale.

Deruelle, T. and Cairó, E. R. (2021). The EU Health Emergency Response and Preparedness Authority (HERA): Institutional impact. *EU Law Live*, November. https://eulawlive.com/analysis-the-eu-health-emergency-response-and-preparedness-authority-hera-institutional-impact-by-thibaud-deruelle-and-elisabet-ruiz-cairo/.

Deruelle, T. and Engeli, I. (2021). The COVID-19 crisis and the rise of the European Centre for Disease Prevention and Control (ECDC). *West European Politics*, 1–25. https://doi.org/10.1080/01402382.2021.1930426.

Deruelle, T. and Greer, S. L. (2022). Will the COVID-19 crisis make the European Health Union? *EuroHealth, 28*(3), 7–9.

Deverell, E. (2009). Crises as learning triggers: Exploring a conceptual framework of crisis-induced learning. *Journal of Contingencies and Crisis Management, 17*(3), 179–188. https://doi.org/10.1111/j.1468-5973.2009.00578.x.

Droogers, M., Ciotti, M., Kreidl, P., Melidou, A., Penttinen, P., Sellwood, C., Tsolova, S., and Snacken R. (July 2019). European pandemic influenza preparedness planning: A review of national plans. *Disaster Medicine and Public Health Preparedness, 13*(3), 582–592. https://doi.org/10.1017/dmp.2018.60.

Duchesne, V. (2018). L'agence, le contrat, l'incitation. Les Agences régionales de santé fer-de-lance administratif de la politique de santé. *Journal de gestion et d'économie médicales, 36*(4), 159–80. https://doi.org/10.3917/jgem.184.0159.

Ekdahl, K. (2016). ECDC support for strengthening capacity for preparedness in the member StatesKarl Ekdahl. *European Journal of Public Health, 26*(suppl_1). https://doi.org/10.1093/eurpub/ckw168.049.

European Centre for Disease Prevention and Control (2020). *Rapid Risk Assessment: Outbreak of Novel Coronavirus Disease 2019 (COVID-19): Increased Transmission Globally — Fifth Update.* Stockholm, Sweden: ECDC. https://www.ecdc.europa.eu/sites/default/files/documents/RRA-outbreak-novel-coronavirus-disease-2019-increase-transmission-globally-COVID-19.pdf.

European Commission (2020). Coronavirus response. Text. European Commission. https://ec.europa.eu/info/live-work-travel-eu/health/coronavirus-response_en.

Fauvelle, M. (2020). Interview de Mme Sibeth Ndiaye, secrétaire d'État, porte-parole du Gouvernement, à France Info le 9 avril 2020, sur le port du masque, l'avenir de l'hôpital public, le dépistage du coronavirus et les mesures de chômage partiel. France Info. https://www.vie-publique.fr/discours/274880-sibeth-ndiaye-09042020-masques-hopital-public-depistage-chomage-partiel.

Freeman, R. (2000). *The Politics of Health in Europe.* Manchester: Manchester University Press.

Gottlieb, D.-K. (dir.). (2021). European health union, now! https://open.spotify.com/episode/2J4U61a8SJ4EAmSMPIefIq.

Greer, S. L., Rozenblum, S., Falkenbach, M., Löblová, O., Jarman, H., Williams, N., and Wismar, M. (2022). Centralizing and decentralizing governance in the COVID-19 pandemic: The politics of credit and blame. *Health Policy,* Lessons learned from the COVID-19 pandemic, 126(5), 408–417. https://doi.org/10.1016/j.healthpol.2022.03.004.

Guarascio, F. (2020). Europe could face more drug shortages as coronavirus squeezes supplies. *Reuters,* March 5. https://www.reuters.com/article/us-health-coronavirus-eu-idUSKBN20S1R2.

Hassenteufel, P. (2020). Handling the COVID-19 crisis in France: Paradoxes of a centralized state-led health system. *European Policy Analysis, 6*(2), 170–179. https://doi.org/10.1002/epa2.1104.

Hornung, J. (2022a). Health policy institutions in France and Germany. *The Institutions of Programmatic Action,* 113–120. https://doi.org/10.1007/978-3-031-05774-8_4.

Hornung, J. (2022b). Programmatic action in French health policy. In J. Hornung (Ed.), *The Institutions of Programmatic Action: Policy Programs in French and German Health Policy* (pp. 121–57). International Series on Public

Policy. Cham: Springer International Publishing. https://doi.org/10.1007/978-3-031-05774-8_5.

Jugl, M. (2022). Administrative characteristics and timing of government's crisis responses: A global study of early reactions to COVID-19. *Public Administration,* online version. https://doi.org/10.1111/padm.12889.

Lee, S., Hwang, C., and Jae Moon M. (2020). Policy learning and crisis policy-making: Quadruple-loop learning and COVID-19 responses in South Korea. *Policy and Society,* 39(3), 363–381. https://doi.org/10.1080/14494035.2020.1785195.

LOI N° 2009-879 Du 21 Juillet 2009 Portant Réforme de l'hôpital et Relative Aux Patients, à La Santé et Aux Territoires (1). 2009.

McCubbins, M. D. and Schwartz, T. (1984). Congressional oversight overlooked: Police patrols versus fire alarms. *American Journal of Political Science,* 28(1), 165–79. https://doi.org/10.2307/2110792.

Michalopoulos, S. (March 6, 2020). Coronavirus puts Europe's solidarity to the test. *Www.Euractiv.Com* (blog). https://www.euractiv.com/section/coronavirus/news/coronavirus-puts-europes-solidarity-to-the-test/.

Milon, A. (June 24, 2020). Rapport fait au nom de la commission des affaires sociales sur la proposition de résolution tendant à créer une commission d'enquête pour l'évaluation des politiques publiques face aux grandes pandémies à la lumière de la crise sanitaire de la COVID-19 et de sa gestion. Social Afairs Committee, Sénat.

Ministère de l'Europe et des Affaires étrangères (May 18, 2020). *European Union — French-German Initiative for the European Recovery from the Coronavirus Crisis.* Paris, France: Diplomacy — Ministry for Europe and Foreign Affairs. https://www.diplomatie.gouv.fr/en/coming-to-france/coronavirus-advice-for-foreign-nationals-in-france/coronavirus-statements/article/european-union-french-german-initiative-for-the-european-recovery-from-the.

Ministère des solidarités et de la santé (2022). La Statistique annuelle des établissements de santé. Minsitère des solidarités et de la santé. https://data.drees.solidarites-sante.gouv.fr/explore/dataset/708_bases-statistiques-sae/information/ (Accessed October 27, 2022).

Naumann, E., Möhring, K., Reifenscheid, M., Wenz, A., Rettig, T., Lehrer, R., Krieger, U., *et al.* (2020). COVID-19 policies in Germany and their social, political, and psychological consequences. *European Policy Analysis,* 6(2), 191–202. https://doi.org/10.1002/epa2.1091.

Nicoll, A. and McKee, M. (2010). Moderate pandemic, not many dead — Learning the right lessons in Europe from the 2009 pandemic. *European*

Journal of Public Health, 20(5), 486–488. https://doi.org/10.1093/eurpub/ckq114.

Pacces, A. M. and Weimer, M. (2020). From diversity to coordination: A European approach to COVID-19. *European Journal of Risk Regulation,* 1–14. https://doi.org/10.1017/err.2020.36.

Pasquier, R. (2016). Crise économique et différenciation territoriale. Les régions et les métropoles dans la décentralisation française. *Revue internationale de politique comparée, 23*(3), 327–353. https://doi.org/10.3917/ripc.233.0327.

Paun (2020). Former French PM, Health Ministers to be investigated for pandemic response. *POLITICO,* July 3. https://www.politico.eu/article/former-french-pm-health-ministers-to-be-investigated-for-pandemic-response/.

Pedrot, F. (July 20, 2020). COVID-19: Les alertes ignorées de la veille sanitaire. AOC.

Pierru, F. (2020). Agences régionales de santé: Mission impossible. *Revue française d'administration publique, 174*(2), 385–403. https://doi.org/10.3917/rfap.174.0089.

Pullano, G., Di Domenico, L., Sabbatini, C. E., Valdano, E., Turbelin, C., Debin, M., Guerrisi, C., *et al.* (2021). Underdetection of cases of COVID-19 in France threatens epidemic control. *Nature,* 590(7844), 134–139. https://doi.org/10.1038/s41586-020-03095-6.

Reiter, R. and Kuhlmann, S. (2016). La décentralisation du système de protection sociale français: Entre « Big Bang » et « débrouillardise », Decentralization of the French welfare state: From 'big bang' to 'muddling through.' *Revue Internationale des Sciences Administratives, 82*(2), 269–287. https://doi.org/10.3917/risa.822.0269.

Renda, A. and Castro, R. (April, 2020). Towards stronger EU governance of health threats after the COVID-19 pandemic. *European Journal of Risk Regulation,* 1–10. https://doi.org/10.1017/err.2020.34.

Rozenblum, S. D. (2021a). Pandemic response credit-claiming and blame-avoidance in France. *European Journal of Public Health, 31*(Supplement_3), ckab164.462. https://doi.org/10.1093/eurpub/ckab164.462.

Rozenblum, S. D. (2021b). France's multidimensional COVID-19 response: Ad Hoc committees and the sidelining of public health agencies. In S. L. Greer, E. J. King, E. Massard da Fonseca, and A. Peralta-Santos (Eds.) *Coronavirus Politics* (pp. 264–279). The Comparative Politics and Policy of COVID-19. University of Michigan Press. https://www.jstor.org/stable/10.3998/mpub.11927713.17.

Sánchez Nicolás, E. and Zalan, E. (May 19, 2021). The EU's vaccine strategy — The key points. *EUobserver*. https://euobserver.com/coronavirus/150747.

Sciences Po CEVIPOF (April 5, 2018). Le Baromètre de la confiance politique. https://www.sciencespo.fr/cevipof/fr/content/le-barometre-de-la-confiance-politique.html.

Stern, E. (1997). Crisis and learning: A conceptual balance sheet. *Journal of Contingencies and Crisis Management, 5*(2), 69–86. https://doi.org/10.1111/1468-5973.00039.

Stromboni, C. (2022). Hôpital: les sénateurs dénoncent l'insuffisance du Ségur de la santé. *Le* Monde.fr, March 31. https://www.lemonde.fr/societe/article/2022/03/31/hopital-les-senateurs-denoncent-l-insuffisance-du-segur-de-la-sante_6119966_3224.html.

Tidey, A. (2020). More French COVID-19 patients flown to Germany and Switzerland. *Euronews*, March 28, sec. *european-affairs_europe*. https://www.euronews.com/2020/03/28/eight-COVID-19-patients-flown-from-france-and-italy-to-german-hospitals.

Vagionaki, T. and Trein, P. (April 2019). Learning in political analysis. *Political Studies Review*, 1478929919834863. https://doi.org/10.1177/1478929919834863.

Wheaton, S. (2020). 'Nothing would have prevented' virus spread, says Health Agency Chief. *POLITICO*, April 8. https://www.politico.eu/article/ecdc-chief-nothing-would-have-prevented-coronavirus-spread/.

WHO (2000). World Health Organization assesses the world's health systems. https://www.who.int/news/item/07-02-2000-world-health-organization-assesses-the-world's-health-systems.

Willsher, K. (2020). Disruption on streets of France as lockdown tensions rise. *The Guardian*, April 22, sec. *World News*. https://www.theguardian.com/world/2020/apr/22/disruption-france-virus-lockdown-tensions-rise-motorbike-police.

Willsher, K. (2021). Macron tells critics: Vaccine passport will protect all our freedoms. *The Observer*, August 8, sec. *World News*. https://www.theguardian.com/world/2021/aug/08/macron-tells-critics-vaccine-passport-will-protect-all-our-freedoms.

Chapter 7

The United Kingdom

Ollie Bartlett

7.1 Introduction

This volume explores the capacity of states to reform their public health policy following the upheaval of the COVID-19 pandemic. This upheaval reveals opportunities to reform laws and practices, or entrench positive developments that flowed from the shattering and remolding of social norms. There will, of course, always be factors that will impede such reform (Marsden & Docherty, 2021). The United Kingdom (UK) has grappled simultaneously with the COVID-19 pandemic and Brexit. Efforts to leave the European Union had been destabilizing the UK's politics, economy, and society for several years before the COVID-19 pandemic struck and, although COVID-19 became the immediate focus of the government and the public, the problems caused by Brexit did not disappear. In fact, Brexit has directly and indirectly had a negative influence on COVID-19 policies in the UK.

After the emergency phase of the COVID-19 pandemic passed, Brexit reasserted itself as a crisis still in need of a resolution. Although progress has been made in stabilizing the UK's relationship with the EU after its official withdrawal in January 2020, much remains uncertain. Not only is a great deal of government time and resources still required to address the ongoing practical consequences of Brexit, but the approach to governance in the UK has also been fundamentally affected by Brexit. Both of these factors will exert a chilling effect on future public health work and, when combined with the legacy of disastrous COVID-19 policymaking, have likely created a public health landscape that will make implementing the lessons of the COVID-19 pandemic a challenge.

This chapter illustrates this in three parts. It first outlines the institutional structure of public health in the UK both before and after COVID-19 and discusses how drastic reforms to these institutions made during COVID-19 will create challenges for future public health work. Second, it provides a thematic overview of the shortcomings of UK COVID-19 policy and focuses in particular on the legacy of the 2020 *Coronavirus Act* for future public health work. Third, it explores the mechanisms through which Brexit affected (and will affect) public health work during and after the pandemic. It considers in particular the options for public health reform that face the UK post-COVID-19 and post-Brexit.

7.2 Public Health Institutions in the UK

7.2.1 *The institutional structure of UK public health pre- and post-COVID*

The UK has a devolved constitutional structure: certain policy competencies are exercised by the central government, whereas other competencies are exercised by devolved governments in Scotland, Wales, and Northern Ireland, with the central government exercising those devolved competencies for England. Heath, and within that, public health, is a devolved policy area, and England, Scotland, Wales, and Northern Ireland all have their own agencies to carry out public health work for their respective populations. The work carried out by these agencies includes vaccine provision, non-communicable disease prevention, substance use work, mental health work, community interventions and screening, and public health literacy work. Examples of powers exercised by the central government which could be used to promote and protect public health include the

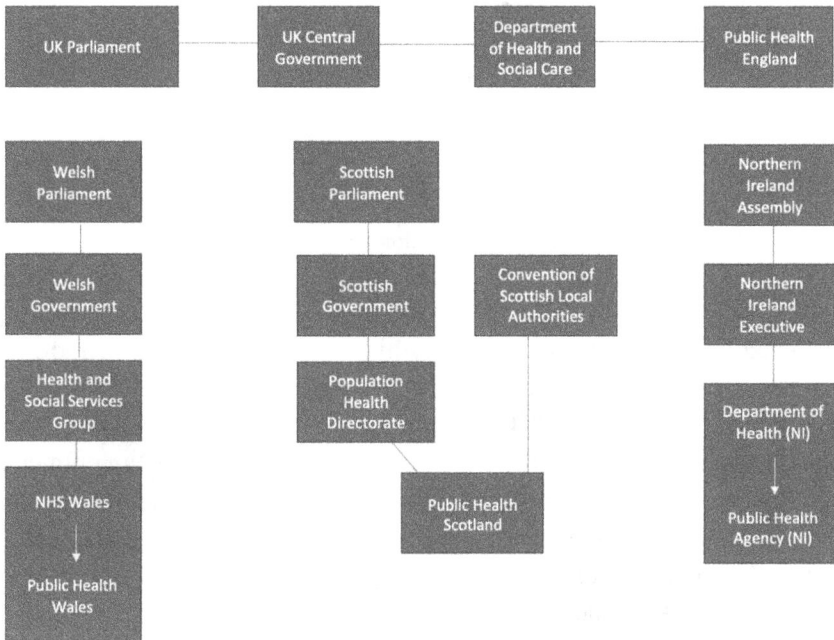

Figure 7.1.   Public health organization across all UK nations.

power to raise taxes and the power to control UK borders. Figure 7.1 identifies the pre-COVID devolved public health agencies and their relationship with the devolved and central governments.

As can be seen, the agencies responsible for public health work in each of the four UK nations have totally different accountability structures. In Scotland and England, public health agencies operate as separate bodies but with accountability to government. In Wales, public health is run as part of the National Health Service in Wales, which itself is accountable to government. In Northern Ireland, the public health agency is *part* of the government. However, following the COVID-19 pandemic, it seems that differences in public health organizations are a minor issue compared to the much more serious impact of the UK's asymmetrical devolution settlement itself upon the adoption of coordinated and effective public health policies. When the COVID-19 pandemic struck, the devolved governments had numerous powers to impose lockdown, organize testing, close businesses, and offer economic support. Some of these

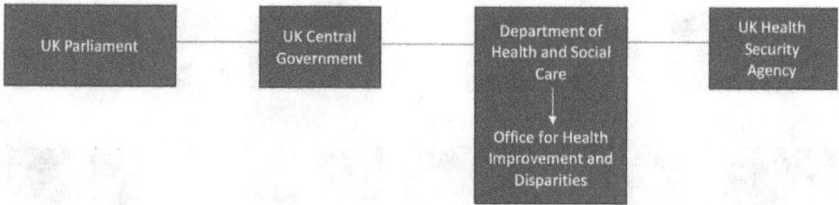

Figure 7.2.   Public health organization for England after COVID-19.

powers were exercised similarly across the UK, but in some respects, the devolved governments took markedly different approaches to each other and the UK central government which exercised such powers for England (Cameron-Blake *et al.*, 2020). These differences arose because of the political choices made by the devolved administrations. Much commentary has since examined the breakdown in political coordination between the UK central government and the devolved governments, and the influence of the tensions of asymmetric devolution upon the UK's ability to plan a coordinated state-wide pandemic response to the aspects of the pandemic that required it (Diamond & Laffin, 2022).

These existing tensions may be further exacerbated by the much-criticized decision of the UK central government to abolish Public Health England and establish in its place the UK Health Security Agency (UKSHA) and the Office for Health Improvement and Disparities (OHID), as illustrated in Figure 7.2.

The UKHSA is a separate body with accountability to government, similar to Public Health England (PHE), while the OHID is fully part of government. The UKHSA will continue to exercise health protection functions for England, but importantly it seems that it also now exercises some health protection functions for the whole of the UK in a way that PHE did not. The relationship between these functions of the UKHSA and the functions of the public health agencies in Scotland, Wales, and Northern Ireland, which have remained intact after the pandemic, is yet to be clarified, and it is uncertain what the political response would be if the exercise of these powers were to conflict with the policies of the devolved administrations.

Before the COVID-19 pandemic, the direction of authority in public health work was toward greater local control of, and accountability for, public health work. Public health functions were moved out of the National Health Service (NHS) by the *Health and Social Care Act* 2012, and many were placed under the control of local authorities and their directors of public health, who were supported by the newly created PHE (Middleton, 2017). The creation of Public Health Scotland also placed more emphasis on local exercise of public health powers (Scottish Government, 2020).

When the COVID-19 pandemic struck, this progress was almost entirely ignored by the UK central government when designing policies for England. Local authorities in England in particular attempted at various points of the pandemic to persuade the UK central government to give them greater control over COVID-19 responses — the standoff between Manchester Metro Mayor Andy Burnham and Prime Minister Boris Johnson over localized lockdown rules and increased local pandemic funding was the most public and embarrassing example for the central government (Kenny & Kelsey, 2020). Ultimately, however, the UK central government largely ignored the calls for a more localized approach and proceeded with centrally designing and implementing COVID-19 response.

7.2.2 Future challenges created by the reform of the UK's public health institutions

Perhaps the most significant challenge will be how to ensure that the UK's new public health institutions work in a positive and productive way. Undoubtedly their rapid creation, without any significant consultation, was influenced both by the desire to shift the blame for poor government policy and by the desire to recentralize public health functions. It appears to have been an unwise move from several perspectives.

Splitting responsibility for health protection and health promotion across two separate agencies, especially when one — the OHID — is fully part of a government department, will clearly reduce the connectedness of public health policymaking and is a development that the public health sector has responded to cautiously (Association of Directors of Public Health, 2021; Royal Society for Public Health, 2021). Health inequalities, for example, persist in both the communicable and non-communicable disease contexts, and the complex job of closing such inequalities requires a whole-of-government response (Ortenzi *et al.*, 2022). Evidence from other jurisdictions demonstrates that strong leadership for this whole-of-government response is required if actions on health inequalities and the social determinants of health are to be effective (Dean *et al.*, 2013). Indeed, evidence from the UK concludes the same thing but finds such leadership lacking (Marmot *et al.*, 2020). Given that PHE struggled with priorities such as the proper funding of non-communicable disease (NCD) prevention activities and connected policy implementation (Hunter *et al.*, 2022), artificially confining responsibility for so-called health "disparities" to one agency which does not appear to have a mandate to reach across the UK government, and which certainly is not empowered to coordinate policy across the devolved governments and their public health agencies, will make it very difficult to achieve this much-needed leadership (Wilkinson, 2021). The rapidity and lack of consultation with which this "distraction" was implemented will likely mean that the failings of PHE regarding policy connectivity will only be reproduced by the UK's new public health agencies (Littlejohns *et al.*, 2022).

Moreover, the use of the term "health disparities", rather than the accepted public health term "health inequalities" (Scally, 2021b), seems to be the latest indication that the current Conservative government (despite recent headline grabbing pledges such as that to create a smoke-free generation and more tightly regulate e-cigarettes) is not entirely committed to the hard work required to eliminate persistent health inequalities within the UK, and may well dilute the ability of the OHID to have a meaningful impact on the UK's widening health inequalities. This lack of commitment became evident in the White Paper on Levelling Up that was published in February 2022, as a much-delayed response to one of Boris Johnson's major campaign pledges. The White Paper was silent on many factors that drive health inequality and contained measures which are unlikely to be effective in addressing health inequality (Ralston *et al.*, 2022). The establishment of the OHID seems to continue in the same vein, since it has initially been tasked with working on neoliberal interventions to promote behavior change rather than interventions that will address the social determinants of health (Oliver, 2021). Moreover, some of those initial priorities have already been changed or canceled (Buck, 2022). This illustrates the dangers of the national agency responsible for addressing health inequalities being wholly accountable to government ministers, whose preferences on health policy are inevitably politically oriented and changeable. In particular, the health policy preferences of the current government seem to be driven not by the evidence but by what the political right of the Conservative party would approve of, as well as by the desire to demonstrate that the UK can come up with innovative health policy as a non-EU state. This has led some commentators to brand the new public health organizations an "ideologically driven distraction" (Scally, 2021a).

Moreover, it seems unwise to create an agency — the UKHSA — that will not only carry out health protection functions for England but will also exercise certain health protection functions for the whole of the UK, in particular functions related to knowledge generation. The devolved agencies in Scotland, Wales, and Northern Ireland were not formally altered following the COVID-19 pandemic, and so it is unclear whether any of their knowledge generation functions have been co-opted by the UKHSA. More likely is that an entirely new remit of knowledge generation for communicable diseases has been created, but this then raises the question of the extent the devolved agencies are entitled to feed into the exercise of these knowledge generation powers. The evidence base strongly suggests a key role for local authorities in improving public health outcomes (Bonner, 2020; Riches *et al.*, 2015). If the findings of the devolved agencies on particular issues conflict with those of the UKHSA, it is unclear whether the devolved agencies would be obliged to follow the evidence generated by the UKHSA. In any event, what is certainly clear is that the OHID was not invested with any such UK-wide powers with respect to its non-communicable disease remit, which raises the question of whether there should be a public authority that is responsible for knowledge generation and coordination on non-communicable disease. This certainly seems like an oversight in this institutional restructuring.

The idea to make knowledge production and dissemination a key aspect of a public health agency's work is a good one; however, the way this has been operationalized in the UK post-COVID-19 leaves much to be desired, and this owes much to the Brexit influence. It is obvious that the UK central government was eager to use the dismantling of PHE to create an institution that contributes to the image of the self-sufficient, global-facing Britain that was promised during the Brexit campaign. The UKHSA was set up as an agency that would produce "world-leading" knowledge and best practices for the whole of the UK, conveniently on a topic that was particularly salient for the public at the time. However, the rhetoric has now collided with reality: a short while after the creation of the UKHSA, the UK government announced that in fact its funding was to be drastically cut, something that apparently was long in the planning (Hill, 2022). At best, this further demonstrates the superficiality of the institutional restructuring exercise. At worst, it is evidence of the cynical use of a major and unnecessary institutional restructuring to advance the political objectives of the government, in full knowledge of the fact that such world-leading work was not possible within the constraints of the resources that the government were willing to allocate. Either way, the UKHSA is now left with a daunting new remit to fulfill, seemingly without the proper resources to achieve this.

It also seems very unwise to unwind, through the establishment of both UKHSA and OHID, the gains achieved through the prior establishment of PHE and the Directors of Public Health. This, largely, was a greater focus on supporting local public health functions (Buck, 2021). Maintaining and strengthening local control over public health is agreed to be a key feature of future public health work (Buck *et al.*, 2018). However, the establishment of the UKHSA and OHID have recentralized public health functions, a move which reflected the government's populist agenda. Keeping health policy functions close to central government and linking them with the private sector (clearly not learning from the disastrous impact of privatizing COVID-19 response policies (Monbiot, 2020)) ensures that central government can control the public health policy narrative if it risks becoming unpopular and especially can steer it in directions that are perceived to avoid paternalism. Unfortunately, this neoliberal approach to public health is clearly not the best strategy not just in light of existing evidence but also of the UK's particular COVID-19 experience (Jones & Hameiri, 2022). Avoiding the perceived unpopular decisions in long-term public health strategy, especially when the UK's high level of health inequality was so starkly revealed during the COVID-19 pandemic, is a profound mistake. Moreover, centralization will risk delocalizing public health work in the UK, something which those working at this level point out must be avoided to prevent distinctly negative impacts upon the protection of community health (Ogden, 2021).

7.3 The Response of the UK Government to COVID-19

It is now well documented that the COVID-19 policies adopted by the UK central government spectacularly failed to contain the spread of the virus. At the time of writing, over 220,000 people have died from COVID-19 in the UK, which is the largest death toll in Europe and the 6th largest in the world (*Statistia*, 2023). To put this in context, this is greater than the entire population of the city of Newcastle. UK COVID-19 policies have breached fundamental rights, bred mistrust, and created difficulties for public health work in the future. The reasons for this failure can be summarized under three themes: policy responses were slow and hypocritical, policy responses were disorganized and lacked transparency, and policy responses were overly politicized. The following subsections expand upon these themes.

7.3.1 *Policy responses were slow and hypocritical*

At the start of the pandemic, the UK government decided not to impose a national lockdown, based on the justification that building "herd immunity" was a superior strategy. Although the government claimed the backing of scientific evidence, the evidence collected was largely based on mathematical models and did not reflect how the disease was actually progressing, thus providing a misleading picture of the necessity of a national lockdown (Bowsher *et al.*, 2020). Moreover, the government's claim that a lockdown would be ineffective because people would get tired of adhering to it — so-called behavioral fatigue — lacked a basis in behavioral science (Sibony, 2020; Mahase, 2020). When a lockdown was eventually imposed, nearly two weeks after most European countries, the level of social contact that had already occurred was the seed for an enormous first wave of disease. Even then, the government was reluctant to clearly communicate the obligatory nature of the lockdown, and the police were reluctant to use their enforcement powers (Cairney & Wellstead, 2021). The UK government was also slow to respond to high-profile breaches of the lockdown. Dominic Cummings, the then-senior advisor to Prime Minister Boris Johnson, drove several hundred kilometers to meet with family, yet was neither punished nor publicly rebuked by the government. Research subsequently showed that this undermined trust in the government and contributed to non-adherence to the lockdown (Fancourt, 2020). Boris Johnson also refused to remove Health Minister Matt Hancock from office after he admitted to kissing his aide in his parliamentary office during lockdown, judging his apology to be sufficient accountability. Scotland's Chief Medical Officer Dr. Catherine Calderwood was defended by Scottish First Minister Nicola Sturgeon, after she also traveled extensively during lockdown. Both were eventually pressured into resignation. Housing Minister Robert Jenrick was allowed to publicly defend his 150 mile round trip to deliver supplies to relatives and did not resign. The most damaging example of rule breaking was, however, the "Partygate" scandal. Parties were held within 10 Downing Street and attended by officials and ministers across government, including the Prime Minister and Chancellor. Both apologized, made excuses, and were eventually fined by the Metropolitan Police alongside over 100 others but only after the extent and nature of the parties had been kept secret for several months. Research now demonstrates that the series of poor judgments by UK politicians surrounding rule-breaking seriously eroded trust in government and undermined public health measures in later phases of the pandemic (Weinberg, 2022; Samuel *et al.*, 2022).

7.3.2 *Policy responses were disorganized and lacking in transparency*

Exercise Cygnus, conducted in 2016 to simulate government response to an influenza outbreak, concluded that the UK was not prepared to deal with a major pandemic (Pegg, 2020). However, the lessons of this exercise were not implemented. The reasons included the following: the culture of political decision-making in the UK, where a small number of decision-makers in central government are quite disconnected from the public health frontline; the lack of agility resulting from the devolution of health policy responsibility to individual UK nations (more on devolution in the following in relation to government communication) resulting in an inability to agree consistent plans across the UK; a neglect to invest sufficient resources and write concrete contingency plans with a resulting lack of capacity to exercise public health functions on a large scale; and a tendency toward overreliance on private providers and cronyism in public procurement (Pollock & Coles, 2021; Jones & Hameiri, 2022). Two of the most notable policy failings occurred in contact tracing and the procurement of personal protective equipment (PPE). These were failures generated by a lack of preparedness but also exacerbated by decisions made once that lack of preparedness had been revealed.

After scrapping the initial program of contact tracing very early in the pandemic without any published explanation, and without considering the role of local authorities (Pollock & Coles, 2021), the UK government created NHS Test and Trace (which was run by private companies and not the NHS) to organize COVID-19 testing and contact tracing. This system was an expensive failure, which did not test an adequate number of people or adequately trace their close contacts, the details of which were starkly revealed by the investigation performed by the House of Commons Committee of Public Accounts (2021). Moreover, the government scrapped their initial contact tracing program very early on. In fact, after the replacement central program — NHS Test and Trace — also failed to noticeably reduce disease levels, the UK's devolved administrations began operating their own contact tracing systems with far greater success, while the leaders of local authorities in England pressed unsuccessfully for greater contact tracing powers (Diamond & Laffin, 2022). The contact tracing debacle was fueled by the subcontracting of component services to private firms with connections to government but little expertise in public health service delivery. Despite the courts holding that the government's procurement of these services was unlawful (Dyer, 2021), the government was never truly held accountable for poor service delivery in several other aspects of its pandemic response (Diamond & Laffin, 2022) that stemmed from extensive cronyism in the procurement of these services (Sian & Smyth, 2022).

Another major organizational failure was the inability to procure sufficient PPE. In 2020, the UK was still in a transitional phase in the Brexit process — it was no longer a Member State but continued to be part of the EU single market and customs union, and to follow EU rules. As a result, the UK had the opportunity to take part in the EU's joint PPE procurement scheme. The government refused, in the belief that it could independently achieve the same purchasing goals (Glencross, 2020). While the EU scheme was far from perfect (for instance, in relation to the time delays involved), it afforded Member States the purchasing power to secure sufficient PPE stock at a lower cost than could be achieved through independent purchasing (McEvoy & Ferri, 2020). The UK by contrast had to engage its own extremely underprepared health procurement system — NHS Supply Chain — which predictably could not cope with the demand for PPE (Sanchez-Graells, 2021). This meant that a number of frontline public servants confronted the COVID-19 pandemic without appropriate PPE — not only NHS staff (Hoernke, 2021) but also the police force (de Camargo, 2022) and social care workers (Rajan et al., 2020), for example.

The way in which the UK government sought scientific advice to guide its COVID-19 policies was also disorganized and lacking in transparency and, in particular, the way in which the government relied upon the Scientific Advisory Group for Emergencies (SAGE). A core group of SAGE insiders were usually consulted on pandemic policies, to the exclusion of other sources of scientific advice (Cairney, 2021b). It is now widely known that SAGE did not offer independent advice but answered the questions that the government sent them (Thacker, 2020). Moreover, some SAGE members both produced the science and were responsible for communicating it to the government within the political frame in which it was requested (Pearce, 2020). As a result, SAGE's policy advice was not always scientifically objective, a situation that prompted the creation of several expert groups, such as "Independent SAGE", which published alternative public health advice. The perception of a lack of independence was not helped by the fact that some SAGE members potentially had financial conflicts of interest over the awarding of public health services contracts to private companies (Thacker, 2020). Nor was it helped by the decision to keep the membership and meeting minutes secret for a long time (Freedman, 2020). Of course, the UK was far from unique in conflating science with politics during the pandemic. However, unlike in most other countries, UK government ministers began to publicly downplay the seriousness of the scientific advice they received from SAGE as the pandemic wore on, when they started disliking the answers to the questions they asked (Hodges et al., 2022). This had the effect of both shattering the previous rhetoric of "following the science" and further undermining trust in both SAGE and the government.

7.3.3 *Communication of policy was overly politicized*

The UK government's public communication strategy during the COVID-19 pandemic was orchestrated and delivered by politicians who were preoccupied with the perception of their policies. Boris Johnson's government never escaped "campaign mode" after the Brexit referendum and general election and has relied upon rhetoric to persuade the population to buy into its approach to COVID-19 policy (Lilleker & Stoeckle, 2021). Indeed, the wartime rhetorical theme has consistently characterized government communication, partly to justify authoritarian leadership and partly to divert attention away from government ineptitude (Spyridonidis, 2022). The public were usually informed of rules and policies by the Prime Minister or Secretary of State for Health in a press briefing, with core members of SAGE in attendance to add scientific credibility. This contrasts sharply with the approach in other countries. In Ireland, for example, rules were usually communicated by the government's scientific advisors, who appeared alone in press briefings, with government ministers only stepping in to communicate key changes in policy direction (Colfer, 2020).

The substance of government communications demonstrated a lack of appreciation for how people behaviorally react to information, was undermined by deteriorating credibility of the source of information (i.e. the government or its advisors), and was inconsistent or vague in terms of its substance (Dagnall *et al.*, 2020). However, not only was communication poorly executed, but it was also deliberately misleading. The government never publicly admitted to any mistakes, either in terms of its policy substance or policy communication (Sanders, 2020). Communications were commonly employed to construct a "truth" about the spread of the virus that diverted attention away from policy mistakes (Sim & Tombs, 2022), and sometimes the government even communicated false information when it was faced with particularly embarrassing mistakes (Newton, 2020). A majority of the UK population unsurprisingly perceived government communications to be low in honesty, credibility, and empathy

(Abrams *et al.*, 2021). This lack of trust may well have translated into a certain level of non-adherence to the rules. It certainly meant that the population sourced much of their information on COVID-19 from the media (Newton, 2020), who added detail and critical commentary to the vagueness of many government messages, particularly in relation to pandemic statistics (Lawson & Lugo-Ocando, 2022).

Communication of COVID-19 policies in the UK was also complicated by devolution. The UK devolves many government functions to administrations in Scotland, Wales, and Northern Ireland. Health policy is devolved, but other powers relevant to tackling COVID-19, such as those concerning economic policy and border policy, are reserved to the central government. Moreover, since there is no devolved administration in England, the central government makes health policy for England. Differences in policy choices between the devolved administrations and the central government caused some confusion for people in Scotland, Wales, and Northern Ireland as to their exact obligations, worsened by media reporting that was not sensitive to the nature of the devolved governments and which government had made which announcement (Cushion *et al.*, 2020).

7.3.4 *Future challenges created by the legislative approach to COVID-19*

Some of the criticism leveled at the UK government's COVID-19 policy response was naïve and perhaps unfair in light of the difficulties inherent in policymaking under conditions of uncertainty (Cairney, 2021a). Some interventions — particularly the economic supports for those who lost their jobs (Brewer & Gardiner, 2020; Brewer & Tasseva, 2021) and the roll-out of the vaccine (Baraniuk, 2021) — achieved their objectives well. In particular, the UK's organization of vaccine trials exceeded that of the EU in terms of the reach and efficiency (Tani, 2022). It is entirely possible that these successes gave the UK government an inflated sense of their overall success in handling the pandemic. They certainly provided rhetorical ammunition that has been employed at every opportunity to defend the government's COVID-19 record.

The great majority of commentary on the UK government's COVID-19 policy has, however, fairly and accurately pointed out a startling lack of competence, which some have claimed amounts to human rights failings (Montel, 2020; Frowde *et al.*, 2020). The next major communicable disease outbreak must be handled radically differently. Heavy investment should be made in public health institutions and the health care system generally, and public health officials must be instructed to design concrete protocols for how public health services will be delivered under pressure. A clear and independent scientific advisory structure should be created, with clear protocols for how government ministers will seek policy advice. Policy communication must be detailed and transparent. Ministers should seek to collaborate with other states and international organizations as much as possible. Many of these failings and lessons are now being articulated in the wide-ranging public enquiry, led by Baroness Hallett, into the UK government's COVID-19 response.

Above all else, however, the legislative approach to the next public health emergency must be different. The doctrine of parliamentary sovereignty means that any element of the UK's public health legal framework can be altered by Parliament at any time. Moreover, this power is unconstrained by judicial review, which is limited to checking that procedures set out in legislation have been properly followed by public bodies. More recent developments in UK law will further reduce the possible scrutiny of changes to how public health is organized. The proposed Bill of Rights aims to substantially limit the influence of the European Court of Human Rights on UK law and has the effect of making it harder for individuals to bring rights-based claims to court (Law Society, 2022). Currently, the application of the European Convention of Human Rights is the only way to exercise a measure of judicial scrutiny over the adoption of public health legislation, such as through the application of Article 5 on liberty of the person to the Coronavirus Act 2020 (Pugh, 2020). Driven by the desire to remove all vestiges of Europe (whether related to the EU or not) from UK law, if the government is successful in getting the Bill of Rights bill enacted, legislation such as the Coronavirus Act 2020 will be all but untouchable. This manner of legislative power can of course be a powerful tool for public health — the ability to adopt effective public health law free from concern of legal challenge would certainly be useful where strong vested interests attempt to prevent such laws. However, such power could also be used to adopt ineffective, unethical, or rights-restrictive public health laws.

The Coronavirus Act 2020 (henceforth "the Act") is a good example of the latter use of power. The Act has been broadly criticized in the academic literature, which generally agrees that the use of a large government majority to quickly and without consultation adopt a piece of legislation that made sweeping and sometimes ineffective restrictions made a counterproductive contribution to the UK's COVID-19 response (Grez Hidalgo et al., 2020; Hickman et al., 2020). The Act did not only have implications in the short term but may have impacts that extend beyond the COVID-19 pandemic. Researchers have already explored the fact that the Act was problematic largely because of the mindset of legislators (Grez Hidalgo et al., 2020). The risk for UK public health is that this mindset will become entrenched through the influence of Brexit upon governance and that the Act sets a precedent for future public health legislating.

The lack of consultation is a particularly worrying precedent to set, as is the lack of any suitable monitoring or accountability mechanisms. Every piece of public health legislation should be built upon a foundation of stakeholder consultation and legislative monitoring, not only to ensure it is effective but also to ensure it meets ethical standards of transparency. The review mechanism added to the Act well after its adoption as a concession to critics was far from acceptable (Lock et al., 2021) and stood more as an illustration of the distain of the current government for accepted or "establishment" governance norms.

Moreover, the precedent of making certain public health rules through delegated legislation is also worrying. Delegated (or "secondary") legislation is made by government ministers through powers granted by Acts of Parliament ("primary" legislation). Delegated legislation is not debated or voted on in the same way that primary legislation is and is usually employed for articulating details of policies which have been democratically debated and enacted through primary legislation. In principle, the use of delegated legislation in public health policy is a useful way of flexibly adding details to a general legal framework, especially to accommodate changes in the evidence base. However, such delegated legislation should not create new restrictions or offenses, as the Act provided powers to do. It is arguable that an extraordinary public health situation demands an extraordinary response — however, since it is difficult to define when a public health threat becomes an emergency, emergency public health legislation should be designed with caution to guard against the imposition of unwarranted strong restrictions. Such design might include the circumspect allocation of delegated powers that would allow government ministers to impose restrictions with limited oversight. The fact that the UK government retained the delegated emergency public health powers given by the Act long after the plausible existence of a state of public health emergency was therefore highly concerning (Grogan, 2020). Parliament should in the future take note that there are ways of enacting emergency public health legislation which limit the potential abuse of emergency powers (Cormacain, 2020).

7.4 Post-COVID Public Health Reform in the UK in the Context of Brexit

Pandemics open a policy window (Kingdon, 1984): weaknesses inherent in public health and health care services crystallize clearly and stakeholders are mobilized, while policymakers have both the political opportunity to address these weaknesses as well as an understanding of possible solutions (Amri & Logan, 2021; Auener *et al.*, 2020; Mintrom & True, 2022; Harris & McCue, 2022). Policy windows opened by pandemics ideally facilitate great leaps in public health policy and will be seized when stakeholders are willing to engage in multilevel, multisectoral collaboration while paying close attention to the scientific evidence base. Most public health issues are too complex in both their causes and their impact for one actor to solve alone. While not resulting from a pandemic, the adoption of the Framework Convention on Tobacco Control is a good example of a public health policy window being seized. A new Director General of the World Health Organization, for whom tobacco control was a priority, drove a highly motivated international coalition of stakeholders, who together mobilized the accumulating evidence on both smoking harm and the practices of the tobacco industry to achieve global political consensus on strengthened tobacco control. At the national level, the adoption of the Public Health (Alcohol) Act 2018 in Ireland is another example of a policy window being seized. This major piece of public health legislation was possibly due to the convergence of increased public attention on the problem of alcohol-related harm in Ireland, institutional developments, and increasing political pressure, which opened a policy window that was capitalized upon by political leaders who were personally committed to reducing alcohol-related harm (Lesch & McCambridge, 2021).

The ongoing Brexit project will largely prevent the UK from capitalizing on the policy window opened by the COVID-19 pandemic. Now that the emergency phase of the pandemic is over, Brexit-related issues have reasserted themselves. The UK is no longer an EU Member State, but the work to replace or change the policies and institutions that the UK participated in or benefited from during its membership will continue for some time, as will the efforts to plug the gaps left by the hastily negotiated Trade and Cooperation Agreement. With respect to health policy in particular, the agreement does not come close to replicating the benefits of EU membership. Moreover, it is clear that the changes to the UK's approach to governance brought about by the Brexit project will persist. Governance in the UK has become more nationalist, more centralized, and more populist, which will make it harder to engage in the multilevel, multisectoral collaboration and evidence-based policymaking that is necessary for meaningful public health reform.

7.4.1 *Brexit has caused practical distractions for health policymakers*

Some have argued that the pandemic will shock the UK out of the turbulent and tribal politics of Brexit (Leonard, 2020). Two changes in Prime Minister and three changes in Chancellor within a few months of Boris Johnson being ousted as Prime Minister by his own MPs suggests that UK politics is still turbulent. The substance of Liz Truss' successful campaign to replace Boris Johnson as Prime Minister — radical conservatism, reassertion of nationalist and isolationist ideas, and the not-so-subtle suggestion that Boris Johnson had been "stabbed in the back" — suggests that UK politics is also still tribal. So too do the multiple threatened rebellions by a group of MPs on the Conservative right against Rishi Sunak's flagship policy to send migrants crossing the English Channel in small boats to Rwanda, on the basis that the implementing legislation was not extreme enough. Experiences from elsewhere demonstrate that political instability will not provide the conditions in which effective public health reform can be easily achieved (Hamdan *et al.*, 2003; Edwards *et al.*, 2022; Wise & Darmstadt, 2016). While the political instability prevailing in the UK is not the result of conflict or deep corruption, it is similarly a departure from a state of predictable and reliable governance. In such circumstances, it is difficult to generate the political will to engage in reform projects that are complex, multisector, and long-term (Cohen, 2022), which is certainly true for the reforms that UK healthcare and public health structures require after COVID-19.

The obsession with "taking advantage of the freedoms of Brexit" has distracted policymakers from thinking about public health reform issues logically. Indeed, it was reported that the goals which the government set for PHE in spring 2019 were topped by Brexit and did not even include pandemic preparedness (Vize, 2020). It has also created the unnecessary task of reinventing public health protections that were provided by EU membership. In early 2022, the government published a report called *The Benefits of Brexit*, which alleges that the government can now do more in tobacco, alcohol, and obesity policy than it could while an EU Member State. On the contrary, EU tobacco policy is already very advanced, and Member States can adopt strong alcohol control and obesity prevention policies under EU law, even though the EU's own alcohol and obesity policy is not extensive. In some respects the UK was already going beyond the EU's efforts on alcohol and obesity while a Member State. The report also discusses the UK's Global Health Insurance Card (GHIC), a new initiative to replace the protections once offered by the European Health Insurance Card (EHIC). Since most UK citizens obtaining healthcare abroad would do so within the EU, the GHIC seems to be a lesser replacement for the EHIC, something which is underlined by the fact that the UK has felt the need to trademark and "market" the GHIC, which is not yet accepted in many countries outside the EU. The efforts to better or replace public health policies that already existed while an EU Member State are diverting the UK government's health policy capacity away from improving the UK's deficient communicable disease preparedness. The report says nothing about the fact that the UK government must also now develop regulatory functions once performed by EU agencies, such as the European Centre for Disease Control, European Medicines Agency, and European Food Safety Authority.

The pursuit of Brexit has also resulted in the removal of established health protections in a number of areas. Food safety standards have been relaxed to facilitate trade deals with other countries that have weaker standards. Occupational health and safety standards in the haulage industry have been relaxed in an effort to reverse the workforce losses caused by Brexit. There will likely be more regression in the health protection enjoyed by UK citizens in the coming years, including in the area of communicable disease protection. At a time when the UK government should be thinking of how to improve communicable disease policy, the pressures of Brexit may well force a reversal of some of these protections.

Finally, it is now evident that Brexit has directly contributed to the cost-of-living and economic crises (Middleton, 2022), which cannot be a positive development for health policy. Research conducted by the Centre for European Reform has found that the UK's Gross Domestic Product at the end of 2021 was 5.2% smaller than a modeled UK that never left the EU, which equates to £31bn in lost GDP (Springford, 2022). Of course it is impossible to say with certainty how much of this, if any, would or could have been spent on improving healthcare and public health services. However, if the proportion of UK GDP that was spent on health in 2021 — 11.9% — is applied to the figure of £31bn, then it is at least plausible to suggest that £3.7bn could have been spent on health but now cannot.

7.4.2   Brexit has caused a governance ideology not conducive to public health reform

As Jarman and colleagues explain, the absence of a written constitution and a dominant executive permits "constitutional casualism" in the UK (Jarman *et al.*, 2020). To enable the pursuit of a hard Brexit, Boris Johnson's government altered several of the prevailing characteristics of UK governance. These alterations will be difficult to undo while British politics remains tribal and turbulent.

Power was consolidated within the central government and in particular in the Prime Minister's Office. This facilitated several policy decisions on COVID-19 that were not only bad COVID-19 policy but which may have lasting implications upon the capacity for public health reform in the UK. The response to the failed contact tracing program was to unilaterally abolish PHE, which was responsible for public health delivery in England, and replace it with two other bodies. These — the UKHSA and the OHID — are less independent than PHE and were designed in haste without adequate consultation. It is clear to all observers that the abolition of PHE was an uninformed scapegoating exercise that would have been unimaginable before the Brexit-driven centralization of power. The new institutions will need time to establish their identities and methods of working. This will evidently prevent them from focusing as fully as possible on efforts to improve the UK's communicable disease preparedness.

Government decision-making also became populist. Several COVID-19 policy decisions were taken because they appealed to the sentiments of many within the population but were simply contrary to the weight of evidence. An excellent example is the Eat Out to Help Out scheme, spearheaded by Chancellor Rishi Sunak. This scheme subsidized restaurant bills as part of a strategy to move quickly away from the unpopular lockdown when COVID-19 cases declined in the summer of 2020, using policies that boosted public mood and injected cash into the hospitality sector (Bale, 2023). However, the scheme predictably led to a significant number of new COVID-19 cases (Fetzer, 2022). Its economic impact was marginal and short lived (González-Pampillón *et al.*, 2022), and it also had the effect of widening social inequality (Power *et al.*, 2020).

The greater impact though of Brexit-inspired populism will be the weakening of public health reform capacity. To counter the market-crashing impact of Liz Truss's 2022 mini-budget of unfunded tax cuts and energy subsidies, as well as the larger deficit in public finances exacerbated by the impact of Brexit, Chancellor Jeremy Hunt declared that all government departments would have to find significant cost savings. This inevitably means a reduction in health spending, at a time when governments should be increasing health spending to increase the resilience and capacity of the public health and healthcare systems.

The UK government's shift toward populism has also shifted it away from evidence-based policymaking. While an exclusive focus on science will lead to public health policy that is insensitive to often equally important competing policy imperatives (Bylund & Packard, 2021), public health policy should be firmly based in scientific evidence, especially during a public health emergency. While Boris Johnson's government declared (at least initially) that they were "following the science", in reality they often ignored expert advice, especially if the advice was perceived to come from "the establishment". During the pandemic, this resulted in some poor policy choices. At the start of the pandemic, the government ignored the early evidence from other jurisdictions about the spread of the virus, and the resulting delay in introducing lockdown led to an enormous first wave of disease. The government also ignored advice from SAGE in September 2020 to impose a short lockdown and revise the existing tiered system of restrictions. The justification was that "science was divided" and a "balanced judgement" was required — a thinly veiled statement that "following the science" was now less important than keeping the population on side (Wardman, 2020). The result was a heavy second wave of disease. The government's public distain for expert advice could be even more harmful though in the long term. Research has found that areas of the UK that voted most heavily for Brexit tended to suffer the heaviest death rates from COVID-19, suggesting that embracing the populist narrative of Brexit encouraged a rejection of advice from the public health authorities (Phalippou & Wu, 2023). This is particularly concerning because these areas of heaviest death rates also tended to be the more socioeconomically deprived parts of the UK. The implication from this research is that promoting a rejection of "establishment" advice will have the effect of widening health inequities, which are already wide in the UK.

The UK government has also turned toward isolationist policies and was particularly keen to avoid the perception that it relied upon external powers in its COVID-19 response. This led to the government ignoring the data from other countries that experienced high rates of infection before the UK, ignoring WHO advice to implement a solid test and trace system, and refusing to join the EU's PPE procurement scheme. It also led to rushed regulatory approval for the Oxford-AstraZenica COVID-19 vaccine, a decision that provided a short-lived opportunity to proclaim a British-made success story, but ultimately resulted in a series of medical and political controversies that led to the vaccine being used far less in the UK than was intended (Walsh, 2022). The greatest impact of Brexit-induced isolationism will be felt in the longer term. The overriding lesson of the COVID-19 pandemic was that international collaboration is essential to managing a disease spreading freely across national borders. Of course, the UK government was part of a group of nations which spearheaded the initiation of discussions for a new global pandemic preparedness treaty (WHO, 2023). However, the UK's new isolationist approach will work against efforts to learn that collaborative lesson. The declining attractiveness of the UK as a destination for non-British health care professionals, who do not feel welcome within the country (Milner *et al.*, 2021), will prevent the UK from attracting the best overseas talent. Taking an even wider view, the UK is now disconnected from EU research institutions and organizations, and the increased difficulty in accessing UK research in health will weaken the overall ability of Europe to respond to public health threats in the future (Hervey *et al.*, 2021). Given the cross-border nature of communicable disease threats, this will also put the UK in a weaker position.

7.4.3 *Post-Brexit options for public health reform*

It is clear that uncertainties created by the upheaval to legal frameworks following Brexit were detrimental to the UK's COVID-19 response specifically (Dayan, 2020) and will be detrimental to future public health work in general (Dayan *et al.*, 2020). It is furthermore clear that leaving the EU single market will reduce the government's economic power, which will make it even harder to take the (expensive) action necessary to reduce the UK's widening health inequalities (McCarey, 2021). Moreover, it is clear that Brexit will not just affect UK public health policy directly but will have indirect impacts through weakening public health capacity outside the UK (Hervey *et al.*, 2021).

What is now crucial for the public health community, including researchers of public health law, to address, is how the development of public health policy in the UK as a non-EU Member State can best improve the protection of public health. The public health community in the UK began considering these issues immediately after the Brexit referendum (Middleton & Weiss, 2016), and leading figures in UK public health called then for Brexit to represent an opportunity to evolve and improve the UK's public health work (Crisp *et al.*, 2016). In particular, attention focused on headline policies that the UK would have to redevelop post-Brexit, such as its trade policy: the Faculty of Public Health released its own vision of a "healthy" trade policy for the UK (Faculty of Public Health, 2019), as have various researchers (Freund & Springmann, 2021; van Schalkwyk *et al.*, 2021).

However, nobody who is experienced in the public health field has called for a wholesale reinvention of the public health protections that have developed in the UK throughout its decades as an EU Member State. As explored in the section earlier, this is precisely what the UK government seems determined to do. Some of the options proposed as necessitated by Brexit, such as the UK Global Health Insurance Card, are a waste of time and resource that could have been spent advancing public health protections rather than replacing ones that UK nationals already enjoyed when they were EU citizens. Some of the proposed options, such as changes to food safety standards (Merrick, 2022), may lower the levels of public health protection that the UK population enjoyed while the UK was a Member State and obliged to implement EU food safety standards. This is all the more concerning given reports that the UK Food Safety Authority are not close to being ready to replace EU law with UK alternatives that will protect health to the same level (Gonçalves, 2023). Moreover, it is clear that the much touted regulatory agility that Brexit would allegedly bring has largely not resulted in better public health outcomes for the UK, and indeed the withdrawal of the UK from EU regulatory bodies may leave the UK dangerously exposed in some respects. For example, the UKHSA has not replicated the capacity of the European Centre for Disease Control to provide early warning of further novel infectious diseases and likely never will (Solomon, 2019; Topping, 2020). Moreover, the Medicines and Healthcare products Regulatory Agency has not been able to approve as many new medicines as the European Medicines Agency (McCarey, 2022). On the other hand, some of the options proposed, such as stronger legislation to tackle obesity, will increase levels of public health protection. However, strong non-communicable disease policies have always been possible within the limits of EU law (Alemanno & Garde, 2015) — leaving the EU will not change this. Another such proposal is the extension of alcohol minimum unit pricing to the rest of the UK, following its adoption in Scotland (Middleton & Weiss, 2016). However, this is something that was prevented in England by intensive alcohol industry lobbying, not the application of EU law.

Brexit does not completely wreck the prospects for public health development in the UK. Although it will be very difficult to conceive of a novel UK institution or process that could improve upon the protections enjoyed as an EU Member State, there are several options open to the UK government to maintain cooperation with EU institutions and agencies, thus preserving an existing level of health protection. One of the most important is the deal to secure access for UK researchers to the EU's Horizon research funding program. The importance of properly funding public health research was starkly illustrated during the COVID-19 pandemic — the development of safe and effective vaccines would have been impossible without significant investment in research. The UK has thankfully taken the opportunity to maintain access to the multibillion euro Horizon funding program. This is welcome, after the protracted and destabilizing brinkmanship the UK employed during negotiations (Sample, 2023). It would be impossible for the UK to replicate the hugely significant level of funding which UK-based researchers have traditionally won from the Horizon program, and the loss of this funding would undoubtedly damage the ability of UK researchers to advance the frontiers of public health knowledge in the manner for which they have until now been renowned. Even now the deal is closed, the damage may already have been done (Sample, 2023), with the collapse in research funding from Europe to the UK in the aftermath of Brexit driving many leading researchers from the UK and eroding trust in the government's ability to secure the future of the UK research industry. Indeed, comments by the UK's Secretary of State for Science to the effect that the UK can do without EU research funding have been rightly called out as shortsighted and dangerous (Nature Editors, 2023).

Whatever proposals are taken forward, the post-Brexit public health landscape in the UK will present challenges for their successful implementation. For example, the proliferation of bodies, organizations, and stakeholders that have claimed input into post-Brexit public health decision-making, such as the Brexit Health Alliance and the UK Alliance for International Health Policy (NHS Confederation, 2023), will risk making the decision-making process more convoluted. Stakeholder input into decision-making is of course essential for effective and legitimate public health work, and certainly a plurality of suggestions for post-Brexit public health development should be seen as positive. However, a greater range of visions inevitably means that deciding upon the most appropriate will become a more complex and even more politicized task. Moreover, the politics of the Brexit campaign has more generally eroded trust in UK institutions and in the politicians which design and run them. Any significant institutional or system reform requires buy-in not just from stakeholders but also from the general public.

7.5 Conclusion

It is somewhat difficult to draw useful conclusions for the future of public health in the UK when the political landscape is still quite volatile. The latest Prime Minister at the time of writing, Rishi Sunak, appears to have brought some stability to the top of UK politics, although this has not necessarily watered down the shift toward populist governance. With a change in government to the Labour Party, many of the concerns relating to populist policymaking may diminish, although the practical legacy of both Brexit and the disastrous pandemic response will remain. It is difficult to draw inspiration from elsewhere — the context of the UK's entry and exit from the COVID-19 pandemic was uniquely conditioned by Brexit, and the UK government has for a while been in the position of having to make unprecedented decision after unprecedented decision. However, there are some reasons for optimism. The UK public health community of practitioners, academics, and political leaders is resilient and outward-looking — this community will continue to provide a critical appraisal of government policy and will continue to work to understand the implications of doing public health work in post-COVID-19 and post-Brexit Britain.

References

Abrams, D., *et al.* (2021). *Public Perceptions of UK and Local Government Communication about COVID-19.* Manchester: Belong Network. https://www.belongnetwork.co.uk/wp-content/uploads/2021/08/Belong_Public Perceptions_paper_V5.pdf.

Alemanno, A. and Garde, A. (2015). *Regulating Lifestyle Risks: The EU, Alcohol, Tobacco and Unhealthy Diets.* Cambridge: Cambridge University Press.

Amri, M. and Logan, D. (2021). Policy responses to COVID-19 present a window of opportunity for a paradigm shift in global health policy: An application of the multiple streams framework as a heuristic. *Global Public Health, 16*(8–9), 1187–1197.

Association of Directors of Public Health (2021). *Statement: Responding to the launch of the Office for Health Promotion.* London: Association of Directors of Public Health. https://www.adph.org.uk/2021/03/statement-responding-to-the-launch-of-the-office-for-health-promotion/.

Auener, S., *et al.* (2020). COVID-19: A window of opportunity for positive healthcare reforms. *International Journal of Health Policy and Management, 9*(10), 419–422.

Bale, T. (2023). Populists and the pandemic: How populists around the world responded to COVID-19. In N. Ringe and L. Rennó (Eds.), *The United Kingdom: The Pandemic and the Tale of Two Populist Parties* (pp. 68–78). Oxon: Routledge.

Baraniuk, C. (2021). Covid-19: How the UK vaccine rollout delivered success, so far. *BMJ, 372,* n421.

Bonner, A. (ed.). (2020). *Local Authorities and the Social Determinants of Health.* Oxford: Oxford University Press.

Bowsher, G., *et al.* (2020). A health intelligence framework for pandemic response: Lessons from the UK experience of COVID-19. *Health Security, 435,* 435–443.

Brewer, M. and Gardiner, L. (2020). The initial impact of COVID-19 and policy responses on household incomes. *Oxford Review of Economic Policy, 36*(S1), 187–199.

Brewer, M. and Tasseva, I. (2021). Did the UK policy response to Covid-19 protect household incomes? *Journal Econ Inequal, 19,* 433–458.

Buck, D., *et al.,* (2018). *A Vision for Population Health: Towards a Healthier Future* London: Kings Fund.

Buck, D. (2021). A qualified success: A personal reflection on the passing of Public Health England. *kingsfund.org.uk,* 5 August.

Buck, D. (2022). The office for health improvement and disparities: One year on. *kingsfund.org.uk.* 13 October.

Bylund, P. and Packard, M. (2021). Separation of power and expertise: Evidence of the tyranny of experts in Sweden's COVID-19 responses. *Southern Economic Journal, 87*(4), 1300–1319.

Cairney, P. (2021a). The UK government's COVID-19 policy: Assessing evidence-informed policy analysis in real time. *British Politics, 16*, 90–116.

Cairney, P. (2021b). The UK government's COVID-19 policy: What does "guided by the science" mean in practice? *Frontiers in Political Science, 3.* doi.org/10.3389/fpos.2021.624068.

Cairney, P. and Wellstead, A. (2021). COVID-19: Effective policymaking depends on trust in experts, politicians, and the public. *PDP, 4*(1). doi.org/10.1080/25741292.2020.1837466.

Cameron-Blake, E., *et al.* (2020). Variation in the response to COVID-19 across the four nations of the United Kingdom. BSG Working Paper Series, No. 35.

Cohen, N. (2022). Public administration reform and political will in cases of political instability: Insights from the Israeli experience. *Public Policy Administration,* doi.org/10.1177/09520767221076059.

Colfer, B. (2020). Herd-immunity across intangible borders: Public policy responses to COVID-19 in Ireland and the UK. *European Policy Analysis, 6*, 203–225.

Cormacain, R. (2020). Keeping Covid-19 emergency legislation socially distant from ordinary legislation: Principles for the structure of emergency legislation. *Theory and Practice of Legislation, 8*(3), 245–265.

Crisp, N. *et al.* (2016). Manifesto for a healthy and health-creating society. *Lancet, 388*(10062), E24–E27.

Cushion, S., *et al.* (2020). Different lockdown dules in the four nations are confusing the public. *LSE COVID 19 Blog,* 22 May.

Dagnall, N., *et al.* (2020). Bridging the gap between UK government strategic narratives and public opinion/behavior: Lessons from COVID-19. *Frontiers in Communication, 5,* doi.org/10.3389/fcomm.2020.00071.

Dayan, M. (2020). *How Will Brexit Affect the UK's Response to Coronavirus?* London: Nuffield Trust.

Dayan, M., *et al.* (2020). *Understanding the Impact of Brexit on Health in the UK.* London: Nuffield Trust.

Dean, H., *et al.* (2013). From theory to action: Applying social determinants of health to public health practice. *Public Health Reports, 128*(Suppl 3), 1–4.

de Camargo, C. (2022). The postcode lottery of safety: COVID-19 guidance and shortages of personal protective equipment (PPE) for UK police officers. *Police Journal, 95*(3), 537–561.

Diamond, P. and Laffin, M. (2022). The United Kingdom and the pandemic: Problems of central control and coordination. *Local Government Studies, 48*(2), 211–231.

Dyer, C. (2021). Covid-19: Hancock's failure to publish contracts was unlawful. *BMJ, 372*(n511). DOI: 10.1136/bmj.n511.

Edwards, L., *et al.* (2022). An assessment of the Libyan baccalaureate nursing education during political turmoil. *Public Health Nursing, 39*(4), 831–838.

Faculty of Public Health (2019). *Negotiating a 'Healthy' Trade Policy for the UK.* London: Faculty of Public Health.

Fancourt, D. (2020). The Cummings effect: Politics, trust, and behaviours during the COVID-19 pandemic. *Lancet, 396*(10249), 464–465.

Fetzer, T. (2022). Subsidising the spread of COVID-19: Evidence from the UK'S eat-out-to-help-out scheme. *The Economic Journal, 132*(643), 1200–1217.

Freedman, L. (2020). Scientific advice at a time of emergency. SAGE and Covid-19. *The Political Quarterly, 91*(3), 514–522.

Freund, F. and Springmann, M. (2021). Policy analysis indicates health-sensitive trade and subsidy reforms are needed in the UK to avoid adverse dietary health impacts post-Brexit. *Nature Food, 2*(7), 502–508.

Frowde, R., *et al.* (2020). Fail to prepare and you prepare to fail: The human rights consequences of the UK government's inaction during the COVID-19 pandemic. *Asian Bioethics Review, 12*(4), 459–480.

Glencross, A. (2020). The importance of health security in post-Brexit EU-UK relations. *European View, 19*(2), 172–179.

Gonçalves, M. (2023). Food safety at 'huge risk' as EU laws set to expire. *thegrocer.co.uk,* 3 February.

González-Pampillón, N., *et al.* (2022). The economic impacts of the UK's eat out to help out scheme. *Centre for Economic Performance Discussion Paper,* No. 1865.

Grez Hidalgo, P., *et al.* (2020). Parliament, the pandemic, and constitutional principle in the United Kingdom: A study of the coronavirus Act 2020. *MLR, 85*(6), 1463–1503.

Grogan, J. (2020). Parliament still does not have the power to scrutinise the Coronavirus Act 2020 properly. *blogs.lse.ac.uk,* 30 October.

Hamdan, M., *et al.* (2003). Organizing health care within political turmoil: The Palestinian case. *The International Journal of Health Planning and Management, 18*(1), 63–87.

Harris, M. and McCue, P. (2022). How a COVID-19 "policy window" changed the relationship between urban planning, transport, and health in Sydney, Australia. *JAPA, 89*, 240–252.

Hervey, T., *et al.* (2021). Health "Brexternalities": The Brexit effect on health and health care outside the United Kingdom. *Journal of Health Politics, Policy and Law*, *46*(1), 177–203.

Hickman, T., *et al.* (2020). Coronavirus and civil liberties in the UK. *Judicial Review*, *25*(2), 151–170.

Hill, J. (2022). UKHSA job cuts could leave UK 'seriously exposed' to health threats. *lgcplus.com*, 27 April.

Hodges, R. *et al.* (2022). The role of scientific expertise in COVID-19 policy-making: Evidence from four European Countries. *Public Organization Review*, *22*(2), 249–267.

Hoernke, K. (2021). Frontline healthcare workers' experiences with personal protective equipment during the COVID-19 pandemic in the UK: A rapid qualitative appraisal. *BMJ Open*, *11*(1), e046199.

House of Commons Committee of Public Accounts (October 27, 2021). Twenty-third report of session 2021–22, test and trace update (HC 182). London.

Hunter, D. *et al.* (2022). Reforming the public health system in England. *Lancet Public Health*, *7*, e797.

Jarman, H. *et al.* (2020). Brexit is just a symptom: The constitutional weaknesses it reveals have serious consequences for health. *Journal of Public Health*, *42*(4), 778–783.

Jones, L. and Hameiri, S. (2022). COVID-19 and the failure of the neoliberal regulatory state. *RIPE*, *29*(4), 1027–1052.

Kenny, M. and Kelsey, T. (2020). Devolution or delegation? What the revolt of the metro mayors over lockdown tells us about English devolution. *blogs.lse.ac.uk*, 12 November.

Kingdon, J. (1984). *Agendas, Alternatives, and Public Policies.* Boston: Little, Brown.

Law Society (2022). Human rights act reforms and the Bill of rights Bill. *lawsociety.org.uk*, 8 November.

Lawson, B. and Lugo-Ocando, J. (2022). Political communication, press coverage and public interpretation of public health statistics during the coronavirus pandemic in the UK. *European Journal of Communication*, *37*(6), 646–662.

Leonard, M. (2020). *The Brexit Parenthesis: Three Ways the Pandemic is Changing UK Politics.* London: European Council on Foreign Relations.

Lesch, M. and McCambridge, J. (2021). Waiting for the wave: Political leadership, policy windows, and alcohol policy change in Ireland. *Social Science & Medicine*, *282*, 114116.

Lilleker, D. and Stoeckle, T. (2021). The challenges of providing certainty in the face of wicked problems: Analysing the UK government's handling of the COVID-19 pandemic. *Journal of Public Affairs*, *21*(4), e2733.

Littlejohns, P., *et al.* (2022). *Lessons from the Demise of Public Health England: Where Next for UK Public Health?* London: National Institute for Health and Care Research.

Lock, D., *et al.* (2021). Parliament's one-year review of the Coronavirus Act 2020: Another example of parliament's marginalisation in the Covid-19 pandemic. *The Political Quarterly*, *92*(4), 699–706.

Mahase, E. (2020). Covid-19: Was the decision to delay the UK's lockdown over fears of "behavioural fatigue" based on evidence? *BMJ*, *370*, m3166.

Marmot, M., *et al.* (2020). *Health Equity in England: The Marmot Review 10 Years on.* London: The Health Foundation.

Marsden, G. and Docherty, I. (2021). Mega-disruptions and policy change: Lessons from the mobility sector in response to the Covid-19 pandemic in the UK. *Transp Policy*, *110*, 86–97.

McCarey, M. (2021). A real risk that Brexit will damage public health. *blogs.bmj.com*, 1 June.

McCarey, M. (2022). *Health and Brexit: Six Years on.* London: Nuffield Trust.

McEvoy, E. and Ferri, D. (2020). The role of the joint procurement agreement during the COVID-19 pandemic: Assessing its usefulness and discussing its potential to support a European Health Union. *EJRR*, *11*(4), 851–863.

Merrick, R. (2022). Food safety and hygiene standards 'in danger' from tearing up of EU law, experts warn. *independent.co.uk*, 8 October.

Middleton, J. (2017). Public health in England in 2016 — The health of the public and the public health system: A review. *British Medical Bulletin*, *121*(1), 31–46.

Middleton, J. (2022). President's summer message July 2022: Brexit is bad for your health. *aspher.org*, 1 August.

Middleton, J. and Weiss, M. (2016). Still holding on: Public health in the UK after Brexit. *Eurohealth*, *22*(4), 33–36.

Milner, A., *et al.* (2021). Brexit and European doctors' decisions to leave the United Kingdom: A qualitative analysis of free-text questionnaire comments. *BMC Health Services Research*, *21*(1). DOI: 10.1186/s12913-021-06201-0.

Mintrom, M. and True, J. (2022). COVID-19 as a policy window: Policy entrepreneurs responding to violence against women. *Policy and Society*, *41*(1), 143–154.

Monbiot, G. (2020). Tory privatisation is at the heart of the UK's disastrous coronavirus response. *theguardian.com*, 27 May.

Montel, L., *et al.* (2020). The right to health in times of pandemic: What can we learn from the UK's response to the COVID-19 outbreak? *Health and Human Rights*, *22*(2), 227–241.

Nature Editors (2023). UK, please drop the rhetoric and fight for collaboration with Europe. *Nature*, *614*(7948), 390.

Newton, K. (2020). Government communications, political trust and compliant social behaviour: The politics of Covid-19 in Britain. *The Political Quarterly*, *91*(3), 502–513.

NHS Confederation (2023). The UK alliance for international health policy. *nhsconfed.org*.

Ogden, P. (2021). A 'local first' public health system. *local.gov.uk*, 24 February.

Oliver, D. (2021). Renaming government agencies won't improve population health. *BMJ*, *373*, n1004.

Ortenzi, F., *et al.* (2022). Whole of government and whole of society approaches: Call for further research to improve population health and health equity. *BMJ Global Health*, *7*(7), e009972.

Pearce, W. (2020). Trouble in the trough: How uncertainties were downplayed in the UK's science advice on Covid-19. *Humanities and Social Sciences*, *7*. doi.org/10.1057/s41599-020-00612-w.

Pegg, D. (2020). What was exercise Cygnus and what did it find? *theguardian.com*, 7 May.

Phalippou, L. and Wu, B. (2023). The association between the proportion of Brexiters and COVID-19 death rates in England. *Social Science & Medicine*, 323. DOI: 10.1016/j.socscimed.2023.115826.

Pollock, K. and Coles, E. (2021). Mind the gap: From recommendation to practice in crisis management. Exploring the gap between the "lessons identified" during exercise cygnus and the UK government response to COVID-19. *Journal of Emergency Management*, *19*(7), 133–149.

Power, M., *et al.* (2020). COVID-19 and low-income families: Why the Chancellor's 'Eat Out to Help Out' offer is hard to stomach. *British Politics and Policy at LSE Blog*, 10 July.

Pugh, J. (2020). The United Kingdom's Coronavirus Act, deprivations of liberty, and the right to liberty and security of the person. *Journal of Law and the Biosciences*, *7*(1). DOI: 10.1093/jlb/lsaa011.

Rajan, S., *et al.* (2020). Did the UK government really throw a protective ring around care homes in the COVID-19 pandemic? *Journal of Long-Term Care*, 185–195.

Ralston, R., *et al.* (2022). Levelling up the UK: Is the government serious about reducing regional inequalities in health? *BMJ, 377*, e070589.

Riches, N., *et al.* (2015). *The Role of Local Authorities in Health Issues: A Policy Document Analysis.* London: PRUComm.

Royal Society for Public Health (2021). *Response to Transforming the Public Health System: Reforming the Public Health System for the Challenges of Our Times.* London: Royal Society for Public Health.

Sample, I. (2023). UK ready to snub key EU science research scheme if Brexit row not resolved. *theguardian.com*, 12 February.

Samuel, G. *et al.* (2022). COVID-19 contact tracing apps: UK public perceptions. *Crit Public Health, 32*(1), 31–43.

Sanchez-Graells, A. (2021). Pandemic legalities: Legal responses to COVID-19 — Justice and social responsibility. In D. Cowan and A. Mumford (Eds.), *COVID-19 PPE Extremely Urgent Procurement in England: A Cautionary Tale for an Overheating Public Governance.* Bristol: Bristol University Press.

Sanders, K. (2020). British government communication during the 2020 COVID-19 pandemic: Learning from high reliability organizations. *CC&C, 5*(3), 356–377.

Scally, G. (2021a). A new public health body for the UK. *BMJ, 373*, n875.

Scally, G. (2021b). England's new office for health improvement and disparities. *BMJ, 374*, n2323.

Scottish Government (2020). About public health Scotland. *publichealthreform. scot*, 24 February.

Sian, S. and Smyth, S. (2022). Supreme emergencies and public accountability: The case of procurement in the UK during the Covid-19 pandemic. *Accounting, Auditing & Accountability Journal, 35*(1), 146–157.

Sibony, A. (2020). The UK COVID-19 response: A behavioural irony? *EJRR, 11*(2), 350–357.

Sim, J. and Tombs, S. (2022). Narrating the coronavirus crisis: State talk and state silence in the UK. *Justice, Power and Resistance, 5*(1–2), 67–90.

Solomon, D. (2019). Brexit and health security: Why we need to protect our global networks. *Journal of Public Health Policy, 40*(1), 1–4.

Springford, J. (2022). *What Can We Know About the Cost of Brexit So Far?* London: Centre for European Reform.

Spyridonidis, D. (2022). Leadership configuration in crises: Lessons from the English response to COVID-19. *Leadership, 18*(5), 680–694.

Statistia (2023). Number of novel coronavirus (COVID-19) deaths worldwide as of May 2, 2023, by country and territory. *statista.com,* 2 May.

Tani, C. (2022). EU health policy taking shape post-COVID-19, *Sciencebusiness. net*, 8 December.

Thacker, P. (2020). Conflicts of interest among the UK government's covid-19 advisers. *BMJ, 371*, m4716.

Topping, A. (2020). Health alliance warns Brexit can leave UK exposed to global outbreaks. *theguardian.com*, 10 February.

van Schalkwyk, M., *et al.* (2021). Brexit and trade policy: An analysis of the governance of UK trade policy and what it means for health and social justice. *Global Health, 17*, doi.org/10.1186/s12992-021-00697-1.

Vize, R. (2020). Controversial from creation to disbanding, via e-cigarettes and alcohol: An obituary of Public Health England. *BMJ, 371*, m4476.

Walsh, F. (2022). AstraZeneca vaccine: Did nationalism spoil UK's "gift to the world"? *bbc.com*, 7 February.

Wardman, J. (2020). Recalibrating pandemic risk leadership: Thirteen crisis ready strategies for COVID-19. *Journal of Risk Research, 23*(7–8), 1092–1120.

Weinberg, J. (2022). Trust, governance, and the Covid-19 pandemic: An Explainer using longitudinal data from the United Kingdom. *The Political Quarterly, 93*(2), 316–325.

Wilkinson, E. (2021). What the new health security agency means for public health. *BMJ, 373*, n996.

Wise, P. and Darmstadt, G. (2016). The grand divergence in global child health: Confronting data requirements in areas of conflict and chronic political instability. *JAMA Pediatrics, 170*(3), 195–197.

World Health Organization (WHO) (2023). Pandemic prevention, preparedness and response accord. *who.int*, 24 February.

Chapter 8

The European Union

Scott L. Greer

8.1 Introduction

The European Union is fundamentally unlike the other polities discussed in this book, and its surprising public health response to the COVID-19 virus reflects this difference in its advances and its limitations. Specifying the nature of the EU is a theoretical challenge, since while it is clearly not a nation-state, there are various theoretically productive and unproductive ways to frame it, i.e. to ask what it is a case of (Ragin, 1992). Accordingly, there are endless debates, some productive, some pettifogging, about whether it should be called supranational, international, federal, confederal, unique, or something else. These decisions about framing can have consequences. For example, viewing the EU as a federation and comparing it to Canada or Australia makes it look like an unusual federation with strong legal and weak fiscal and execution powers (Greer, 2020), while viewing it as a regional international organization and comparing it to ASEAN or the African Union make it a strikingly successful case of integration (Greer *et al.*, 2022a). Whatever else it resembles, it is not like its member states, for what it does is not what a state does, and many states do not do what it does (Dehousse, 1994). Whether that changes is a long-term question.

The confusion grows from the fact that the EU combines features of different regimes in a manner that is probably unique. It is a voluntary arrangement that pools the sovereignty of 27 member states to a varying degree in various policy areas. As Brexit showed, departure is possible but not a good idea for the departing country. The EU has an extraordinarily strong legal system, with member state courts not just enforcing but actively developing EU law in a dialog across legal systems of the continent (Kelemen, 2019). Notably, this legal system is often far harder on barriers to trade within the EU than the legal system of established federations, such as Australia, Canada, or the US (Matthijs *et al.*, 2019; Parsons & Springer, 2018). It has strong policy capacity across its institutions, including the European Parliament, but very little implementing capacity. Even some of its most powerful policy tools such as the medicines authorization regime or agricultural policy turn out to work primarily through member state agencies and ministries (Hauray, 2013). Its workforce is, by the standards of member states or even their larger local governments, trivial (and much of its total head count are translators).

Furthermore, and perhaps in contradiction to the impression one might have that political activity on the continent revolves around seeking EU grants or European Investment Bank loans, its budget (around 1% of EU GDP) is far from the share of GDP member states spend on healthcare, let alone the public sector in general. As discussed in the following, it had very limited debt-raising powers. The result is that it cannot and does not redistribute effectively or even provide effective insurance to its member states. That would take far more money, and debt issuance powers, than it has in 2023. It should not be surprising, therefore, that the EU has wider economic disparities between its states than any rich federation, or that there has been little evidence of economic convergence for nearly two decades.

On the other hand, it is deeply involved in the financial and fiscal architecture of the continent through its powerful and (by design) democratically unaccountable central bank, the ECB, which has, in concert with member central banks, overturned governments and effectively forced entire countries into receivership. It has a remarkably intrusive and ambitious fiscal surveillance regime that tries to compensate for the

EU's trivial fiscal stabilization abilities by forcing member states to avoid deficits and bubbles (Greer & Jarman, 2016, 2018). Finally, it has large investment bank resources which can support investments outside the obvious decisions in the EU budget.

This makes the EU an intriguing combination of clear formal strength, clear formal weakness, and informal strength. Clear formal strength: its legal system above all, but also specific powers in areas such as trade and animal health. Clear formal weakness: its lack of a serious budget, territorial redistribution, or implementation capacity, but also the endless challenges of implementing any policy in a coherent way across 27 countries and legal systems. Informal strength: in many areas the EU and its agencies such as the European Food Safety Authority or the European Medicines Agency provide a default technical standard for decisions and structure regulatory networks that are often influential worldwide. Countries such as Norway or Switzerland, which are very clearly not member states, implement EU policy and explicitly work to shape it; a putatively non-coercive EU is a major actor in coordinating border security, notably through its Frontex agency and even military expeditions, and EU policy advice which seems to have no teeth at all can have more impact than EU policy that is supposedly obligatory.

Public health contains all these contradictions and perhaps showcases them particularly well. The EU has many powers which clearly contribute to avoidable morbidity and mortality, notably in animal health and food safety, environmental health, occupational health and safety, and consumer protection. It has fewer powers with any clear identification as public health; the treaty section called "Public health" has one article, 168 TFEU, and that article is an *omnium gatherum* of ways treaty language can limit EU action. It had, in 2019, one public health agency as such, the European Centre for Disease Prevention and Control (ECDC), primarily focused on dissemination of data and capacity-building. The EU has next to no formal powers over healthcare systems, though its extensive market-making powers have erected a legal edifice that regulates access to healthcare services and important elements of healthcare policy, such as the regulation of medicines, devices, and professionals. It is therefore possible to look at the EU from a strictly institutional perspective and see almost no public health powers since Article 168 and an agency or two make up a very small quota of power. It is also possible to look at the EU from a broader regulatory perspective and see an enormous contribution to public health improvement from its environmental, labor, occupational health and safety, and consumer protection regimes. And it is possible to focus more on its contribution to healthcare, via courts' application of internal market law and endless attempts to institutionalize austerity, and see a force that is hostile to health.

The EU, in spring 2020, did not look like a polity likely to become a major health policy actor. The phrase "European Health Union" seemed so ambitious as to be naive. By September 2020, a European Health Union was an explicit goal of the institutions, one backed up by policies that would have been hard to imagine a year earlier. This chapter is about why that happened and what lessons we might draw.

8.2 Public Health Responses

The EU's response to COVID-19 can perhaps be best understood in light of its multiple faces (Greer, 2014). Its first face, explicit public health policy, was its least important. Article 168 is tightly constraining, the Health Program' was being eliminated ("mainstreamed") in 2020, and the only statutory agency grounded in Article 168, the ECDC, was small and had limited and largely soft power. The real sources of power over health policies and outcomes in the EU had been elsewhere, particularly in the second face of EU health policies: the policies by which the EU can affect health but whose politics and legal bases are elsewhere. These second-face policies include pharmaceutical regulation, healthcare workforce regulation (framed as a question of professional regulation), investment in healthcare systems through loans and regional aid, environmental regulation, food safety regulation, and workplace health and safety regulation. The third face is fiscal governance: the fiscal surveillance regime that the EU operates, vetting member state budgets and budgetary priorities and often making very detailed recommendations to member states that in some cases are theoretically backed by a fine. This regime, justified by the argument that member state profligacy endangered the Eurozone in 2010, attempts to institutionalize austerity and is accordingly under constant and often effective attack from opponents of austerity.

In other words, the EU had three faces but none were ideally positioned to face COVID-19. The first face was relevant but, by design, not very important. Despite ECDC's work during the pandemic, it had extremely limited technical resources and guidance for member states, which often looked elsewhere for international and scientific advice. The second face, the management and regulation of the internal market, has easily been the source of the EU's biggest effects on health policies and outcomes, but again it was not immediately relevant to combatting the pandemic. It was, rather, important in fending off or legalizing member state actions taken in the pandemic that endangered the unity and consistency of the EU internal market. This meant everything from working against blockages on transfer of personal protective equipment (PPE) to ensuring quick evaluation of vaccines and therapeutics to relaxing rules on state aid as member states bailed out companies, such as airlines. In particular, the Council adopted Recommendations to limit border controls (partly in response to ECDC arguments that they did no good) and, even more clearly, developing the European Digital Certificate which, from July 2021, allowed member states to issue widely accepted digital certificates that the holder was unlikely to spread the disease (Deruelle, 2022). This system was adopted, and recognized, by countries outside the EU and provided an especially stark contrast to the impractical US alternative of small pieces of cardboard. Preserving the internal market and its law in a 2020 wave of national egotism and panic was no easy task, but it did not directly address the pandemic or its economic consequences.

Finally, the third face of austerity and fiscal surveillance was irrelevant, though it is almost certain that the austerity agenda of which it was part had weakened southern and central European health systems that were about to be overwhelmed by illness. Member states recognized its irrelevance by invoking the "general escape clause," which effectively suspended the surveillance process; when the fiscal surveillance system returned to the health politics agenda, it was in a very different context (described as follows).

The EU's response was substantially in the first face, explicit health policies, and it was big. Perhaps the most important element of its response in terms of health outcomes was the decision to adopt joint advance purchase agreements for vaccines. By early 2021, the EU had signed agreements with six vaccine manufacturers. The advance purchase agreements and their results produced some controversies. The UK, which had opted out of the EU arrangements, and other rich non-EU countries, such as the United States and Australia, had signed agreements which gave them earlier access to vaccines. The European approach focused, more than those countries, on price and liability. That focus slowed negotiations and meant countries willing to pay more and write weaker liability rules into contracts with the pharmaceutical companies were ahead of it in the companies' priorities. Notably, the EU ended up in legal action with AstraZeneca after the company did not deliver the promised number of doses in time.

The vaccine acquisition program can be seen as a major success, especially from the point of view of the smaller and poorer member states, which would have had difficulties in securing either a good price or priority from the companies. The large European market meant that it was possible to negotiate both rapid delivery and a relatively low price. The public image of the EU's vaccine purchasing approach was not so positive, however. This is in part because of a correct public understanding that the EU member states were not receiving vaccines as quickly as a few other countries, for all that the AstraZeneca problem was eventually solved by a huge purchase of mRNA vaccines from Pfizer that were probably better vaccines as well. It is also in part because of the well-known blame avoidance strategy of member state governments, which tried to shift blame for local problems onto "Europe." Slow vaccine distribution was a problem in a number of member states, and blaming Europe was an attractive political strategy. The result, however, is that what looks like a broadly successful European action is not universally perceived as such. This gap between qualified but real policy success and a memory of bad headlines means that the shape of future EU vaccines production and acquisition policies is unclear and will depend on whether its benefits (particularly to smaller countries) and the expertise that the Commission acquired in the procurement balance out the vague bad taste it left many voters and political elites.

The key movement in EU broader health politics, especially by the standards of EU health politics to date, came at the European Council meeting on June 17–21, 2020. Formally, the European Council, which unites heads of government, has long had a weak position. The EU's formal structures attribute the Council's decision-making powers to the particular ministers who meet in particular formations (such as health and social policy or economic and financial affairs). Informally, European Council meetings are crucial because they are the venues in which national heads of government decide what issues they prioritize and what policies they want. Given that heads of government tend to also speak for governments and legislative majorities in their member states, their meetings tend to predict (and influence) political decisions further down the line and their communiques are taken as decisions that the Commission and other institutions will implement.

The highlight of the June 2020 Council meeting, later turned into Commission proposals and legislation, was the decision to substantially increase the resources dedicated to health, in particular health emergencies preparation and response. The Commission would later dub the whole package the "European Health Union." The Health Programme, a small funding vehicle run by DG SANTE, had been performing the time-honored role of developing a constituency for EU health policy action and evidence to inform it. The Juncker Commission, backed by a Council with a majority of governments of the right, had successfully zeroed it out in proposals for the next 7-year budget (MFF), instead "mainstreaming" it into larger funding programs. June 2020 reversed that, renaming it Europe4Health and massively increasing its budget. The policy and political impact of any grant-making program will take time to emerge, as they cumulate out of individual decisions which reveal the sustainable priorities of the Commission in its implementation, but it could be an epochal change in the composition, resources, and focus of the European Union health policy community.

The EU's quantitative change in its public health policies was so dramatic as to be effectively qualitative. The tiny Health Programme budget increased by almost 20 times as it was transformed into the EU4Health Program. It is never clear when a quantitative, parametric, change becomes a qualitative, policy, change, but a nearly twentyfold increase in budget seems like it might be above the threshold.

Member states also agreed to improve European capacity in public health surveillance and response, building resources such as expertise, networks, and data systems to complement money. The ECDC, which was regarded as performing well, received additional powers and resources. The Council also agreed to create a new "agency," Health Emergency and Response Agency (HERA) charged with pandemic preparedness and preparedness for more general health threats. HERA's birth and development were more confused, with expectations ranging from a European equivalent to the US Biomedical Advanced Research and Development Authority (BARDA) through to a division of the Commission used primarily as a purchasing vehicle (a good guide to the debate is Anderson *et al.*, 2021). HERA's legal status, activities, and budget all remained uncertain years after the decision to create it, and as the pandemic receded in policymakers' minds the likelihood that it would become anything like BARDA also receded.

RescEU, finally, is not part of EU health policy. It is legally and organizationally part of civil protection, an oddly configured area that substantially grew from the outside in as externally focused disaster response organizations began to acquire roles within the EU. RescEU, which is the key element of implementation of the civil protection system, began in 2019 and is essentially a co-financing scheme with member states designed to expand Europe-wide access to key resources for disasters as well as deploy surge capacity, such as medical experts or firefighting equipment. Member states were slow to activate it in the egotism of spring 2020, and it did not have much relevant material at that time anyway, but the June 2020 Council meeting supported a vast expansion of its budget. The EU will have substantially better stockpiles of equipment for health emergency response through the end of the 2020s. It is a different question whether its budgeting and policy process, and member state partners, will remain committed to the upkeep and maintenance of the stockpiles as the time comes for their renewal and COVID-19 fades from political memory.

Externally, the EU took what was probably the obvious, if somewhat cynical, approach for a rich major power and chose to participate in the WHO's COVID-19 Vaccines Global Access (COVAX) scheme as a donor rather than purchasing through COVAX. COVAX had launched with what might have been excessive optimism as a global platform for vaccine research support, acquisition, and development, but it rapidly turned into a more conventional example of global health politics in which richer countries, especially the EU, donated money as much as they chose while looking after themselves and total COVAX resources came in at far less than was necessary to achieve its goals, let alone global vaccination. The EU was more generous and far more committed to multilateral action than most other rich powers or its member states, but that is a very low comparative standard.

8.3 Shortcomings and Weaknesses

There are two major kinds of shortcomings that differ in the measuring-stick that we use. One is about the shortcomings of the EU response, measured by the kinds of policy instruments that are available to it or that it could quickly develop in the pandemic. The EU response was recognizably focused, based on key instruments it uses to act in many areas: money (EU4Health, the Pharmaceuticals Strategy, and RescEU); resources, meaning expertise grounded in agencies and their networks of member state agencies (ECDC and HERA); and, a relative novelty, joint purchasing of vaccines. The EU can provide (co-)funding to promote certain goals, strengthen experts and their advice, and, it turns out, negotiate commercial agreements on behalf of its member states.

In each case, it is possible to identify clear shortcomings by the standards of European Union legal and real competence as of the start of 2020. In particular, HERA, much heralded, was established within the Commission, without its own statute, and proceeded to drift as principals argued about what it should actually do. The advance purchasing of vaccines did not just absorb blame for member state failures. It did show some signs that the EU's expertise in strategy for such purchases was flawed. In particular, the focus on company liability and price made some political sense in a political system suspicious of pharmaceutical companies but slowed the purchases and might have contributed to bad relations with companies and supply problems. The EU is formidably good at its processes, but high-level purchasing negotiations with big companies, under pressure, at the behest of more than two dozen governments, went beyond what its processes could do and produced unsurprising problems.

Finally, it is possible that from the perspective of the 2030s, the EU and its leaders will deserve criticism for failure to commit. Personal protective equipment such as masks was in some cases purchased in 2009 as a panic response to pandemic influenza, expired in 2019, and was destroyed without being replaced just as people started to fall ill in Wuhan. Public health preparedness decisions have a strong element of a panic-neglect cycle in any political system, and while the EU's 7-year budget window creates more certainty about public health expenditures than in most countries, it also means that there is a chance that public health expenditures, and the resources they enabled, will be slashed in the 2028–2035 MFF.

The other is about the shortcomings of the EU as it is currently constituted. If we regard the EU as a regional international organization and compare it to ASEAN or the African Union, it entered the pandemic as a tremendously effective organization and left it still stronger (Greer *et al.*, 2022a). No regional international organization comes close to its combination of breadth and effectiveness (Panke & Stapel, 2020). If we regard the EU as a federation comparable to Canada, Germany, or the US, then it looks dangerously imbalanced, with a powerful law-state that enables particular kinds of capitalism and public policy but nowhere near the resources to compensate people and member states which lose in the markets and policy environments configured by the EU (Matthijs *et al.*, 2019; Greer, 2020; Höpner & Schäfer, 2010; Scharpf, 2010).

This reluctance to redistribute seems obvious when we consider that the EU, by the standards of federations, is both extravagantly multinational and faced with enormous territorial inequalities. The gap between GDP in rich and poor member states of the EU is larger than the gap in GDP between, for example, U.S. states, Canadian provinces, or even the states in highly unequal countries, such as Argentina and Brazil. It is hard to imagine just how much money would have to be redistributed within the Union if it were to attain the goals of equalization instituted in rich federations, even ones with major interregional inequalities. It is also probably pointless, given the difficulty the EU has faced in far smaller redistributive measures (many of which are better conceptualized as side payments than as real attempts to equalize). While internal heterogeneity within countries limits the usefulness of country-level comparative data on territorial inequality, it is clear that convergence has been real, though huge disparities remain, and since around 2008 the evidence for ongoing convergence is very unclear (Makszin, 2020; Makszin *et al.*, 2020).

The COVID-19 pandemic and policy responses have exacerbated inequalities (Dauderstädt, 2022; Ladi & Tsarouhas, 2020; Ceron & Palermo, 2022). In the absence of the hoped-for convergence in the size and composition of its economies, the EU continues to have internal strains that its fiscal policies can by no means correct.

What the EU can do, and what has happened in other federations, is some mutualization of debt (Ladi & Tsarouhas, 2020). One of the weakest elements of the whole EU system is the extent to which it does not fulfill the insurance function that most established federations do. If a member state falls into trouble, there is no reliable mechanism to cushion blows to it or its citizens. *Ad hoc* and very expensive responses to debt crises after 2008 were not institutionalized, with member states and European institutions preferring to take the perspective of creditor states and tighten *ex ante* rules on governments. This is not a very credible policy for a variety of reasons, notably that the relationship between fiscal policy and deficits tends to be overshadowed by economic cycles (Ladi & Tsarouhas, 2014), that the economic theories embedded in the fiscal governance system might not have been very robust, and implementation of the process was predictably undermined by people whose interests were opposed to austerity or simply wished to use the momentum of fiscal governance to pursue their own goals (Greer & Brooks, 2020; Verdun & Vanhercke, 2022).

8.4 External Shocks and Policy Change

COVID-19 was in many respects a crisis foretold, whether in policy plans, a best-selling board game, or blockbuster movies. Experts and policy entrepreneurs in communicable disease control had long been arguing that the EU, with its abilities to pool resources and its large, disease-prone common market, should have a stronger ability to influence and coordinate member states in a crisis, though other experts had insisted that the WHO and member state agencies should be the key actors.

Crises, often crises foretold, are nonetheless a big part of the history and characteristic explanation of European integration. Most scholars rightly explain these odd combinations by examining the politics of the EU — the way its institutions and characteristic agenda — setting mechanisms put some issues on different planes than others, and the way the apparatus of EU law, including member state as well as EU courts, creates issues and diffuses policies. But the EU and its relatively unusual pattern of self-sustaining integration also come about because the EU is necessary to so many key policymakers, a scholarly thesis called "neo-functionalism" in the EU studies literature. In part, the global geopolitical environment is one in which smaller countries have cause to band together if their voices are to be heard and their economies strong. In part, as well, integration has its own self-sustaining momentum; once an area is inte-grated, it is costly to disintegrate it, as the EU showed in the first months of the pandemic, and it has a way of spreading into over other areas and creating pressure for further integration. In short, the EU becomes more and more needed.

That is why, with almost absurd regularity, crises hitting the EU lead to opinion pieces in English-language media about the threats of EU dis-sension and breakup and then so often lead to further integration. The 2008 financial crisis and the 2010–2012 debt crisis both led to further integration and in fact a new treaty (Jones *et al.*, 2015). The 2015 migra-tion "crisis" led to strong EU borders policy and an executive border guard/coast guard agency with more than twenty thousand staff, whose existence suggests some rethinking of the characterization of the EU as a civilian power might be useful (Micinski, 2022). And the COVID-19 cri-sis, also initially framed by many as a carnival of national egotism and conflict, also led to more integration. The EU has become more politically contested across Europe, but that dissensus can be quite permissive of further integration (Greer & Löblová, 2016).

These arguments, more or less explicitly, and with a wide variety of empirical supports from different policy areas and case studies, argue that integration in the EU tends to advance when member states are suddenly faced with an inescapably large problem for most or all of them; can see no other way out; and face costs of inaction or regression that are unset-tlingly large. A commonsensical neofunctionalist perspective suggests that this is when they realize the scale of their integration and shared problems and, forced to end their denial, update their governance to match their problems. Two decades of argument about whether the integration of the EU was best characterized by intergovernmentalism (the EU as the tool of member states) and neofunctionalism (which made integration at least partially endogenous) sputtered out as scholars realized that member states are powerful but also trapped by a logic of endogenous integration, often visible in exogenous shocks, that is unacceptably costly to exit. The EU is, frequently, the mechanism for the "rescue of the nation-state" when it faces problems it cannot manage alone (Milward, 1999). The experience of Greece, whose government stayed in the Eurozone despite a ruinous price, showed how greatly policymakers can estimate the costs of disintegration. The experience of Brexit then showed just how immense those costs can indeed be (Greer & Laible, 2020).

Perhaps the best current take on these issues is the "failing forward" thesis (Jones *et al.*, 2015). In this analysis, the EU does have endogenous pressures toward integration, e.g. a common currency creates pressure for common fiscal policies of some sort, or shared borders create pressure for shared border rules and enforcement. But member states, eager to maintain both their sovereignty and their preference for consensus in the Council, respond with the least possible integration relative to the size of this crisis. These half-measures are both integrative, moving the EU forward, and responsive to failure while also creating the conditions for new failures and crises.

The EU and health literature is no exception to the crisis-driven narrative, in which crises make salient the problems of integration that will often be answered with further integration (Greer *et al.*, 2021). There is a longstanding trope of writing about the European Union, and in particular the development of its public health policies, which frames them as crisis response. Thus, the development of EU public health policy in any narrative will feature the variant Creutzfeldt-Jakob disease (vCJD) ("mad cow") crisis of the 1990s, and perhaps the French tainted blood scandal, the 2001 anthrax attacks in the US, 2003, SARS outbreak, the 2009 swine flu pandemic, and, of course, COVID-19. This can be a usefully simplifying way to write, and done with a great deal of sophistication and knowledge, it can be productive (Riddervold *et al.*, 2021), but it has some serious theoretical challenges. The definition of a crisis is far from fixed or easy to apply even in mid-crisis (were all of these perceived as crises at the time or afterwards, and by whom?). "Crisis" is, in fact, one of the many elements of politics that are socially constructed by political and media actors that might be very strategic. It is also a problem to argue that crises produce action, since some do not, or to argue that the action takes a particular direction, such as further European integration (Lefkofridi & Schmitter, 2015; Brooks *et al.*, 2023). Member states might buy into (or once again think of and accept) the logic of integration and opt to fail forward, but they also might not, or they might come up with integrative but counterproductive policies. They also might fail to fail forward enough, in a sense — not do enough to even address their current crisis (Cox & Kurzer, 2024). To sum up, the existence of a crisis can be hard to determine, responses might not result, and the fact or nature of the crisis might not point to a particular resolution.

Perhaps the way out is simply to accept the probabilistic nature of policy. Member state governments are powerful and jealous of their sovereignty, but they also have a long-established consciousness of their shared fate, and so they will often take an integrative step forward when confronted with clear evidence that their existing level of shared governance is not adequate to manage their shared problems. Their step might be integrative but wrong-headed in the eyes of policy analysts, and almost certainly viewed as inadequate, but that sets up the conditions to fail forward again. If this is the case, and it is the failing-forward hypothesis, then it might be fruitful to use Kingdon's multiple-streams theory more often in order to understand how and why items get on the agenda, particularly the European Council agenda, and how problems come to be matched with solutions (Kingdon, 2003; Page, 2006; Princen, 2009; Greer, 2015).

8.5 Futures of European Union Public Health Policy

The EU's window of opportunity for major public health policy change closed in 2020, and the window for smaller changes (e.g. in the debates over exactly how HERA would work and what it would do) was largely closed by the end of 2022. As any good theory of agenda-setting would predict, the opportunity to make big changes in response to a crisis does not last long and in this case it is reasonable to argue that the big decisions were past, and the agenda moving on, by autumn 2020.

But the EU's institutional rhythm also locks in the effects of those changes for a predictable period of time. Much of what we have discussed by way of public health policy is changes in budgets and spending programs, and even capacities for e.g. ECDC or HERA are substantially driven by their budgetary support. In the EU, the key budget document is the Multiannual Financial Framework (MFF) for 2021–2028. The EU has what amounts to a 7-year budget cycle, setting the priorities and sums out for 7 years instead of setting annual budgets; these 7-year budgets, which are generally fulfilled, are the MFFs. The current MFF sets the EU budget for effectively that whole time frame and is the source for the numbers reported here; eventual spending will almost certainly match the MFF well.

This means that the EU faces a new, wholly endogenous, window of opportunity for policy change in about 2026–2027. The MFF structure means that it will be hard to cut back public health budgets or ambition in the EU over that time but also that there will come a defined moment of intense intergovernmental and interinstitutional bargaining during which public health budgets will be under close scrutiny. There is a well-known panic-neglect cycle of public health politics, a phenomenon well known for a long time but named by journalist Ed Yong before being adopted by everybody from scholars to think tanks to McKinsey (Yong, 2022). The regularity of the panic-neglect cycle suggests that, barring another major emergency, member states could be deep into the neglect phase of the cycle and the next MFF could endanger the EU public health commitment as well as enhance it. The result is that advocates of any particular EU public health have a defined period of time to build their supporting coalitions, prove their value, and convince the member states of the value of specific public health investments. The window of opportunity for big change has been closed for years, but the next MFF could be a reckoning for the whole project that was agreed in 2020.

8.6 Conclusion

In 2019, I was part of a group that published the second edition of a guide to EU health policy at the end of the Juncker Commission (Greer *et al.*,

2019). That Commission, dominated by politicians of the right, was broadly hostile to health policy as such and deemphasized consideration of health problems or health consequences of other policies. DG SANTE (the directorate-general for health within the Commission) itself was lucky to have survived into the new von der Leyen Commission, rescued mainly because an increasingly fragmented European Parliament had parties on the left which supported an EU public health role. But the Health Programme was being eliminated ("mainstreamed"), there was only one open legislative dossier and it was going nowhere (health technology assessment), civil society and policy forums were being abandoned, and Juncker's Commission had openly entertained the idea of ceasing to have any positive health policy. We accordingly emphasized the second face of health policy, such as environmental, consumer protection, and workplace law, because there had been so little new action on the first face of EU health policy and the third face was losing its ambition. Suggesting ways health advocates could make headway in consumer protection or workplace safety was a way to find health impact in the absence of an overt health policy.

In 2022, we had to publish a substantially revised edition (Greer *et al.*, 2022b). The *quantitative* changes to existing EU health policies, notably budgets, were so great as to look like a *qualitative* change in the nature of EU health policy. Quantity has a quality of its own, and increasing the health program budget, due to be zeroed out, or RescEU, by more than an order of magnitude makes each a different kind of a program. It is instructive, perhaps, to see what we had to do. A section on explicit EU public health, the core of the first face, expanded into its own section, not just because of the pandemic response but also because of, for example, a more explicit health policy role in medical devices regulation and food safety (Jarman *et al.*, 2021). The other change, driven by practical editorial considerations of chapter length but also EU political movements, was an increasing attention to EU global health policy, and the extent to which the pandemic, decisions about vaccine development and distribution worldwide, and other issues such as the Russian invasion of Ukraine and various migration "crises" had made clear the scale of the EU's health impact; the EU was apparently thinking along the same lines and published a global health strategy of its own in early 2023.

Authors reflecting on the ever-increasing page counts of their books might not seem so interesting, but our practical problem of updating a primer reflected real changes. The EU is failing forward in health. It is therefore unsatisfying to many, but from the perspective of integration, it has taken a big step forward. It also has taken this step in a direction that many in public health institutions can approve, which is not the case for other major integrative steps, such as fiscal governance and migration policy. It has, in not just public health but also the creation of mutualized debt, potentially taken a baby step toward the kind of interregional insurance that every sustainable federation operates. It was, after all, impossible to pretend that profligacy was the cause of the pandemic or austerity the cure. Our local problem is perhaps an index of a real change in the EU, a quantitative change in some areas that is so big as to be qualitative and, maybe, prefigure an even bigger change in the direction of resembling a viable federation. The next key data point will probably be the budget negotiations in 2027.

References

Anderson, M., Forman, R., and Mossialos, E. (2021). Navigating the role of the EU Health Emergency Preparedness and Response Authority (HERA) in Europe and beyond. *Lancet Regional Health, 9,* 100203. DOI: 10.1016/j.lanepe.2021.100203.

Brooks, E., de Ruijter, A., Greer, S. L., and Rozenblum, S. (2023). EU health policy in the aftermath of COVID-19: Neofunctionalism and crisis-driven integration. *Journal of European Public Policy, 30*(4), 721–739.

Ceron, M. and Palermo, C. M. (2022). Structural core–periphery divergences in the EU: The case of responses to the COVID-19 crisis in 2020. *European Politics and Society,* 1–20. DOI: 10.1080/23745118.2022.2037209.

Cox, R. H. and Kurzer, P. (2024). For want of a champion: Why the EU won't be ready for the next public health crisis. *Journal of European Public Policy, 31*(2), 610–631.

Dauderstädt, M. (2022). We are not (at) all in the same boat: Covid-19 winners and losers. In B. Vanhercke and S. Spasova (Eds.), *Social Policy in the European Union: State of Play 2021* (pp. 11–38). ETUI/OSE.

Dehousse, R. (1994). Comparing national and EC law: The problem of the level of analysis. *The American Journal of Comparative Law, 42*(4), 761–781.

Deruelle, T. (2022). Covid-19 as a catalyst for a European Health Union: Recent developments in health threats management. In B. Vanhercke and S. D. *Spasova* (Eds.), *Social policy in the European Union: State of Play 2021: Re-emerging Social Ambitions as the EU Recovers from the Pandemic* (pp. 127–144).

Greer, S. L. (2014). The three faces of European Union health policy: Policy, markets and austerity. *Policy and Society, 33*(1), 13–24.

Greer, S. L. (2015). John W. Kingdon, *Agendas, Alternatives, and Public Policy*. In S. J. Balla, M. Lodge, and E. C. Page (Eds.), *The Oxford Handbook of Classics of Public Policy and Administration* (pp. 417–432). Oxford: Oxford University Press.

Greer, S. L. (2020). Health, federalism and the European Union: Lessons from comparative federalism about the European Union. *Health Economics, Policy and Law*, 1–14. DOI: 10.1017/S1744133120000055.

Greer, S. L. and Brooks, E. (2020). Termites of solidarity in the house of Austerity: Undermining fiscal governance in the European Union. (8706615). *Journal of Health Politics, Policy and Law*. DOI: 10.1215/03616878-8706615.

Greer, S. L. and Jarman, H. (2016). Reinforcing Europe's failed fiscal regulatory state. In B. Dallago, G. Guri, and J. McGowan (Eds.), *A Global Perspective on the European Economic Crisis* (pp. 122–143). Abingdon: Routledge.

Greer, S. L. and Jarman, H. (2018). European citizenship rights and European fiscal politics after the crisis. *Government and Opposition, 53*(1), 76–103.

Greer, S. L. and Laible, J. (Eds.). (2020). *The European Union After Brexit*. Manchester: Manchester University Press.

Greer, S. L. and Löblovà, O. (2016). European integration in the era of permissive dissensus: Neofunctionalism and agenda-setting in European health technology assessment and communicable disease control. *Comparative European Politics*. DOI: 10.1057/cep.2016.6.

Greer, S. L., Amaya, A. B., Jarman, H., Legido-Quigley, H., and McKee, M. (2022a). Regional International Organizations and Health: A framework for analysis. *Journal of Health Politics, Policy and Law, 47*(1), 63–92.

Greer, S. L., de Ruijter, A., and Brooks, E. (2021). The COVID-19 pandemic: Failing forward in public health. In M. Riddervold, J. Trondal, and A. Newsome (Eds.), *Palgrave Handbook of EU Crises* (pp. 747–764).

Greer, S. L., Fahy, N., Rozenblum, S., Jarman, H., Palm, W., Elliott, H. A., & Wismar, M. (2019). *Everything You Always Wanted to Know About European Union Health Policy But were Afraid to Ask*. (2nd, revised edn.). Brussels: European Observatory on Health Systems and Policies.

Greer, S. L., Rozenblum, S., Fahy, N., Brooks, E., de Ruijter, A., Palm, W. I., and Wismar, M. (2022b). *Everything You Always Wanted to Know About European Union Health Policy But were Afraid to Ask* (3rd, completely revised edn.). Brussels: WHO/European Observatory on Health Systems and Policies.

Hauray, B. (2013). The European regulation of medicines. In S. L. Greer and P. Kurzer (Eds.), *European Union Public Health Policy: Regional and Global Trends* (pp. 81–93). Abingdon: Routledge.

Höpner, M. and Schäfer, A. (2010). Polanyi in Brussels? Embeddedness and the three dimensions of European economic integration. *MPIfG Discussion Paper*, 10/8. https://hdl.handle.net/11858/00-001M-0000-0012-428A-5.

Jarman, H., Rozenblum, S., and Huang, T. J. (2021). Neither protective nor harmonized: The crossborder regulation of medical devices in the EU. *Health Economics, Policy and Law, 16*(1), 51–63.

Jones, E., Kelemen, R. D., and Meunier, S. (2015). Failing forward? The Euro crisis and the incomplete nature of European integration. *Comparative Political Studies, 49*(7), 1010–1034. DOI: 10.1177/0010414015617966.

Kelemen, R. D. (2019). Is differentiation possible in rule of law. *Comparative European Politics, 17*(2), 246–260. DOI: 10.1057/s41295-019-00162-9.

Kingdon, J. W. (2003). *Agendas, Alternatives, and Public Policies*. New York: HarperCollins.

Ladi, S. and Tsarouhas, D. (2014). The politics of austerity and public policy reform in the EU. *Political Studies Review, 12*(2), 171–180.

Ladi, S. and Tsarouhas, D. (2020). EU economic governance and Covid-19: Policy learning and windows of opportunity. *Journal of European Integration, 42*(8), 1041–1056. DOI: 10.1080/07036337.2020.1852231.

Lefkofridi, Z. and Schmitter, P. C. (2015). Transcending or descending? European integration in times of crisis. *European Political Science Review, 7*(1), 3–22.

Makszin, K. (2020). The East-West divide: Obstacles to further integration. In S. L. Greer and J. Laible (Eds.), *The European Union after Brexit* (pp. 128–145). Manchester: Manchester University Press.

Makszin, K., Medve-Bálint, G., and Bohle, D. (2020). North and South, East and West: Is it possible to bridge the gap. In R. Coman, A. Crespy, and V. Schmidt (Eds.), *Governance and Politics in the Post-Crisis European Union* (pp. 335–357). Cambridge: Cambridge University Press.

Matthijs, M., Parsons, C., and Toenshoff, C. (2019). Ever tighter union? Brexit, Grexit, and frustrated differentiation in the single market and Eurozone. *Comparative European Politics, 17*(2), 209–230. DOI: 10.1057/s41295-019-00165-6.

Micinski, N. R. (2022). *Delegating Responsibility: International Cooperation on Migration in the European Union.* University of Michigan Press.

Milward, A. (1999). *The European Rescue of the Nation State.* London: Routledge.

Page, E. C. (2006). The origins of policy. In M. Moran, M. Rein, and R. E. Goodin (Eds.), *The Oxford Handbook of Public Policy* (pp. 207–226). Oxford: Oxford University Press.

Panke, D. and Stapel, S. (2020). *Comparing Regional Organizations: Global Dynamics and Regional Particularities.* Bristol: Policy Press.

Parsons, C. and Springer, B. (2018). Just how wrong is the Brexiteer view of an anti-market EU? *Ask Canada or Australia-LSE Brexit Blog*, 15 October. http://eprints.lse.ac.uk/91924/.

Princen, S. (2009). *Agenda-Setting in the European Union.* Basingstoke: Palgrave Macmillan.

Ragin, C. C. (1992). "Casing" and the process of social inquiry. In C. C. Ragin and H. S. Becker (Eds.), *What is a case?: Exploring the Foundations of Social Theory* (pp. 217–226). New York: Cambridge University Press.

Riddervold, M., Trondal, J., and Newsome, A. (Eds.) (2021). *The Palgrave Handbook of EU Crises.* Cham: Springer.

Scharpf, F. W. (2010). The asymmetry of European integration, or why the EU cannot be a 'social market economy'. *Socio-Economic Review*, 8(2), 211–250. DOI: 10.1093/ser/mwp031.

Verdun, A. and Vanhercke, B. (2022). Are (some) social players entering European recovery through the Semester back door. In B. Vanhercke and S. Spasova (pp. 107–130). The European Trade Union Institute (ETUI).

Yong, E. (2022). America is zooming through the pandemic panic-neglect cycle. *The Atlantic.* https://www.theatlantic.com/health/archive/2022/03/congress-covid-spending-bill/627090/.

Chapter 9

Croatia and Slovenia

Tomislav Sokol

9.1 Introduction

The COVID-19 pandemic has severely influenced public health systems across the entire world. The enormous strain it has placed on healthcare systems globally is obvious,[1] including testing capacity; functioning of supply chains for personal protective equipment; specimen-collection swabs; supplies and equipment, including ventilators, for patients requiring hospital care; and organization of vaccines and vaccinations (Guest *et al.*, 2020, p. 1). The same holds true for Croatia and Slovenia, as is the case for other EU member states. This has resulted in a very complex set of public policy responses by the state authorities, influencing the organization and management of public health protection, but also all other aspects of peoples' lives. In Croatia, more than 16,000 people died from COVID-19 by 2022 with more than one million cases reported (Government of the Republic of Croatia, 2022a), while in Slovenia, the number of

---

[1] On the impact of COVID-19 on healthcare systems in general, see, for example, (Chang *et al.*, 2020, p. 1; Frawley *et al.*, 2021; Haldane *et al.*, 2021).

deaths stands at more than 7,000, with the number of reported cases also exceeding one million (World Health Organisation (WHO), 2022).

This chapter analyzes the impact COVID-19 pandemic has had on the public health systems of these two countries and the lessons which can be learned from this development in terms of opportunities and obstacles to the reform of healthcare systems. It is divided into three parts. First, it presents a short description of the national healthcare systems in Croatia and Slovenia, with a special emphasis on organization, regulation (including the special rules on public health crises), and coverage of the population, followed by a description of policy and regulatory responses to the pandemic which were undertaken. The second part revolves around the identified shortcomings and points of contention related to the (public) response to COVID-19, especially in the regulation of decision-making powers and the role of healthcare providers (with a focus on primary care) and vaccination. Finally, the third part evaluates the opportunities and impediments to public health reform highlighted by COVID-19 and the measures undertaken to fight the pandemic.

9.2 Public Health Responses to COVID-19

The Croatian healthcare system is regulated through acts enacted by the Croatian Parliament (Hrvatski Sabor) and statutory instruments enacted by the minister in charge of health (who also conducts supervision and monitoring), Health Insurance Institute of Croatia (HIIC), and other designated institutions. The protection of public health in Croatia is organized via a network of public health institutes, with the Croatian Institute of Public Health (CIPH) and 21 county institutes which are supervised and coordinated by the CIPH. CIPH is responsible, *inter alia*, for the collection, analysis, and publication of epidemiological data and public health statistics; health education; maintenance of health registers; and disease prevention and control (*Health Care Act*, Official Gazette 100/18 to 147/20, art. 130, 221). Every resident of Croatia is under a duty to acquire social insurance with the HIIC on one of the prescribed grounds (*Compulsory Health Insurance Act*, Official Gazette 80/13 to 98/19, art. 4, 7), which cover essentially 99% of the population (Džakula *et al.*, 2021, p. 119).

Healthcare delivery is organized through primary, secondary, and tertiary providers (*Health Care Act*, art. 29).

Primary healthcare is the first point of contact between an individual and the public healthcare system. Importantly, it fulfills a gate-keeping role for the secondary providers since access to secondary care is conditional upon obtaining a referral from a primary healthcare provider. Primary healthcare consists predominantly of private providers who enter into contracts with the HIIC (Džakula *et al.*, 2021, p. 25, 89). Secondary care providers in Croatia include primarily public providers like polyclinics and general county hospitals who enter into contracts with the HIIC. More complex tertiary health treatments are provided by a small number of clinics, clinical hospitals, and clinical hospital centers owned by the state (*Health Care Act*, arts. 32–35; Džakula *et al.*, 2021, p. 94). Finally, it is important to mention that a special body entitled Civil Protection Headquarters of the Republic of Croatia (Civil Protection Headquarters) is provided by the *Civil Protection System Act* (see Figure 9.1). It is established by the Government which also determines its composition (*Civil Protection System Act*, Official Gazette 82/15 to 20/21, arts. 22–22a). It is composed of representatives of several ministries and state institutions and is headed by the minister in charge of interior (Ordinance on the Composition, Mode of Operation and Requirements for the Nomination of the Head, Deputy and Members of the Civil Protection Headquarters, Official Gazette 126/19, art. 2).[2] During the pandemic, its mandate has been expanded to include adoption of compulsory decisions in response to the said public health threat, including those which limit fundamental rights like freedom of movement and assembly (*Act on the Protection of the Population from Infectious Diseases*, Official Gazette 79/07 to 143/21, art. 47).

The Slovenian healthcare system is regulated through acts enacted by the Slovenian Parliament (Državni zbor Slovenije) and statutory

---

[2] According to the Ordinance, art. 4–5, local and regional headquarters are established by the local self-government and are subordinated to the national Headquarters in cases of emergencies, as prescribed by the Civil Protection System Act, art. 22a. On the legal nature of the Headquarters and its measures, see also Ofak (2021, pp. 465–467).

CROATIA

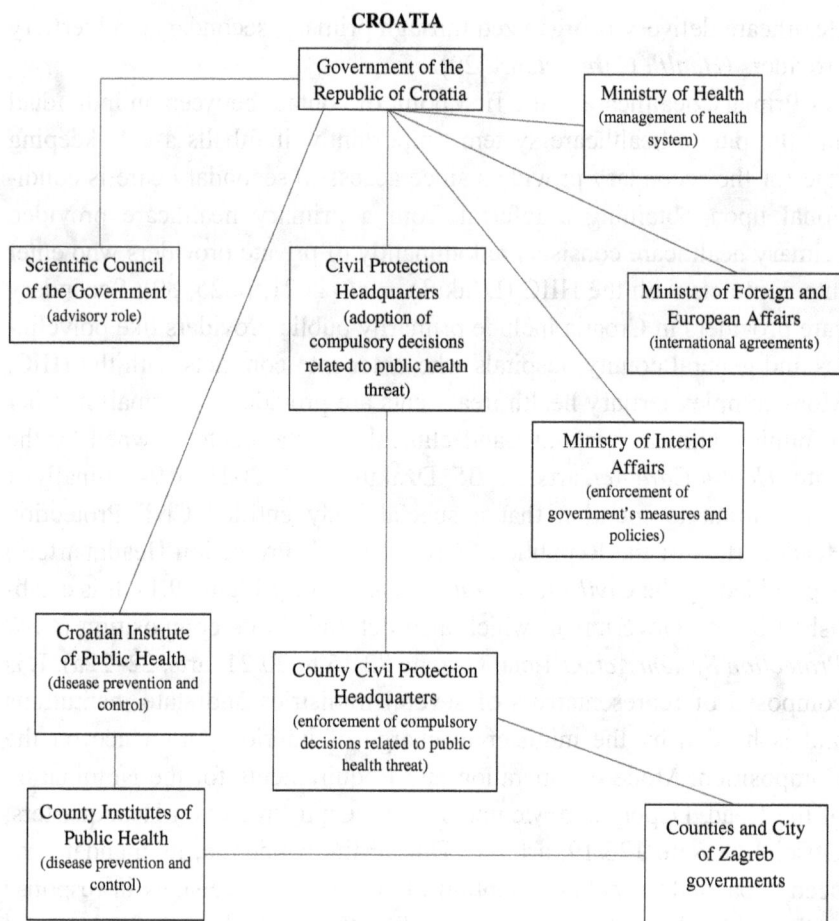

Figure 9.1. Organization of public health in Croatia.

instruments enacted by the minister in charge of health (who also conducts supervision and monitoring), Health Insurance Institute of Slovenia
(HIIS), and other designated institutions. Protection of public health in
Slovenia is organized via a network of public health institutes, with the
National Institute of Public Health of Slovenia (NIPH) and its nine
regional units (see Figure 9.2). NIPH is responsible, *inter alia*, for surveillance of communicable diseases, maintaining important health statistics
databases, health education and disease prevention and control (*Health
Services Act,* Official Gazette 9/92 to 196/21, art. 23a; Albreht *et al.*,

SLOVENIA

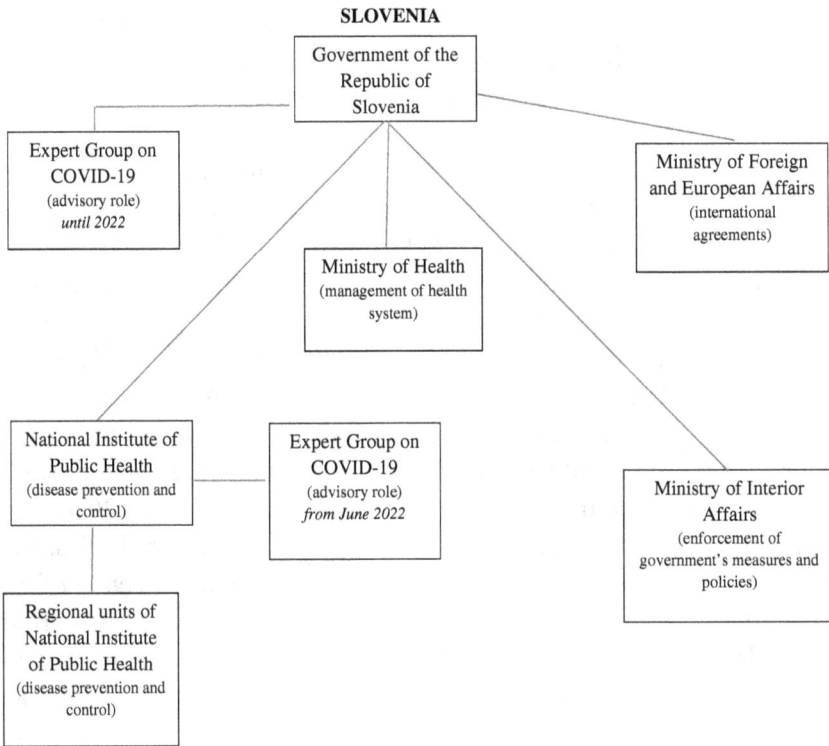

Figure 9.2.   Organization of public health in Slovenia.

2021, pp. 90–93). Prescribed categories of persons are socially insured *ex lege*, resulting in 99% of the population being covered (*Health Care and Health Insurance Act*, Official Gazette 9/92 to 43/22, art. 15; Albreht *et al.*, 2021, p. 147). Healthcare delivery is organized through primary, secondary, and tertiary providers (Health Services Act, art. 2). Primary healthcare is the first point of contact between an individual and the public healthcare system. As in Croatia, it fulfills a gate-keeping role for the secondary providers since access to secondary care is conditional upon obtaining a referral from a primary healthcare provider. Unlike in Croatia, the majority of primary care is provided by health centers owned by local communities (Albreht *et al.*, 2021, p. xxiii, 19). Secondary care providers in Slovenia include primarily state-owned providers like hospitals who enter into contracts with the HIIS and more complex tertiary health treatments are provided by a small number of state-owned clinics and specialized institutions (*Health Services Act*, arts. 13–18; Albreht *et al.*, 2021, p. 16). The power to adopt compulsory decisions under pandemics, including the ones limiting fundamental rights and freedoms, has rested with the government since the beginning of the pandemic in 2020; before that it rested with the minister in charge of health (*Communicable Diseases Act*, Official Gazette 69/95 to 178/21, art. 39).

The Croatian Minister of Health declared the epidemic on the basis of the *Act on the Protection of the Population from Infectious Diseases*, art. 2., on March 11, 2020 (Decision on Declaring the Epidemic of Disease COVID-19 caused by virus SARS-CoV-2, March 11, 2020).[3] After that, a number of measures were adopted aimed at preventing and supressing the spread of COVID-19 by the Minister of Health (for example, Decision on the Introduction of Quarantine, February 21, 2020) and (mainly) the Civil Protection Headquarters. In case of epidemics, the Headquarters is entitled, on the basis of the *Act on the Protection of the Population from Infectious Diseases*, art. 47 (as amended after the start of the epidemic in 2020), to adopt measures including, for example, establishment of quarantine; the ban on travel to countries in which there is an epidemic of a disease; the ban on the movement of persons or the restriction of such movement in infected or directly endangered areas; the prohibition or restriction of certain types of products; the prohibition of the use of equipment, facilities, and means of transport; the isolation of persons in their own home or other appropriate spaces (self-isolation); compulsory use of face-masks; and the prohibition or restriction of public gatherings as well as other special measures.

The said provision and the *Civil Protection System Act*, art. 22a were used to adopt, *inter alia*, the Decision on Limiting Social Gatherings, Retail, Services, Sporting and Cultural Events (Official Gazette 32/20), the Decision on the Ban on Leaving One's Permanent Residence in the Republic of Croatia (Official Gazette 35/20), the Decision on

---

[3] This power has since, by the subsequent amendment of the Act on the Protection of the Population from Infectious Diseases, been transferred to the government (Act Amending the Act on the Protection of the Population from Infectious Diseases, Official Gazette 47/20, art. 1).

the Necessary Measure of Compulsory Use of Face-masks or Medical Face-masks During the COVID-19 Epidemic (Official Gazette 80/20), the Decision on the Organization of Public Transport During the COVID-19 Epidemic (Official Gazette 143/20), the Decision on the Temporary Ban on Crossing the Borders of the Republic of Croatia (Official Gazette 32/20), and the Decision on the Working Hours and the Organization of Retail During the COVID-19 Epidemic (Official Gazette 51/20). The strongest restrictions were in force during spring of 2020, including the prohibition of public gatherings, limitation of freedom of movement, limitation of the right to work, property rights, closure of bars and restaurants, and the like. After that, there were several new cycles of strengthening and relaxing restrictions, but these restrictions never reached the level of the ones imposed during the first wave. Additionally, compulsory use of the EU COVID Certificate was prescribed for certain sectors when admitting service recipients, including healthcare (Decision on the Introduction of Special Safety Measure of Compulsory Testing for Health Institutions, Companies Providing Health Services and Private Health Workers When Admitting Patients, Official Gazette 105/21). All restrictions, apart from the compulsory use of face-masks in healthcare and social welfare sectors, were revoked in spring of 2022 (Government of the Republic of Croatia, 2022b). Some of the measures were challenged in front of the Constitutional Court, which is further analyzed in the following section.

In addition to restrictions, an important measure in the area of public health was obviously vaccination. The government did not opt for compulsory vaccination but left the decision on whether to get vaccinated or not to the citizens. The pressure which was exerted was related to the use of the EU COVID Certificate for certain categories of people, namely for those employed in state, public, and local administration (Decision on the Introduction of Special Safety Measure of Compulsory Testing for State, Local and Regional Officials, Persons Employed in Public Services, Companies and Institutions, Official Gazette 121/21) in November of 2021, meaning that people employed in public sector who had not received a vaccination or survived the disease needed to get tested two times a week when arriving at work. This measure was also revoked in the spring of 2022. As of July 23, 2022, 2,246,105 people were fully vaccinated (Government of the Republic of Croatia, 2022a).

In terms of the organization of the healthcare system, COVID-19 resulted in important temporary measures. Certain facilities were designated as COVID-19 facilities and special isolation units were created in several hospitals. At the same time, many elective procedures and tests were canceled, especially during periods when the inflow of new COVID-19 patients was the highest and access to all services apart from emergency treatments was severely reduced. The work of health professionals was also reorganized in a way that a large disparity arose between the workload of healthcare professionals treating COVID-19 patients and those who did not treat COVID-19 patients (Džakula *et al.*, 2022, pp. 459–461).

The government of Slovenia declared the pandemic and the end of the pandemic several times. The first time was on the basis of the *Communicable Diseases Act* (art. 7), on March 12, 2020 (Order on the Declaration of the COVID-19 Epidemic in the Territory of the Republic of Slovenia, Official Gazette 19/20).[4] It then adopted in the spring of 2020 several measures to prevent and suppress the spread of COVID-19. This included the adoption, in March 2020, of the first Decision on the Temporary General Prohibition of Movement and Public Gathering in Public Places and Areas in the Republic of Slovenia (Official Gazette 30/20), replaced by the Decision on the Temporary Prohibition of the Gathering of People at Public Meetings at Public Events and Other Events in Public Places in the Republic of Slovenia and Prohibition of Movement Outside the Municipalities (Official Gazette 38/20) and subsequent measures. Other measures like the Decision on the Temporary Prohibition of Offering and Selling Goods and Services to Consumers in the Republic of Slovenia (Official Gazette 25/20) were also adopted. The strongest restrictions were in force during spring of 2020, including the prohibition of public gatherings, limitation of freedom of movement, limitation of the right to work, property rights, closure of bars and restaurants, and so on. After that, there were several new cycles on strengthening and relaxing restrictions, but these restrictions never reached the level of the ones imposed during the first wave. All restrictions were revoked in the beginning of 2022 (Government of the Republic of Slovenia, 2022a) with

---

[4]The end of epidemic was, for the first time, declared in May 2020 (Decision on the Revocation of the COVID-19 Epidemic, Official Gazette 68/20).

an exception of use of face-masks in healthcare and social welfare sectors (Decision on the Temporary Measures for the Prevention and Control of Infectious Disease COVID-19, Official Gazette 68/22). Several of the measures adopted were also deemed unconstitutional by the Constitutional Court of Slovenia, which are analyzed in more detail in the following section.

Another important measure in the area of public health was vaccination. The government did not opt for compulsory vaccination, similarly to Croatia, but left the decision on whether to get vaccinated or not to the citizens. The pressure which was exerted concerned the use of the EU COVID Certificate for employed and self-employed persons. An additional pressure was imposed on persons employed in state administration since it was prescribed that employees in the bodies of the state administration had to fulfill the recovered-vaccinated requirement to perform tasks at their workplace on the premises of the employer or on the premises of another body of the state administration (Decision on the Manners of Complying with the Recovered-Vaccinated-Tested Requirement to Contain the Spread of Infection with the SARS-CoV-2 Virus Official Gazette 147/21). This was also revoked in the first half of 2022. The provision of the said decision related to persons employed in state administration was also deemed unconstitutional, which is further analyzed in the following section. As of July 23, 2022, 1,205,608 people were fully vaccinated (WHO, 2022).

Relating to the organization of the healthcare system, the pandemic has resulted in the focus of the healthcare system on COVID-19 treatment, resulting in the suspension of many elective health services (Albreht *et al.*, 2021, p. 148). In the area of oncology, for instance, significant drops in first oncological referrals, first outpatient visits, mammograms, x-rays, and ultra-sounds during the beginning of the crisis in 2020 were reported, pointing to a delay in treatment and diagnosis of cancer for some patients during the COVID-19 epidemic in Slovenia (Zadnik *et al.*, 2020, p. 334).

9.3 Problems Related to the Public Health Responses to COVID-19

There has been substantial criticism (as well as legal challenges) regarding how the Croatian authorities have handled the COVID-19 epidemic. It has been stated in the literature, for example, that "(A)lmost all decisions became politically influenced, and the interventions proposed by the experts were also considered political choices" and "information provided by national authorities became vague, unclear, and ambiguous, and more and more concerns were raised about the accuracy of official information and the accountability of national authorities. The resulting politicization of COVID-19, as well as politicians not being up to the task and putting their interests first, undermined public trust in public health advice and interventions" (Džakula *et al.*, 2022, p. 461). The decision to relax measures in the summer of 2020 was stated to be the result of "the increasing public tensions arising from the restrictive measures and their negative effects on the economy, along with the upcoming tourist season" (Džakula *et al.*, 2022, p. 459). It is true that measures in Croatia were relaxed in both summers of 2020 and 2021 which can be explained by declining numbers of infected persons but also the need to maintain the tourist season as a major source of state income. The explanation given by Prime Minister Plenković on several occasions has been that the government needs to balance public health considerations with economic and broader societal ones (Government of the Republic of Croatia, 2020a, 2020b). It is also important to note that the ruling majority decided to hold general elections at the beginning of July 2020 when the measures were relaxed, a few months before the constitutional end of the mandate. The ruling Croatian Democratic Union (HDZ) won 66 out of 151 seats and quickly formed a new ruling majority with the same center partners as before. The way it handled the epidemic in its initial stage (especially the relaxation of measures) definitely influenced the outcome, which can be seen from the fact that Minister of Health Vili Beroš, not well known to the public before the COVID-19 outbreak, won more preferential votes (35.678) than Prime Minister Plenković who is also the head of HDZ (State Electoral Commission of the Republic of Croatia, 2020).

There were several legal challenges against government measures in front of the Constitutional Court, primarily focused on the authority of the Civil Protection Headquarters to adopt measures restricting fundamental rights (to free movement, assembly, and so on) and the scope of these measures. The main question was whether the measures aimed at tackling COVID-19 should be based on art. 16 or art. 17 of the Constitution.

According to art. 16, freedoms and rights may only be restricted by law in order to protect the freedoms and rights of others, public morals, the legal order, and health with such restrictions having to be proportionate to the nature of the need for such restriction in each individual case. According to art. 17, individual constitutionally guaranteed rights and freedoms may be restricted, *inter alia*, in the event of a natural disaster, with the decision having to be made by a two-thirds majority of all Members of Parliament or, if the Parliament is unable to convene, at the proposal of the government, by the President of the Republic. Hence, the application of art. 17 would have meant that consent of the main opposition parties (dominated by the center-left) would have been required for adopting legislation relating to COVID-19. Since the President of the Republic also comes from a center-left political background, the potential inability to convene the Parliament would have also made opposition unavoidable in case of application of art. 17.

Since the amendments to the relevant *Civil Protection System Act* and *Act on the Protection of the Population from Infectious Diseases*, giving the Headquarters the power to make binding decisions related to COVID-19, were enacted on the basis of art. 16, these amendments were challenged and ultimately settled by the Constitutional Court. The Court stated that the Parliament may, in exercising its legislative power when restricting certain human rights and freedoms, act on the basis of two constitutional grounds, art. 16 and art. 17. The Court held that the decision on whether the public health measures to combat the COVID-19 epidemic will be taken either by the application of art. 16 or art. 17 is in the exclusive domain of Parliament since the Constitution itself gave this alternative to Parliament as a legislative body. The Court thus stated that it is not authorized to order Parliament which of the two constitutional options to choose. Therefore, the fact that the impugned laws (and measures) were not enacted on the basis of art.17 did not in itself make those laws unconstitutional. Furthermore, the Court held that decisions enacted by the Headquarters can be subject to Constitutional Court review because they represent "other regulations" prescribed by art. 125 of the Constitutions which are capable of being subject to that review (U-I-1372/2020, Constitutional Court of the Republic of Croatia, September 14, 2020). Several decisions made by the Headquarters were indeed challenged in front of the Court, but the Court was generally reluctant to deem them unconstitutional, with very few exceptions.[5] The approach of the Constitutional Court was severely criticized by the President of the Republic who stated that the Court got scared and that it is a political body making political decisions (President of the Republic of Croatia, 2020).

Another problem visible in Croatia relating to COVID-19 concerns vaccination. As noted in the previous section, less than 60% of the entire population was vaccinated: one of the lowest percentages in the European Union (European Centre for Disease Prevention and Control, 2022). Even though there is a need for additional studies, some of the reasons highlighted by the studies already carried out show that the strongest reason for hesitation was perceived low danger of COVID-19 infection. It has been suggested in the literature that previous public communication about the dangers and the course of the pandemic has failed since a significant part of the population refused to accept the severity of the disease. Some of the reasons mentioned include "dissonant tones between different actors in the media and in the public about the suitability of epidemiological measures and the need for vaccination. Public discourse also primarily emphasized certain groups as being vulnerable (older people and persons with existing health conditions). This may have contributed to the failure of previous public communication by constructing a low risk perception in certain social groups." It has been stated that the narrative of emphasizing social solidarity (namely, toward the elderly) was not successful within certain social groups. Finally, distrust toward institutions and, to a large extent, scientists has also been mentioned as an important factor to be considered (Bagić *et al.*, 2022, pp. 95–96).

---

[5] For example, the Constitutional Court upheld the decision to prescribe compulsory use of EU COVID Certificate for persons employed in state, public, and local administration, with the exception of the provision which gave the higher education institutions the possibility to decide the opposite (U-II-7149/2021, Constitutional Court of the Republic of Croatia, February 15, 2022). Also, the Court found, *post festum*, the restriction of Sunday trading to be unconstitutional. See U-II-2379/2020, Constitutional Court of the Republic of Croatia, September 14, 2020. It was stated in the literature that the latter represents the "single significant finding of unconstitutionality" in the jurisprudence by the Court (Barić and Miloš, 2022, p. 444).

Strong opposition to some of the public health measures was also visible within the healthcare system. That opposition was not necessarily caused by the measures themselves but had more to do with the role the authorities (Ministry of Health) envisaged for some of the actors within the system for implementation of the measures. This mainly applies to primary healthcare providers. A concrete example here is what arose at the beginning of 2022, when the Ministry of Health decided that rapid antigen tests would be accepted as proof of infection with SARS-CoV-2 virus and that the tests would be administered by all primary healthcare providers contracted by HIIC (Ministry of Health of the Republic of Croatia, 2022). This decision caused a strong backlash among the primary healthcare providers, whose representatives stated that they are overstretched, lacking resources to carry out such a task and that they have not received any instructions or organizational support from the Ministry (*Croatian Television*, 2022). When the testing began, there was a lot of organizational and technical problems with its implementation (*NOVA TV*, 2022). Also, it should be mentioned that a decision by the Ministry that primary care providers should promote and carry out vaccination among the elderly was challenged in front of the Constitutional Court. The decision by the Court is important since it clearly stated that private primary healthcare providers contracted by HIIC are under a duty to carry out tasks related to protection of public health in case of emergencies, like epidemics. The Court's reasoning was based on art. 197 of the Health Care Act, which empowers the minister in charge of health to adopt extraordinary measures, including the ones relating to the organization of work of private primary healthcare providers who are contracted by HIIC. The decision of the Minister was finally upheld (U-II-6278/2021, Constitutional Court of the Republic of Croatia, April 12, 2022).

When one speaks of the scientific basis of the relevant decision-making, it should be noted that the decisions made during the pandemic were essentially policy decisions which took into account various factors, including not just epidemiology and virology but also economy (addressed by Croatian Prime Minister Plenković in a statement cited above), public security, mental health of the population, etc. Hence, there is no overwhelming authority of one scientific field or authority which has to be respected but different points of view which needed to be taken into account.

In Croatia, the crucial body within the system, the Civil Protection Headquarters, as noted earlier, consists of representatives of a wide array of state institutions, including the CIPH and the Croatian Institute of Emergency Medicine (Decision on the Nomination of a Member of the Civil Protection Headquarters, Official Gazette 37/20), which should represent the point of view of medical science within the process. All the decisions of the Headquarters have been published in the Official Gazette and the official website and regular press conferences were held. It is important to note that, at first, these decisions generally did not contain reasoning or explanation, which made it very hard to determine which scientific evidence was used by the Headquarters, especially when changing its practice by reversing previous decisions. However, this did change, as the Constitutional Court declared in December 2021 that the Civil Protection Headquarters decisions should contain reasoning, for the sake of transparency and especially to make sure that the principle of proportionality is respected (U-I-5781/2021, Constitutional Court of the Republic of Croatia, December 21, 2021). Therefore, the decisions made since the start of 2022 contained reasoning, making the system much clearer and more transparent in terms of rationale used by the Headquarters. Importantly, the decisions now often contain references to the situation and practices in other European countries making it easier to make the relevant comparisons. A good example of a rather elaborate reasoning is the Decision on the Necessary Epidemiological Measure of Use of Face-masks or Medical Face-masks (Official Gazette 44/22) which limited the categories of persons required to wear face-masks, by making references to the decisions already made in other EU member states (Belgium, Germany, and Scandinavian countries) and third countries (Israel and the UK), but also to the concrete numbers of vaccinated and newly infected persons. The evolving situation with the Omicron variant made it possible to change the practice and revoke many restrictions which were previously in force.

Another body created because of the pandemic is the Scientific Council of the Government, chaired by the Prime Minister. The Council, consisting of 15 members, was established in March 2020 on the basis of the *Government of the Republic of Croatia Act* (Official Gazette 150/11 to 80/22, art. 23) to provide a forum for exchanging opinions between the renowned scientists and the policymakers on the fight against COVID-19 (Government of the Republic of Croatia, 2020c; *Net*, 2020). This body does not have power to adopt decisions or recommendations but has contracted much public attention due to public statements by individual members reflecting their different positions on the measures adopted against COVID-19. One member was removed from the Council after public speculations about his statements downplaying the benefits of vaccination and other disagreements with the majority of the Council members (Jutarnji list, 2021) and calling for public demonstration against the use of EU COVID Certificates (Index, 2021). Thus, it can be stated that the plurality of opinions was allowed to a large degree but not to an extent which was considered to jeopardize public health and security.

As in Croatia, there has been considerable criticism of (and legal challenges to) the way in which Slovenian authorities have handled the COVID-19 epidemic. Those criticizing the center-right government, which took office in the beginning of the pandemic, were saying the government was tackling the epidemic wrongly and unsuccessfully by, for example, forcing people to receive vaccination and discriminating against persons who had not been vaccinated, as well as by introducing measures that, according to these persons, unduly restricted their fundamental rights. They particularly accused the government of "destroying democracy and the rule of law and attacking independent journalism" (Flander, 2022, p. 28). Additionally, they accused the government of "hate policies against ideological and political opponents, xenophobia and discrimination against refugees, corruption" (Flander, 2022, p. 28) and similar sentiments. The overall public pressure on the government relating to the direction in which the country was going was argued to have been a major factor in the ruling coalition's electoral loss in 2022 (*Washington Post*, 2022), where a newly formed Freedom Movement (GS) won and easily formed a new government (State Election Commission of the Republic of Slovenia, 2022).

One of the political battlegrounds was the jurisprudence of the Constitutional Court. The first important decision concerned the prohibition of movement outside the municipality of one's permanent or temporary residence introduced in early 2020. In this early case, the Court upheld the measure, since it deemed it appropriate for achieving the pursued objective because there existed the requisite probability that — according to the data available at the time of the adoption of the challenged measure — it could have contributed toward slowing down or reducing the spread of COVID-19, primarily by reducing the number of contacts between those persons living in areas with a higher number of infections and those persons living in areas with a lower number of infections. The Court also deemed it necessary for achieving its objective since previously adopted measures (like suspension of public transport and general prohibition of public gatherings) were not considered enough to prevent the spread of infection to such an extent that adequate healthcare could be provided to every COVID-19 patient. Finally, the Court conducted a proportionality test *stricto sensu* and concluded that "the demonstrated level of probability of a positive impact of the measure on the protection of human health and life outweighed the interference with the freedom of movement". The fact that several exceptions to the prohibition were prescribed played an important role in the Court's assessment (U-I-83/20, Constitutional Court of the Republic of Slovenia, August 27, 2020).

After this initial period,[6] the Constitutional Court has proven to be less supportive of the government's legal arguments, especially related to the power of the government itself to adopt measures limiting fundamental rights in Slovenia, quite the opposite to the Croatian situation. The crucial decision was made in relation to the *Communicable Diseases Act* (art. 39 par. 2 and 3) which empowered the government to restrict or prohibit the movement in infected or directly endangered areas and prohibit gathering of people in public places in order to prevent the introduction and spread of a communicable disease if the said objective cannot be accomplished by other measures prescribed by the *Communicable Diseases Act*. Several public health measures adopted by the government on the basis of the said provisions were also challenged (U-I-79/20, Constitutional Court of the Republic of Slovenia, May 13, 2021).

---

[6] The Court also refused to suspend the implementation of a decision imposing a curfew (U-I-426/20, Constitutional Court of the Republic of Slovenia, December 21, 2020) until the final judgment was made.

The Court first explained the main principles which needed to be taken into account when assessing the possibilities to empower government to make decisions limiting fundamental rights. It stated that, whenever the legislature empowers the executive to adopt a statutory instrument implementing legislation, it must first by itself clearly prescribe the content that is to be the subject of the statutory instrument and determine the guidelines and framework for regulating the content in more detail by way of a statutory instrument. There can be no blanket empowerment of the executive, especially in cases dealing with fundamental rights. Thus, a general act which directly interferes with fundamental rights of an indeterminate number of individuals can only be enacted in a form of a law. In case of restrictions on free movement and the right of association and assembly of people in order to prevent the spread of a communicable disease, the legislature may exceptionally leave it to the executive to prescribe measures by which these rights and freedoms are directly curtailed. However, the law must precisely determine the purpose of these measures (or the purpose must be clearly evident therefrom), the scope, admissible types and conditions concerning the restriction of the freedom of movement and of the right of association and assembly and association, as well as contain other appropriate safeguards against the arbitrary restriction of fundamental human rights (U-I-79/20, Constitutional Court of the Republic of Slovenia, May 13, 2021).

According to the Court, the challenged provisions of the *Communicable Diseases Act* did not fulfill the aforementioned constitutional requirements, since they allowed the government to choose, in a discretionary manner, the scope, types, and duration of restrictions, which curtailed the freedom of movement of (possibly all) residents in the territory of Slovenia. The legislature also gives autonomy to the government

> to freely assess, throughout the entire period while the threat of the spread of the communicable disease lasts, in which instances, for how long, and in how extensive an area in the state it will prohibit the gathering of people in those public places where, according to the Government's assessment, there exists a heightened risk of spreading the communicable disease. The regulation also lacks safeguards that could limit the discretion of the Government, such as the duty to consult or cooperate with the expert community and to inform the public of the circumstances and opinions of

experts that are important for deciding on such measures (U-I-79/20, Constitutional Court of the Republic of Slovenia, May 13, 2021).

On basis of these findings, the Court decided that the *Communicable Diseases Act* (art. 39 par. 2 and 3) was contrary to the constitution (arts. 34 and 42) which prescribes that freedom of movement and the right of assembly and association may be limited by law and ordered that the legislator prescribe new relevant rules within 2 months from the publication of its decision in the Official Gazette. At the same time, it decided that the unconstitutional provisions of the *Communicable Diseases Act* will continue to apply until the new provisions were adopted. The challenged government decisions were also deemed to be unconstitutional, but the government order declaring the epidemic was upheld (U-I-79/20, Constitutional Court of the Republic of Slovenia, May 13, 2021).[7]

As in Croatia, another problem visible in Slovenia relating to COVID-19 concerned vaccination. As noted in the previous section, less than 60% of the entire population is vaccinated, one of the lowest percentages in the European Union and just a fraction (two percentage points) above the Croatian result (European Centre for Disease Prevention and Control, 2022). Even though there is a necessity for additional studies, some of the reasons highlighted by the studies already carried out show that important factors of hesitation related to the unstable political situation, trust in alternative sources, and distrust in government while, obviously, people having more trust in official sources of information, such as public health institutions and experts, are more likely to get vaccinated. Additionally, open-ended question responses which were part of the relevant studies revealed that vaccine hesitancy was clearly related to the rapid vaccine development and scepticism about its efficiency (Petravić *et al.*, 2021, pp. 12–13).

---

[7] The Court made a similar decision relating to Communicable Diseases Act, art. 39 par. 4 (U-I-155/20, Constitutional Court of the Republic of Slovenia, October 7, 2021) where it held that the legislature granted the government a very wide margin of discretion to determine the scope and duration of the measures by which business activities and the right to work of all natural persons and legal entities on the territory of the Slovenia can be curtailed. Thus, Communicable Diseases Act, art. 39 par. 4 was contrary to the freedom of work determined by Constitution art. 49 and free economic initiative prescribed by Constitution art. 74.

It should be noted that the Constitutional Court held that a decision on the use of EU COVID Certificates related to persons employed in state administration was not adopted in conformity with the statutory requirements prescribed by the *Communicable Diseases Act* art. 22 (in conjunction with art. 25) for the determination of the vaccination of employees. Thus, it decided that the said provisions of the decision were inconsistent with the Constitution (art. 120) which prescribes that the executive performs its activities on the basis of the Constitution and laws. The Court did not decide whether the assessed measure — had it been adopted on the correct statutory basis — would have been constitutionally admissible from the viewpoint of the principle of proportionality and the principle of equality before the law (U-I-210/21, Constitutional Court of the Republic of Slovenia, November 29, 2021), for some patients during the COVID-19 epidemic in Slovenia (Zadnik *et al.*, 2020, p. 334).

As far as the use of scientific evidence goes, it should be emphasized that decisions on fighting COVID-19 were made by the government itself and published in the Official Gazette. These decisions generally did not contain reasoning, which made it very hard to determine which scientific evidence was used by the government, especially when changing its practice by reversing previous decisions. According to the Government of the Republic of Slovenia Act (Official Gazette 24/05 to 163/22, art. 20), the National Security Council is the government's body responsible for making recommendations and proposals to the government in times of crises but also for coordination. However, at the start of the pandemic, coordination and decision-making were completely taken over by the government itself. Additionally, to advise the government, the Expert Group on COVID-19 was created, consisting of scientific and medical experts providing advice to the relevant institutions on issues related to the COVID-19 pandemic; "their task was to prepare opinions and proposals for measures, verify their justification, and propose their application, amendment or abolition, and monitor the epidemiological situation" (Government of the Republic of Slovenia, 2020a; Ferlin *et al.*, 2021, pp. 640–641).[8]

After revocation of the restrictions in 2022, the Expert Group was dissolved and its roles taken over by NIPH, which created its own expert

---

[8] Before that, the Crisis Management Headquarters was created but abolished just a few days later (Government of the Republic of Slovenia, 2020b; Ferlin *et al.*, 2021, p. 647).

group in June 2022 (Government of the Republic of Slovenia, 2022b; NIPH, 2022). Interestingly enough, the NIPH expert group is now led by an epidemiologist who left the government's Expert Group two times because its decisions were, in his opinion, contrary to NIPH opinion and standard epidemiological protocols (Dnevnik, 2022). It can be stated that the system in Slovenia during the pandemic tried to achieve clarity and transparency in terms of scientific evidence used and the rationale behind the decisions made by the government mostly by communicating with the general public through press conferences and other channels such as Twitter (Ferlin *et al.*, 2021, pp. 642–643) and the official website. It has been stated in the literature, however, that the restrictive measures have been communicated in an authoritarian way, supported with little research to prove their effectiveness (Ferlin *et al.*, 2021, p. 645). Centralization of the decision-making within the government itself and lack of publicly transparent reasoning also made it hard to challenge the decisions in a public debate.

9.4 Barriers and Opportunities for Public Health Reform

COVID-19 has highlighted the need to conduct public healthcare system reforms in several areas in Croatia and Slovenia, as demonstrated in the previous section. Organization and management of the system are particularly important, especially in the need to better utilize capacities in the hospital sector; increase the number of healthcare professionals (especially in the primary sector), better balance their workload, improve the salary system and other working conditions; tackle long waiting times in certain areas (Albreht *et al.*, 2021, pp. 127–142; Džakula *et al.*, 2021, pp. 107–116; U-I-25/22, Constitutional Court of the Republic of Slovenia, March 17, 2022) which have increased during the pandemic due to the focus of the healthcare systems on COVID-19; and strengthen digitalization. In areas like digitalization, the pandemic has resulted in strong improvements (even though the processes started before COVID-19; see, for example, Albreht *et al.*, 2021, pp. 78–80; Džakula *et al.*, 2021, pp. 136), but there are many other problems which remain in need of improvement. Problems of defining the role of primary care professionals (especially private) during public health crisis, coupled with their overall deficit (Ombudsman of the Republic of Croatia, 2022) and the general fragmentation and underutilization of primary care services (Džakula *et al.*, 2021, p. 135), have been particularly visible in Croatia.

COVID-19 has highlighted important obstacles to healthcare system reform. One of those is the tendency to maintain the status quo within the system. This was clearly visible during the confrontation between the Croatian Minister of Health and associations of primary care providers over their duties within the overall effort of fighting the epidemic. It can be argued that this conflict was exacerbated by the fact that most primary care providers in Croatia are private ones contracted by the HIIC, which makes them less answerable to orders from the government and more inclined to resist additional workload caused by public health crisis. The opposition to reform was even more clearly manifested by the fact that the representatives of the primary care providers' association left (in June 2022) the working group established by the Minister of Health to prepare healthcare reform. The reason they stated for such behavior was that they opposed the proposal of the Ministry to impose additional obligations on primary care providers of working in emergency medicine (Index, 2022).

The overall political situation in both Croatia and Slovenia can be seen also as not contributing to the reform potential. First, both countries employ a proportional system of electing members of national parliaments (Act on the Election of Members of Croatian Parliament, Official Gazette 116/99 to 98/19, art. 38; National Assembly Election Act, Official Gazette 44/92 to 29/21, art. 92), and such system tends to lead to broad and fragmented coalitions (like in Slovenia during the previous center-right government), which may be less able to change existing policies and initiate reforms than single-party governments (Carey & Hix, 2011, p. 384).

Additionally, the opposition parties especially in Croatia failed to come up with concrete systematic proposals of overall healthcare reform but were almost completely focused on criticizing the government's public health responses to COVID-19, trying to gain political points by advocating more freedom and less restrictive measures. For example, the most important public health initiative of the opposition in Croatia was the support of some opposition parties for conducting a referendum on the public health responses to COVID-19. It should be mentioned here that the Croatian Parliament may call a referendum on any proposal to amend the

Constitution of the Republic of Croatia, act, or any other issue falling within its purview. The Croatian Parliament must call a referendum when so requested by 10% of the total electorate of the Republic of Croatia (Constitution of the Republic of Croatia, Official Gazette 56/90 to 5/14, art. 87). An initiative was organized in 2021 to gather support to obtain two objectives. The first initiative aimed at amending art. 17 of the Constitution so that the pandemic was added to the list of emergencies during which the Parliament, by a two-thirds majority of all Members, could restrict constitutionally guaranteed rights and freedoms. The second initiative aimed at amending the *Act on the Protection of the Population from Infectious Diseases* (art. 47) in a way that the decisions on limiting fundamental rights would have to be made only by the Parliament, instead of the Civil Protection Headquarters. It can be seen here that the main goal of the opposition was to take away the power to make policy decisions from the government (and ruling coalition). The Constitutional Court declared both initiatives to be unconstitutional. Relating to the first one, the Court concluded that the proposed referendum question itself was not in line with the objective of always requiring a two-thirds majority of all Members of Parliament for restricting constitutionally guaranteed rights and freedoms since the way in which it was phrased would still allow the ruling majority to choose whether art. 16 or art. 17 would be used. Thus, the question was contrary to the rule of law prescribed by art. 3. of the Constitution (U-VIIR-2180/2022, Constitutional Court of the Republic of Croatia, May 16, 2022). Relating to the second initiative, the Court held that it aimed at transferring inherently executive powers to the legislature, thereby violating the division of powers prescribed by the Constitution and the principle of the rule of law (U-VIIR-2181/2022, Constitutional Court of the Republic of Croatia, May 16, 2022).

If one looks at the reform proposals from the main opposition parties in Croatia and in Slovenia (now in power in Slovenia after the 2022 elections), it can be seen that they more or less correctly identified certain problems within the healthcare system. Social Democratic Party of Croatia (SDP) produced an 11-page document on the key principles for future reform. These include better access to healthcare, stronger incentives for better performance of the workforce, more efficient organization and management of the system, better equipment and infrastructure (including investments into the omnipresent digitalization), and financial sustainability (Social Democratic Party of the Republic of Croatia, 2022). The electoral program of the new main ruling party in the Slovenia Freedom Movement (GS) headed by Prime Minister Golob, which dominates the coalition in power, is even less detailed on healthcare than the Croatian SDP. The healthcare part is placed at the very end of the overall 24-page program and mentions, *inter alia*, better organization of working time for healthcare workers, better accessibility and reduction of waiting times, better organization of the system, and digitalization (Freedom Movement, 2022). It has also published a more detailed program covering the period until 2030 which contains around 20 pages on healthcare, crucially setting a target of 10% of GDP spending for public health system by 2030 (Freedom Movement 2022b). It can be argued here that the opposition especially in Croatia has not shown capacity for preparing serious reforms of the national healthcare systems and engaging the national governments on this but only for limiting (with more or less success) the activities of the national governments.

Closely intertwined with the political situation, constitutional jurisprudence should also be mentioned as an important factor relating to potential reforms. Here it should be noted that a major role in curtailing the government's power to adopt concrete measures in Slovenia was played by the Constitutional Court, while in Croatia the Constitutional Court was more benevolent toward the government's power to act in the area of public health. This in itself could be seen as an obstacle to the government's possibilities for reforming Slovenian healthcare system, but it is hard to conclude whether such a restrictive approach by the Court was a product of specific circumstances (a ruling coalition heavily criticized from all directions about its fundamental rights track-record) or a more general approach of limiting the power of the executive in the future.

In any case, the analysis has shown that two important legislative changes in Croatia and Slovenia would be required if one wanted to have more clarity and legal certainty within the system. First, a much clearer set of statutory rules regarding the public health obligations of private primary care providers than the ones prescribed by *Health Care Act* (art. 197) is necessary so that potential future disputes are avoided. The same held true for amending the *Communicable Diseases Act* (art. 39) in Slovenia as a consequence of the jurisprudence of the Slovenian Constitutional Court. The new provisions should have been formulated in a way which adheres to the principles set by the Slovenian Constitutional Court: the law must precisely determine the purpose of these measures, the admissible scope, types, and conditions concerning the restriction of the fundamental freedoms in question, and must also contain other necessary safeguards against the arbitrary restriction of the said rights. This was finally accomplished in October 2022 when the amending act enacted by the new ruling majority entered into force (*Act Amending the Communicable Diseases Act*, Official Gazette 125/22, art. 1).

If one looks at opportunities for public health reform in Croatia and Slovenia, one can observe that the list is rather shorter than the list of obstacles. Politically, the main positive thing is that in both countries the elections in 2020 and 2022 resulted in a more overwhelming victory for one party than at any time in the last 20 years. Even though they require coalition partners, the political support and the mandate they received provide them with a much stronger opportunity to make important changes in the healthcare systems than the previous leading parties in power had. This is particularly important since some of the reforms, like better organization of the system, could entail unpopular moves like closing of certain unsustainable local hospital wards and, to do that, a strong electoral mandate is required. In Croatia, after 2 years having passed since the elections, comprehensive reform documents were revealed to the public in the end of 2022 which are described in the following. Since 2024 will be a year of elections, it seems that the autumn and winter of 2022/2023 represent the last opportunity in Croatia to enact a concrete reform that could actually get implemented before the electoral populism takes over.

Finally, the influence of the European Union, through its provision of funding via the Recovery and Resilience Facility, conditioned by carrying out national structural reforms, should also be mentioned. Both Croatian and Slovenian plans for spending the money provided by the EU have been approved by the European Commission (European Commission, 2022). In the area of healthcare, Croatia has dedicated an allocation of around 340 million EUR to improving its healthcare system with a general aim of enabling sustainability, efficiency, quality, and availability of healthcare. When one speaks of reforms, strengthening the long-term financial sustainability of the healthcare system, by assuring joint procurement purchasing for national health facilities, should be mentioned. Next, it is provided that the long-term sustainability of health services and the efficient use of existing human resources will be addressed through the reorganization and restructuring of essential health services via, for example, the functional integration of hospitals and the strengthening of day hospitals at both secondary and tertiary levels, and the development of regional centers of excellence. Also, a new care model for patients concerning crucial health challenges like cancer will be developed. Investments to ensure quality and access to healthcare will focus on developing harmonized standards and fostering the uptake of modern healthcare treatments through such strategies as purchasing modern medical equipment and investing into overall infrastructure. It is also envisaged to promote full territorial availability of primary healthcare, thus improving the resilience and preparedness of the healthcare system while also increasing the quality of life in remote, rural, and insular areas. Furthermore, the introduction of strategic management of the health workforce shows the emphasis placed on the human capital aspect of healthcare by providing specialized medical staff training and increasing number of healthcare professionals. Of course, investments in digitalization are provided to enable remote healthcare services and better utilization of limited resources and treatment capacity (Government of the Republic of Croatia, 2021, pp. 983–1090).

This influence of these EU funding possibilities has significantly contributed to the actual reform proposed by the government and to the passing of the first reading in the Parliament at the end of 2022. It consists of the amendments to two basic laws regulating healthcare in Croatia: the *Health Care Act* and the *Compulsory Health Insurance Act*. One of the main reforms consists of transferring the ownership of the secondary care providers from counties to the state (Bill *Amending the Health Care Act*, art. 19) the purpose of which is to strengthen the long-term financial sustainability of the healthcare system, by assuring joint procurement purchasing, as stated in the national recovery and resilience plan. Financial sustainability is addressed also by doubling the maximum amount of co-payment (the percentage of the treatment cost the patients have to pay out of their own pocket) prescribed by law (Bill *Amending the Compulsory Health Insurance Act*, art. 8). Also, principles of integration and quality are defined (Bill *Amending the Health Care Act*, arts. 4–6) in order to facilitate functional integration of hospitals and more efficient use of limited resources and to increase the quality of healthcare provision. The possibility of creating centers of excellence is expanded to all hospitals (Bill *Amending the Health Care Act*, art. 36). Availability is addressed by establishing a legal basis for the creation of mobile pharmacies (Bill *Amending the Health Care Act*, art. 10) in less developed parts of the country (like remote and rural areas) where access to medicines represents a problem. Availability of primary care is tackled by prescribing that there can be one primary healthcare center per county and defining health services provided by primary healthcare centers in a bit more detail (Bill *Amending the Health Care Act*, arts. 30–31).

Furthermore, the problem of accessibility due to waiting lists is addressed by enabling private providers to be contracted by HIIC (Bill *Amending the Compulsory Health Insurance Act*, art. 35) and by empowering the minister in charge of health to determine maximum waiting times (Bill Amending the Health Care Act, art. 7). On basis of the lesson learned from COVID-19, the power of CIPH to coordinate county public health institutes in emergency situations is explicitly prescribed (Bill *Amending the Health Care Act*, art. 42). Finally, the issue of health workforce is addressed in several provisions, including the ones enabling health workers to work up until the age of 68 and even beyond that (Bill *Amending the Health Care Act*, art. 48), enabling counties to provide incentives for healthcare professionals to work in their territory (Bill Amending the Health Care Act, art. 2) and the new program of including medical doctors without (yet) specialization into the healthcare system (Bill Amending the Health Care Act, art. 52).

In Slovenia, an allocation of EU resources for healthcare in the amount of around 225 million EUR is provided, with an overarching aim of ensuring financial sustainability as well as accessibility and quality of the healthcare system. Structural reforms include a clearer definition of statutory health insurance rights and restructuring of the complementary health insurance, improving the system of incentives (including salaries and general working conditions) for healthcare professionals, and better organization of the system. Concrete investments will focus on training of healthcare workers to address shortages (especially in the area of primary care) by modernizing the secondary professional education in the area of health services and allowing more enrollments in the medical faculties. Also, investments related to improving the healthcare infrastructure (especially concerning the more efficient treatment of communicable diseases) are provided along with those aimed at further promoting digitalization of the system and better organization aimed at improving the accessibility of healthcare services (Government of the Republic of Slovenia, 2021, pp. 395–418). How the implementation of all this will work in practice, especially taking into account the results of recent elections in Slovenia, remains to be seen.

Several legal acts have been adopted adhering to the parts of the national recovery and resilience plan. The main emphasis has been placed on strengthening accessibility by reducing waiting lists and providing additional incentives for healthcare professionals. Relating to workforce, healthcare professionals working directly with COVID-19 patients within the public health system are now entitled to a salary supplement in the maximum gross amount of 900 EUR a month (*Act on the Emergency Measures to Contain the Spread and Mitigate the Consequences of the Infectious COVID-19 Disease in the Field of Health Care*, Official Gazette 141/22, art. 36). Furthermore, a salary supplement for medical doctors starting with a specialization in family medicine (primary care) in 2023 has been prescribed in the gross amount of 1,000 EUR a month (*Act on the Emergency Measures to Contain the Spread and Mitigate the Consequences of the Infectious COVID-19 Disease in the Field of Health Care*, art. 35). It has also been declared that 70 additional specializations in clinical psychology will be funded from the state budget in 2023 and 2024 (*Act on the Emergency Measures to Contain the Spread and Mitigate the Consequences of the Infectious COVID-19 Disease in the Field of Health Care*, art. 34). Additional rules have also been enacted by the government, determining the amounts of supplements for primary health-care professionals in less developed municipalities and for healthcare professionals with an increased workload in primary care (Regulation Determining the Amount of Supplement for Special Working Conditions in the Territory of Less Developed Municipalities, Official Gazette 132/22 and Regulation Determining the Amount of Supplement for Increased Workload for Hazardous Work and the Number of Additional Health Care Staff, Official Gazette 132/22).

Concerning access to healthcare, outpatient clinics for patients without a selected personal general practitioner will be established in order to enable accessibility to health service to all insured persons (*Act on the Emergency Measures to Contain the Spread and Mitigate the Consequences of the Infectious COVID-19 Disease in the Field of Health Care*, art. 18). Special measures to reduce waiting times have also been prescribed, including easier and faster conducting of payments for healthcare delivered, enabling private providers to be contracted by HIIS, and additional payments for healthcare professionals who are prepared to provide more services, including outside their regular hours (*Act on the Emergency Measures to Contain the Spread and Mitigate the Consequences of the Infectious COVID-19 Disease in the Field of Health Care*, art. 14). According to Prime Minister Golob, the real structural reform should be enacted in 2023 and fully implemented in 2024, while the current actions of the government can be described as "extinguishing fires" (*24ur*, 2022).

It can be seen that the strong political mandate coupled with incentives provided by EU recovery and resilience funding are capable of bringing about healthcare reforms. This is especially visible in Croatia which has come up with a rather comprehensive set of reform measures that are strongly reflecting the national recovery and resilience plan. Measures enacted by the new Slovenian Government are not considered a deep reform, which should start in the coming years, but still the priority objectives stated in the national recovery and resilience plan are visible in the measures which have been enacted so far.

9.5 Conclusion

The COVID-19 pandemic has severely influenced public health systems across the entire world. It has placed enormous strain on healthcare systems globally, including Croatia and Slovenia, as in other EU member states. This has resulted in a very complex set of public policy responses by the state authorities, influencing the organization and management of public health protection, but also of many other aspects of people's lives. The measures were challenged in different ways, highlighting problems in defining the powers of the relevant authorities, different approaches to review of the constitutionality of the said measures, but also the lack of trust by one segment of the public in the national governments and institutions in general.

Problems in adopting and implementing public health measures in response to COVID-19 have also highlighted the obstacles and opportunities for conducting healthcare reforms in these countries in general. When one speaks of obstacles, it is possible to mention resistance to reforms within the healthcare sector, lack of political will to carry out unpopular reforms on the part of the governments, lack of political power by the governments to actually carry out reforms due to the limitations imposed by the overall public perception, but also due to constitutional jurisprudence, and lack of capacity of the opposition to constructively engage the government on important healthcare topics. On the other hand, a strong electoral mandate given to the two main ruling parties in Croatia and Slovenia represents an opportunity to make necessary changes within the healthcare system, but that window of opportunity will close quickly, meaning there is no time to lose if one wants to have better national healthcare systems than before COVID-19.

The influence of the European Union, through its provision of funding via the Recovery and Resilience Facility, conditioned by carrying out of national structural reforms, has proven to be promisingly significant so far. Both countries' national plans have been approved by the European Commission as a necessary prerequisite for being able to spend the money provided by the EU. In the area of healthcare, Croatia and Slovenia have defined the overarching objectives of the stated reforms in the same way: sustainability, quality, and availability of healthcare. Concrete investments are mostly focused on health workforce, medical infrastructure, and equipment. Croatia has already come up with a rather comprehensive set of reform measures that strongly reflect the national recovery and resilience plan. Slovenian structural reform is still pending, but the measures enacted so far are already aligned with the plan.

Finally, the public health crisis has shown that two important legislative changes in Croatia and Slovenia were required if one wants to have more clarity and legal certainty within the healthcare system. First, a much clearer set of statutory rules on the public health obligations of private primary care providers than that prescribed by the *Health Care Act* (art. 197) is necessary so that potential future disputes are avoided. The same held true for amending the *Communicable Diseases Act* (art. 39) in Slovenia. The new provisions should have been formulated in a way which adheres to the principles set by Slovenian Constitutional Court: the law must precisely determine the purpose of these measures, the admissible scope, types, and conditions concerning the restriction of the fundamental freedoms in question, and also contain other necessary safeguards against the arbitrary restriction of these rights. This was finally accomplished in October 2022 when the amending act enacted by the new ruling majority entered into force.

References

24ur (2022). Zdravstvena reforma predvidena za leto 2024. Do takrat gasimo požare. https://www.24ur.com/novice/slovenija/zdravstvena-reforma-predvidena-za-leto-2024-do-takrat-gasimo-pozare.html (Accessed on January 6, 2023).

Act Amending the Communicable Diseases Act, Official Gazette 125/22.

Act on the Election of Members of Croatian Parliament, Official Gazette 116/99 to 98/19.

Act on the Emergency Measures to Contain the Spread and Mitigate the Consequences of the Infectious COVID-19 Disease in the Field of Health Care, Official Gazette 141/22.

Act on the Protection of the Population from Infectious Diseases, Official Gazette 79/07 to 143/21.

Albreht, T., Polin, K., Pribaković Brinovec, R., Kuhar, M., Poldrugovac, M., Ogrin Rehberger, P., Prevolnik Rupel, V., and Vracko, P. (2021). *Slovenia Health System Review*. Denmark: World Health Organization.

Bagić, D., Šuljok, A., and Ančić, B. (2022). Determinants and reasons for coronavirus disease 2019 vaccine hesitancy in Croatia. *Croatian Medical Journal, 63*, 89–97.

Barić, S. and Miloš, M. (2022). Mapping the constitutional Terrain of vulnerability in the COVID pandemic: The Croatia case, *Zbornik Pravnog fakulteta Sveučilišta u Rijeci, 43*, 431–451.

Bill Amending the Compulsory Health Insurance Act, 2022.

Bill Amending the Health Care Act, 2022.

Carey, J. M. and Hix, S. (2011). The electoral sweet spot: Low-magnitude proportional electoral systems. *American Journal of Political Science*, *55*, 383–397.

Chang, A. Y., Culler, M. R., Harrington, R. A., and Barry, M. (2020). The impact of novel coronavirus COVID-19 on noncommunicable disease patients and health systems: A review, *Journal of Internal Medicine*, *289*, 450–462.

Civil Protection System Act, Official Gazette 82/15 to 20/21.

Communicable Diseases Act, Official Gazette 69/95 to 178/21

Compulsory Health Insurance Act, Official Gazette 80/13 to 98/19.

Croatian Television (2022). KoHOM: Postanu li ordinacije testna mjesta, tko će raditi naš posao? https://vijesti.hrt.hr/hrvatska/kohom-testiranje-u-ordinacijama-alibi-za-nesposobnost-ugrozava-pacijente-4688918 (Accessed on July 25, 2022).

Decision on Declaring the Epidemic of Disease COVID-19 caused by virus SARS-CoV-2, 11 March 2020.

Decision on Limiting Social Gatherings, Retail, Services, Sporting and Cultural Events, Official Gazette 32/20.

Decision on the Ban on Leaving One's Permanent Residence in the Republic of Croatia, Official Gazette 35/20.

Decision on the Introduction of Quarantine, February 21, 2020.

Decision on the Introduction of Special Safety Measure of Compulsory Testing for State, Local and Regional Officials, Persons Employed in Public Services, Companies and Institutions, Official Gazette 121/21.

Decision on the Introduction of Special Safety Measure of Compulsory Testing for Health Institutions, Companies Providing Health Services and Private Health Workers When Admitting Patients, Official Gazette 105/21.

Decision on the Manners of Complying with the Recovered-Vaccinated-Tested Requirement to Contain the Spread of Infection with the SARS-CoV-2 Virus, Official Gazette 147/21.

Decision on the Necessary Epidemiological Measure of Use of Face-masks or Medical Face-masks, Official Gazette 44/22.

Decision on the Necessary Measure of Compulsory Use of Face-masks or Medical Face-masks During the COVID-19 Epidemic, Official Gazette 80/20.

Decision on the Nomination of a Member of the Civil Protection Headquarters, Official Gazette 37/20.

Decision on the Organisation of Public Transport During the COVID-19 Epidemic, Official Gazette 143/20.

Decision on the Revocation of the COVID-19 Epidemic, Official Gazette 68/20.

Decision on the Temporary Ban on Crossing the Borders of the Republic of Croatia, Official Gazette 32/20.

Decision on the Temporary General Prohibition of Movement and Public Gathering in Public Places and Areas in the Republic of Slovenia, Official Gazette 30/20.

Decision on the Temporary Measures for the Prevention and Control of Infectious Disease COVID-19, Official Gazette 68/22.

Decision on the Temporary Prohibition of Offering and Selling Goods and Services to Consumers in the Republic of Slovenia, Official Gazette 25/20.

Decision on the Working Hours and the Organisation of Retail During the COVID-19 Epidemic, Official Gazette 51/20.

Dnevnik. (2022). Odpravljeni še zadnji epidemični ukrepi, strokovna skupina za covid-19 prenehala z delom. https://www.dnevnik.si/1042990142/slovenija/odpravljeni-se-zadnji-epidemicni-ukrepi-strokovna-skupina-za-covid19-prenehala-z-delom (Accessed on January 4, 2023).

Džakula, A., Banadinović, M., Lukačević Lovrenčić, I., Vajagić, M., Dimova, A., Rohova, M., Minev, M., Scintee, S. G., Vladescu, C., Farcasanu, D., Robinson, S., Spranger, A., Sagan, A., and Rechel, B. (2022). A comparison of health system responses to COVID-19 in Bulgaria, Croatia and Romania in 2020. *Health Policy, 126*, 456–464.

Džakula, A., Vočanec, D., Banadinović, M., Vajagić, M., Lončarek, K., Lukačević Lovrenčić, I., Radin, D., and Rechel, B. (2021). *Croatia Health System Review*. Copenhagen: World Health Organization Denmark.

European Centre for Disease Prevention and Control (2022). COVID-19 vaccine tracker. https://vaccinetracker.ecdc.europa.eu/public/extensions/COVID-19/vaccine-tracker.html#uptake-tab (Accessed on July 25, 2022).

European Commission (2022). Review report on the implementation of the recovery and resilience facility. https://ec.europa.eu/info/sites/default/files/com_2022_383_1_en.pdf (Accessed on August 31, 2022).

Ferlin, A., Malešič, M., and Vuga Beršnak, J. (2021). Preparedness vs. improvisation: A response to the Covid-19 crisis in Slovenia. *Teorija in praksa, 58*, 632–651.

Flander, B. (2022). 'Constitutional unconstitutionality': Constitutional review of the COVID-19 restrictions on fundamental rights in Slovenia. *Law, Identity and Values, 2*, 25–64.

Frawley, T., van Gelderen, F., Somanadhan S., Coveney, K., Phelan, A., Lynam-Loane, P., and De Brún, A. (2021). The impact of COVID-19 on health systems, mental health and the potential for nursing. *Irish Journal of Psychological Medicine, 38*, 220–226.

Freedom Movement (2022a). Zaslužimo si volilni program 2022. https://gibanjes voboda.si/wp-content/uploads/2022/03/SVOBODA_volilni-program.pdf (Accessed on July 27, 2022).

Freedom Movement (2022b). V kakšni Sloveniji želimo živeti v letu 2030. https:// gibanjesvoboda.si/wp-content/uploads/2022/04/SVOBODA_program-Vizija-2030.pdf (Accessed on January 25, 2024).

Government of the Republic of Croatia (2020a). Plenković za CNBC: Pobijedili smo virus u prvom poluvremenu, moguća djelomična turistička aktivnost u Europi. https://vlada.gov.hr/vijesti/plenkovic-za-cnbc-pobijedili-smo-virus-u-prvom-poluvremenu-moguca-djelomicna-turisticka-aktivnost-u-europi/29423 (Accessed on July 25, 2022).

Government of the Republic of Croatia (2020b). Plenković za VL: Pobijedili smo COVID-19 u prvom valu, reaktiviranje gospodarstva podrazumijeva i otvaranje granica. https://vlada.gov.hr/vijesti/plenkovic-za-vl-pobijedili-smo-covid-19-u-prvom-valu-reaktiviranje-gospodarstva-podrazumijeva-i-otvaranje-granica/29832 (Accessed on July 25, 2022).

Government of the Republic of Croatia (2020c). Predsjednik Vlade s hrvatskim znanstvenicima o borbi protiv koronavirusa. https://vlada.gov.hr/vijesti/predsjednik-vlade-s-hrvatskim-znanstvenicima-o-borbi-protiv-koronavi-rusa/29080 (Accessed on January 3, 2023).

Government of the Republic of Croatia (2021). Nacionalni plan oporavka i otpornosti 2021–2026. https://ec.europa.eu/info/sites/default/files/recovery_and_resilience_plan_for_croatia_hr.pdf (Accessed on August 31, 2022).

Government of the Republic of Croatia (2022a). Koronavirus. https://www.koronavirus.hr/ (Accessed on July 22, 2022).

Government of the Republic of Croatia (2022b). Odluke Stožera civilne zaštite za sprječavanje širenja zaraze novim koronavirusom. https://www.koronavirus.hr/odluke-stozera-civilne-zastite-za-sprjecavanje-sirenja-zaraze-novim-koronavirusom/323 (Accessed on July 23, 2022).

Government of the Republic of Croatia Act, Official Gazette 150/11 to 80/22.

Government of the Republic of Slovenia (2020a). 119. dopisna seja Vlade Republike Slovenije. https://www.gov.si/novice/2020-11-05-119-dopisna-seja-vlade-republike-slovenije/ (Accessed on January 4, 2023).

Government of the Republic of Slovenia (2020b). Krizni štab Republike Slovenije o konkretnih ukrepih za zajezitev epidemije. https://www.gov.si/novice/2020-03-14-krizni-stab-republike-slovenije-o-konkretnih-ukrepih-za-zajezitev-epidemije/ (Accessed on January 4, 2023).

Government of the Republic of Slovenia (2021). Načrt za okrevanje in odpornost. https://www.gov.si/assets/organi-v-sestavi/URSOO/01_si-rrp_23-7-2021.pdf (Accessed on August 31, 2022).

Government of the Republic of Slovenia (2022a). Coronavirus disease COVID-19. https://www.gov.si/en/topics/coronavirus-disease-covid-19/ (Accessed on July 23, 2022).

Government of the Republic of Slovenia (2022b). Prenehanje vseh ukrepov za preprečevanje in obvladovanje okužb z nalezljivo boleznijo COVID-19. https://www.gov.si/novice/2022-05-30-prenehanje-vseh-ukrepov-za-prepre-cevanje-in-obvladovanje-okuzb-z-nalezljivo-boleznijo-covid-19/ (Accessed on January 4, 2023).

Government of the Republic of Slovenia Act, Official Gazette 24/05 to 163/22.

Guest, J. L., del Rio, C., and Sanchez, T. (2020). The three steps needed to end the COVID-19 pandemic: Bold public health leadership, rapid innovations, and courageous political will. *JMIR Public Health and Surveillance, 6,* 1–4.

Haldane, V., De Foo, C., Abdalla, S. M., Jung, A-S., Tan, M., Wu, S., Chua, A., Verma, M., Shrestha, P., Singh, S. Perez, T., Tan, S. M., Bartos, M., Mabuchi, S., Bonk, M., McNab, C., Werner, G. K., Panjabi, R., Nordström, A., and Legido-Quigley, H. (2021). Health systems resilience in managing the COVID-19 pandemic: Lessons from 28 countries. *Nature Medicine, 27,* 964–980.

Health Care Act, Official Gazette 100/18 to 147/20.

Health Care and Health Insurance Act, Official Gazette 9/92 to 43/22.

Health Services Act, Official Gazette 9/92 to 196/21.

Index (2021). Vlada: Lauc je izbačen iz Znanstvenog savjeta. https://www.index.hr/vijesti/clanak/vlada-lauc-je-izbacen-iz-znanstvenog-savjeta/2319633.aspx?index_ref=naslovnica_vijesti_najnovije_d (Accessed on January 3, 2023).

Index (2022). "Obiteljski liječnici napustili radnu skupinu koja radi na Beroševoj reformi. https://www.index.hr/vijesti/clanak/obiteljski-lijecnici-napustili-radnu-skupinu-koja-radi-na-berosevoj-reformi/2375956.aspx (Accessed on July 27, 2022).

Jutarnji List (2021). Znanstveni savjet pred raspadom, niz članova želi otići, a razlog je samo jedan čovjek! https://www.jutarnji.hr/vijesti/hrvatska/znanst-veni-savjet-pred-raspadom-niz-clanova-zeli-otici-a-razlog-je-samo-jedan-covjek-15112067 (Accessed on January 3, 2023).

Ministry of Health of the Republic of Croatia (2022). Bolest covid-19 potvrđivat će se brzim antigenskim testovima. https://zdravlje.gov.hr/vijesti/

bolest-covid-19-potvrdjivat-ce-se-brzim-antigenskim-testovima/5564 (Accessed on July 25, 2022).

National Assembly Election Act, Official Gazette 44/92 to 29/21.

National Institute of Public Health of Slovenia (2022). Sklep o imenovanju delovne skupine za spremljanje gibanja virusa SARS-CoV-2. https://nijz.si/ wp-content/uploads/2022/07/sklep_o_imenovanju_ds_za_spremljanje_ gibanja_virusa_sars-cov-2_27.6.2022.pdf (Accessed on January 4, 2023).

Net (2020). Tko, zapravo, donosi mjere i kreira naše živote?/Plenković je okupio znanstvenike, tvrde da su nezavisni, ali glavnu riječ vodi netko drugi. https:// net.hr/danas/hrvatska/tko-zapravo-donosi-mjere-i-kreira-nase-zivote-plenkovic-je-okupio-znanstvenike-oni-tvrde-da-su-nezavisni-ali-glavnu-rijec-vodi-netko-drugi-d7176ff6-b1c5-11eb-8d3e-0242ac130043 (Accessed on January 3, 2023).

NOVA TV (2022). Žestoki odgovor ministru: "Ljudi su krivi jer se ne pridržavaju mjera, iako su gotovo nikakve. Mi smo krivi jer ukazujemo na probleme…". https://dnevnik.hr/vijesti/koronavirus/zavrsio-prvi-dan-testiranja-u-ordinaci-jama-obiteljskih-lijecnika---692488.html (Accessed on July 25, 2022).

Ofak, L. (2021). Pravna priroda mjera usmjerenih na suzbijanje pandemije COVID-19. *Zbornik radova Pravnog fakulteta u Splitu*, *58*, 459–475.

Ombudsman of the Republic of Croatia (2022). "Važnost obiteljskih liječnika u zaštiti prava na zdravlje. https://www.ombudsman.hr/hr/vaznost-obiteljskih-lijecnika-u-zastiti-prava-na-zdravlje/ (Accessed on July 27, 2022).

Order on the Declaration of the COVID-19 Epidemic in the Territory of the Republic of Slovenia, Official Gazette 19/20.

Ordinance on the Composition, Mode of Operation and Requirements for the Nomination of the Head, Deputy and Members of the Civil Protection Headquarters, Official Gazette 126/19.

Petravić, L., Arh, R., Gabrovec, T., Jazbec, L., Rupčić, N., Starešinić, N., Zorman, L., Pretnar, A., Srakar, A., Zwitter, M., and Slavec, A. (2021). Factors affecting attitudes towards COVID-19 vaccination: An online survey in Slovenia. *Vaccines*, *9*, 1–15.

President of the Republic of Croatia (2020). Predsjednik Milanović: Odlukom Ustavnog suda rasprava o radu Stožera neće prestati. https://www.predsjed nik.hr/vijesti/predsjednik-milanovic-odlukom-ustavnog-suda-rasprava-o-radu-stozera-nece-prestati/ (Accessed on July 25, 2022).

Regulation Determining the Amount of Supplement for Increased Workload for Hazardous Work and the Number of Additional Health Care Staff, Official Gazette 132/22.

Regulation Determining the Amount of Supplement for Special Working Conditions in the Territory of Less Developed Municipalities, Official Gazette 132/22.

Social Democratic Party of the Republic of Croatia (2022). Polazne točke za reformu zdravstva u Republici Hrvatskoj Solidarno zdravstvo i zdravlje za sve. http://www.sdp.hr/wp/wp-content/uploads/2021/12/SDP-Polazne-tocke-za-reformu-zdravstva.pdf (Accessed on July 27, 2022).

State Election Commission of the Republic of Slovenia (2022). Volitve v Državni zbor 2022. https://volitve.dvk-rs.si/#/rezultati (Accessed on July 26, 2022).

State Electoral Commission of the Republic of Croatia (2020). Izbori za zastupnike u Hrvatski sabor. https://www.izbori.hr/site/ostalo/opce-informacije/rezultati-izbora-otvoreni-podaci/izbori-za-zastupnike-u-hrvatski-sabor-479/479 (Accessed on July 25, 2022).

U-I-1372/2020, Constitutional Court of the Republic of Croatia, 2020, 14 September.

U-I-155/20, Constitutional Court of the Republic of Slovenia, 2021, 7 October.

U-I-210/21, Constitutional Court of the Republic of Slovenia, 2021, 29 November.

U-I-426/20, Constitutional Court of the Republic of Slovenia, 2020, 21 December.

U-I-5781/2021, Constitutional Court of the Republic of Croatia, 2021, 21 December.

U-I-79/20, Constitutional Court of the Republic of Slovenia, 2021, 13 May.

U-I-83/20, Constitutional Court of the Republic of Slovenia, 2020, 27 August.

U-II-2379/2020, Constitutional Court of the Republic of Croatia, 2020, 14 September.

U-II-6278/2021, Constitutional Court of the Republic of Croatia, 2022, 12 April.

U-II-7149/2021, Constitutional Court of the Republic of Croatia, 2022, 15 February.

U-VIIR-2180/2022, Constitutional Court of the Republic of Croatia, 2022, 16 May.

U-VIIR-2181/2022, Constitutional Court of the Republic of Croatia, 2022, 16 May.

Washington Post (2022). Slovenia voted against an illiberal leader and for an untested party. https://www.washingtonpost.com/politics/2022/04/26/slovenia-jansa-golob-backsliding-democracy/ (Accessed on July 26, 2022).

World Health Organisation (WHO) (2022). Slovenia situation. https://covid19.who.int/region/euro/country/si (Accessed on July 23, 2022).

Zadnik, V., Mihor, A., Tomšić, S., Žagar, T., Bric, N., Lokar, K., and Oblak, I. (2020). Impact of COVID-19 on cancer diagnosis and management in Slovenia — Preliminary results. *Radiology and Oncology*, *54*, 329–334.

Chapter 10

The Russian Federation

Pavitra Paul

10.1 Introduction

Given the extensive size of the Russian Federation, it is unsurprising that the governance structures within which public health is embedded are rather complex. The Russian Federation itself (Figure 10.1) is comprised of six different categories of regional jurisdictions. These include 22 ethnic enclaves with the status of republics (including Crimea since 2014), three cities of federal importance (Moscow, Saint Petersburg, and Sevastopol), four autonomous okrugs (regions), nine krais (territories), and 46 oblasts (provinces). The governors of all these regions have, since 2010, been appointed by the central government, and they represent the Russian President in their respective jurisdictions.

Within the legislative structure of the Russian Federation, local government is determined through elected and other bodies of local self-government. These bodies address matters of local importance, including the ownership, use, and disposal of municipal property. They independently manage municipal property; form, approve, and execute the local

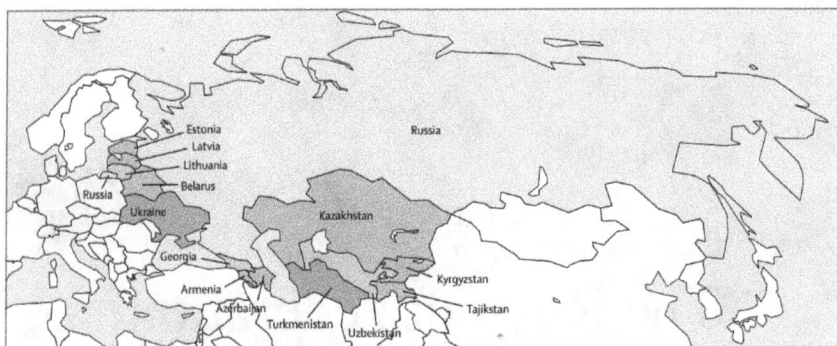

Figure 10.1.   Contemporary Russia.

Source: Michel Kazatchkine, United Nations Secretary-General's Special Envoy for HIV/AIDS in Eastern Europe and Central Asia (2012–2017).

budget; establish local taxes and fees; maintain public order; and resolve other issues of local importance. The relations between the federal center and regional governments have always been an integral part of the political process in Russia and an important factor in its outcomes. However, the existence of a formal structure of responsibility for regional authorities does not necessarily mean autonomy in political and policy decision-making. Local self-government bodies are not included in the system of state authorities: they are, however, independent within the parameters of their formal jurisdiction, and the Russian Federation (at least formally) recognizes and guarantees local self-government.

The Russian legislation regulating the healthcare sector is characterized by a high degree of interconnectedness between regulatory levers. The levers used to regulate healthcare at the federal and municipal levels are both administrative and financial (Nadskakuła-Kaczmarczyk, 2017; Sharafutdinova, 2009). Administrative measures are generally coordinated through the Federal Service for Surveillance in Health Care while financial mechanisms address the allocation of funding for state and municipal bodies. This highly centralized political power greatly contributed to the coordination of measures governing the health system during COVID-19: nonetheless, as discussed in the following, ubiquitous corruption within the healthcare system (and more widely) meant that policy decisions were based on rent-seeking behavior rather than on responses to regional need.

The Federal Service for Surveillance in Health Care maintains its regional presence through Territorial Directorates located in all regions and funded from the federal budget (Healthcare Development Concept, 2020). The Territorial Directorates have local offices at the municipal level, and representatives in hospitals report through the vertical organizational structure (via line departments). The Federal Service for Surveillance in Health Care is also responsible for public health issues like infectious disease control, registration of diseases, food and drinking water safety, and all matters that have an obvious effect on population health. The guidelines and recommendations of the Federal Service for Surveillance in Health care act as "soft law" (quasi-legal instruments) for all activities and functions within the domain of Russian health.

According to WHO rankings, Russia's population exhibits average life expectancy (WHO, 2020). Insufficient funding constrains the appropriateness of medical care, especially in the level of medical technology employed. The availability of modern medicines is also very low, as are healthcare sector wages (Ivanov & Suvorov, 2021). One of the main problems of economic development is the widening of the income gap with an increasing concentration of income within the top 1% of the population (*Davos Agenda*, 2021).

Russia was not spared from the impact of COVID-19. 162,000 deaths were associated with coronavirus infection in 2020 alone (*Rosstat*, 2022), with around 400,000 reported COVID-19 deaths as of August 2023 (Our World in Data, 2023). As a result of this increase in mortality, the average life expectancy has decreased by more than 2 years (to 71.1 years in 2020), returning to 2014 levels (Ivanov & Suvorov, 2022). Excess mortality caused by the coronavirus pandemic in Russia amounted to 350,900 deaths (240 cases per 100,000 people) while deaths from COVID-19 were more than two times higher in Russia than in Austria, the Netherlands, and France during the period between April 2020 and February 2021(*ibid.*).

The relatively high mortality in Russia not only reflects the inefficiency of the Russian healthcare system but also the inadequacy of its policy response to the pandemic. For example, entry to Russia from countries where the epidemic began was not restricted in a timely manner. Despite the fact that in February 2020 cases of infection with COVID-19 were officially registered in many European countries, and quarantine was introduced in 11 regions of Italy, the Russian authorities stopped air traffic with European countries only on March 27, 2020. In the first quarter of 2020, more than a million Russian tourists visited EU countries, including 180,000 thousand visits to Italy (Outbound Tourist Trips, 2020). Neither testing for coronavirus, nor quarantine measures for those arriving in Russia from countries where the epidemic began, was carried out in the Russian Federation. Furthermore, no measures were taken to prevent the spread of infection from Moscow, which is the country's main gateway, to other regions. Not only were the majority of the population not provided with timely personal protective equipment but, alarmingly, neither were many medical workers who had direct contact with those infected with COVID-19.

A unified public system of pandemic measures was, in general, simply non-existent. The responsibility for introducing specific measures to combat COVID-19 remained with the heads of the regions (Ivanov & Suvorov, 2022). This meant that not only did Russia have the same organizational challenges faced by other federal states during the pandemic but these were compounded by limited healthcare resources, poorer population health indicators, and a pervasive culture of rent-seeking.

10.2 The Structure of Healthcare and Public Health Governance in Russia

10.2.1 *The Russian healthcare system*

The Federal Law of 11/21/2011 N 323-ФЗ, *Health of citizens in the Russian Federation* (with amendments subsequently on June 11, 2022, and on July 13, 2022), governs the health system of the country. The healthcare in the Russian Federation is a three-tiered system, involving federal, regional, and municipal levels (Figure 10.2). At the federal level, the Ministry of Health (Minzdrav) is the federal executive body, which implements and develops state policy governing healthcare. It also acts as a legal regulator in healthcare. In addition to the provision of medical care, the Ministry regulates such areas as pharmaceuticals, quality control, drug safety and effectiveness, medical devices, health resort services, and sanitary and epidemiological conditions. A key function of the Ministry is to coordinate and monitor the activities of the Federal Service for Surveillance in Healthcare (Roszdravnadzor) as well as activities of the Federal Mandatory Health Insurance Fund.

At the regional level, health system management is performed by regional departments and ministries (Figure 10.2), which are responsible

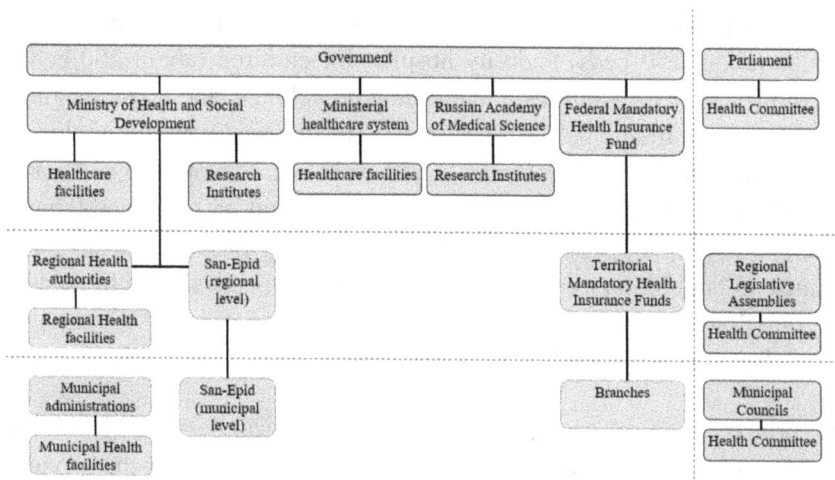

Figure 10.2.   Health system organization.

for the development and realization of regional health programs, the implementation of preventive measures, medical care and expertise, organization of labor protection and social guarantees for medical personnel, and management of medical care in emergency conditions. Regional executive authorities have the power to determine the budget and funding for the provision of specialized medical care. Regional health authorities are subordinate to the regional governments, which in turn are answerable to the regional health ministers. Regional healthcare facilities usually include a hospital with around 1,000 beds as well as a pediatric hospital with about 400 beds. Both include outpatient services. There are also regional specialized healthcare facilities for infectious diseases, tuberculosis, and psychiatric illness.

At the municipal level, local government bodies manage many aspects of the healthcare system. Their functions include monitoring and analyzing citizens' well-being and medical care provision, organizing and coordinating healthcare activities, and developing and implementing municipal healthcare programs. Municipal executive authorities have the power to plan the costs for emergency care, primary medical care in outpatient and inpatient facilities, and medical care for women during pregnancy, delivery, and after childbirth.

Urban rayons (cities) typically have a multifunctional city hospital for adults (about 250 beds) and city hospital for children (about 200 beds). Most primary care facilities, independent polyclinics, and a few diagnostic centers are municipal. In rural rayons, institutions typically include a central hospital with approximately 250 beds, which may also serve as a polyclinic. Some rayons also have a smaller hospital with about 100 beds. There are independent polyclinics (not part of any hospital), small polyclinics or "ambulatory care facilities," and health posts staffed by feldshers (auxiliary health workers, such as physician assistants). Medical care in the Russian health system has three tiers:

- primary medical care, including general medical services (including emergency care) and specialized medical care (except for the services provided within the framework of secondary and tertiary medical care),
- secondary medical care, focusing on general medical services (including emergency care) and specialized medical care (except highly technologically specialized services) provided by health facilities having designated departments and clinics,
- tertiary medical care, comprised of general medical services (including emergency care) and specialized medical care (including advanced care) provided by health facilities that offer high-tech medical services.

In practice, many regions and rayons function in a coordinated manner where local governance remains within the regional Ministry of Health.

Despite a well-developed network of the out-patient-polyclinic facilities, the existing system of primary care remains overloaded and often ineffective. The ineffectiveness of the polyclinics is partly attributable to the mechanism allocating excessive numbers of patients to the polyclinics. The restricted opening hours of the polyclinics also leads to issues of accessibility for the working population.

10.2.2 *Public health governance*

In Russia, as in other states, public health functions incorporate both illness prevention and disease surveillance. The institutional organization of public health in Russia is set out in Figure 10.3.

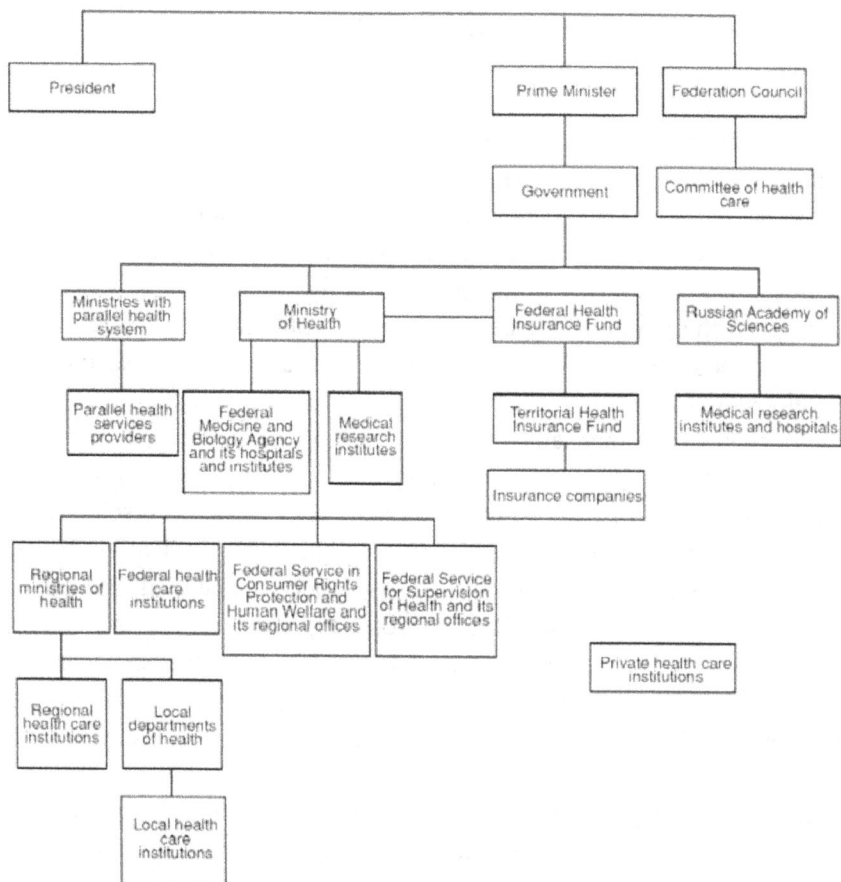

Figure 10.3. Organization of public health.

10.2.2.1 *Disease prevention and health promotion*

The framework of illness prevention has three components. The first includes measures aimed at preventing diseases (including immunization and the promotion of healthy lifestyles), while the second focuses on the early detection of diseases, the mitigation of disease exacerbation and complications, physical capacity decline, and premature mortality. The third element emphasizes rehabilitation and focuses on actions to eliminate, minimize, or compensate disability in order to restore limited functions as much as possible. All preventive actions are performed in both inpatient and outpatient facilities, as well as specialized public health centers (created for this purpose under the *Order of the Ministry of Health of the Russian Federation No. 748n* dated July 28, 2020).

Among the most successful areas where the Russian Federation has made progress toward the realization of Sustainable Development Goals are in the focus on healthy balanced diets across the population and in the promotion of healthy lifestyles and overall well-being. The focus here has been to reduce all forms of malnutrition in the population, as well as to strengthen the agricultural sector (which is politically important as the source of economic growth, increased employment rates, and sustainable development for the country). Measures to overcome excessive food price volatility include a mechanism based on state procurement and commodity interventions. To ensure that children in Russia are well nourished, measures are being implemented to provide free hot meals to schoolchildren, with a particular emphasis on quality and safety indicators. Under the Federal Improvement of Public Health Project, the Federal Service for Surveillance on Consumer Rights Protection and Human Well-being together with the Nutrition and Biotechnology Institute have been working extensively to prevent unhealthy diets in the population and reduce the number of obese and overweight people. The Federal Science and Technology Programme for Agriculture Development (2017–2025) is establishing such policy priorities in this area as the transition to highly productive and environmentally friendly agriculture and aquaculture, the storage and effective processing of agricultural products, as well as the production of safe and quality food. However, integrating the state, the business sector, and wider societal actors to this end remains politically challenging.

To combat the sale of counterfeit or substandard products capable of harming human health, in January 2021, the voluntary labeling of dairy products has begun in order to test the effectiveness of the mechanism of food labeling (which tracks products from the manufacturer to the consumer (WTO, 2021)). Russia has introduced a "State Programme" (*Order No. 207-r of February 13, 2019 of the Government of the Russian Federation*) for the Comprehensive Development of Rural Areas for the period 2020–2025: this is intended to promote the comprehensive, all-round development of agricultural production and rural infrastructure and, importantly, to bring the quality of life of the rural population closer to urban standards. Russia has adopted the Health in All Policies (HiAP) approach emphasizing societal factors and actions that shape everyday living environments, integrating the "health and well-being" of the citizens into the development trajectory of the Russian Federation.

10.2.2.2 *Disease surveillance*

Russia's sanitary and epidemiological surveillance system is represented by both medical authorities (sanitary and epidemiological agencies and health facilities) and non-medical ones. The surveillance system is mandated to collect data and determine trends in epidemic progression, to identify of the root causes and conditions enabling epidemic spread across certain territories, to carry out pre-epidemic diagnostics, and to make epidemiological diagnoses. It forecasts the epidemiological situation based on information flows and takes management decisions and estimates their effectiveness and efficiency. Interestingly, the strategic document describing the development of Russian healthcare (*Decree of the President of the Russian Federation of June 6, 2019 No. 254*) did outline risks similar to the COVID-19 pandemic 6 months prior to the official recognition of the new coronavirus infection. This document is candid about both the emergence of new infections caused by unknown pathogens, requiring continuously maintaining a high level of anti-epidemic preparedness, and the biosecurity needed to carry out a set of prophylactic and anti-epidemic measures to prevent the introduction and spread of infectious diseases with natural foci and zoonotic infections (as well as preparations to respond to natural and intentional biological threats).

The federal Ministry of Health has also developed a concept for the modernization of its infectious disease service that includes creating a multilevel system for laboratory diagnostics of infectious diseases, modernizing the infrastructure of clinics and hospitals, building an applied research center for infectious diseases at the federal level, and improving the infectious disease management system. Russia is now evaluating the establishment of an integrated system for preventing risks and epidemiological threats (*Decree of the President of the Russian Federation "On Strategy for Development of Health care in the Russian Federation until 2025 ")* within the BRICS (the association of five major emerging economies: Brazil, Russia, India, China and South Africa).

To fight against anti-microbial resistance and against the use of antibiotics to promote animal growth, the Russian Federation has embraced a "One Health" approach, a comprehensive concept to address threats to the health of human beings, animals, plants, and environment. The Federal Service for Surveillance on Consumer Rights Protection and Human Well-being (Rospotrebnadzor) in Moscow remains responsible for good hygienic practices in farming activities throughout the whole "farm to fork" process. It also fights against falsified products emerging as a result of a developed trans-border trading activities (Food and Agriculture Organization, 2022).

10.3 The Response to COVID-19

Once the potential threat of COVID-19 was acknowledged, the relatively weak level of parliamentary influence on the political and policy processes in Russia, the President's control of the government, and formal and informal rules governing the mass media facilitated a focused, top-down response to the pandemic. To a large extent, this strategy focused on repurposing medical facilities and reorganizing medical care. Interlevel and interagency cooperation, supported by interconnected regulatory levers, facilitated command-and-control decision-making for combating the crisis. Since regional governors are directly under the authority of the federal government, compliance with the directives of the federal government (i.e. of the President) by the regional (subnational) governments was consistently uniform and free from any institutional constraints across all regions. Nonetheless, the appointment-based system of gubernatorial selection did create a problem of moral hazard, giving some regional leaders unconstrained power in the respective territories (Sharafutdinova, 2009). Because governors are not elected but appointed by the President, loyalty to the President overrides representation of the respective electorates. There exists a "principal–agent" relationship that does not recognize either competence or political autonomy but operates through a form of "delegated power". In consequence, there is an "information asymmetry" between the principal and the agents, which leads to different forms of rent seeking behaviors within the system of governance.

One major impediment to the state's strategy of pandemic management was the low degree of public compliance with restrictive measures. This was further complicated in situations where patients remained responsible for their own referrals and coordination of care pathway between different types and levels of care. The local authorities had introduced a number of punitive measures (e.g. fines for not using personal protective equipment in public places or using it improperly), but these measures were often implemented inconsistently and without any coherent approach across different levels of governance. In some cases, these measures even exceeded the boundaries of legitimate power (Kravchenko & Ivanova, 2021).

10.3.1 *The structural changes triggered by COVID-19*

The federal portion of the basic mandatory health insurance (OMC) program was, through amendments of the OMC law (Federal Law dated 08.12.2020 No. 430 "On Amendments to the Federal Law 'On Compulsory Health Insurance in the Russian Federation'"), introduced to provide additional funding for medical services provided by federal health facilities. Under these amendments, the Federal Mandatory Health Insurance Fund (FOMC) was enabled to distribute and monitor spending directly. In this way, the FOMC became both a fund manager as well as the controller responsible for spending outlays. Because of this, competition between health facilities became restricted and a sub-health system comprising health facilities of federal government developed, making it difficult to coordinate the activities of federal and regional health facilities operating in the same territory. It also meant that patients lost the opportunity to choose between federal and regional health facilities when seeking medical care. Furthermore, the amendment of the OMC law[1] excludes medical insurance organizations (MIOs) from servicing

---

[1] Order of RF Ministry of Health No. 1024n of September 25, 2020 "On Amendments to Rules of Compulsory Medical Insurance, approved by Order of RF Ministry of Health No. 108n of February 28, 2019, and a Standard Form of Contract on Financial Support of Compulsory Medical Insurance, approved by Order of the Ministry of Health and Social Development dated 09.09.2011 No. 1030n.

programs of FOMC fund and debars MIOs' rights to receive the income from savings of the OMC funds. The amendment of the OMC law also limits the volume of activities in private healthcare facilities while guaranteeing medical care for public facilities (including recruiting doctors of private healthcare facilities in public institutions) in an emergency (Galayants, 2020).

Toward the end of November 2019, a bill was submitted to the State Duma mandating approval for the Ministry of Health to appoint heads of health authorities at all levels of governance in the Russian Federation. This established a unified system of remuneration supporting a unified salary system effective from January 1, 2022 for healthcare workers across the country.

10.3.2 *Expanded social support specific to COVID-19*

In general, due to the pandemic, the minimum and maximum amounts of unemployment benefits were increased, and additional payments for the children of unemployed parents were introduced. The specific initiatives included the following:

- eliminating the need for certification of payment toward benefits,
- widening and intensifying the social security net in the form of (1) payment for children from 3 to 7 years to families with low incomes, (2) extension of child benefit, (3) lowering the threshold of sick leave benefit, (4) payment for children between 6 and 18 years old, (5) remote examination for disability confirmation, (6) extension of temporary disability benefits, (7) lump sum payment for pensioners, (8) extension of time periods for fare reimbursement (for the residents of far north) and subsidies for housing and commune services, (9) extension of child care allowance up to 1.5 years, and (10) sick days allowance not below the minimum wage,
- special measures for care workers, including (1) payments to doctors who fell ill with COVID-19, (2) social security guarantees for doctors, middle and junior medical staff, and ambulance drivers, and (3) additional payment to health workers,

- examination of the loss of professional ability to work, retraining of unemployed caused by the pandemics, remote registration for enrollment in the labor market and payments to employees of social institutions, and
- measures targeting non-citizens (disputed residency status): this focused on the amendment of migration legislation (extending the validity of documents for foreigners in the territory of the Russian Federation).

Other measures included extended renewal of licenses and business permits, introduction of distance education (schools and higher education), selective or total closures of public space including business enterprises (except those for emergency services) by the respective regional governments based on the prevailing epidemiological situation, a special procedure for accessing the provision of public services remotely; penalties for violation of quarantine measures, financial support for scientific, educational, and medical institution, and the creation of temporary jobs.

There was also a program of COVID-19 support for trade, industry, and commerce. This included (1) remote provision of financial services, (2) preferential mortgage rates reduced by 70%, (3) extension of the lease of state and commercial real estate for affected industries, (4) expansion of concessional lending programs and microcredit for small and medium enterprises (SMEs), (5) relaxation of eligibility criteria and documentation requirements for agricultural producers to receive loans at 5% per annum, (6) subsidies for loans at the Central Bank rate to maintain working capital and save jobs, (7) special grants to SMEs and non-governmental organization (NGOs) to compensate suspension of work caused by anti-epidemic measures in the regions, (8) preferential loans for the production of critical medical products, (9) cancellation of fines and penalties when postponing the deadline for the execution of a state contract, (10) the provision for receiving up to 50% of the state contract amount in advance, (11) relaxation of conditions for granting subsidies to enterprises of folk art crafts, (12) extension of repayment schedules including introduction of deferment of payments on loans to farmers (including collective investments), (13) restructuring preferential investment and preferential short-term loans to farmers, (14) payroll subsidy (three minimum wages per new employee) to the business for the employment of the unemployed, (15) subsidies for certified exporters' goods and employment support loans, (16) state support with simplified process for electronics industry enterprises, (17) subsidies for measures to prevent COVID-19, (18) subsidies to the airports, (19) special financial support for self-employed citizens, employment support loans for wage payments, and interest-free daily settlement loans, (20) credit payment holidays for up to 6 months for a mortgage or consumer loan, (21) remote account opening for individuals, individual entrepreneurs, and legal entities, (22) a bankruptcy moratorium (for affected industries) and a moratorium on payments of penalties for government contracts, (23) restrictions on the payment of dividends, (24) financial support for cooperatives, Russian car manufacturers, private circuses, and zoos, and (25) reducing the compliance burden on joint-stock companies and for government contracts.

Further, the import taxes (duties) on medical supplies were reviewed, and an extensive list of exemptions including substantial reduction of such taxes on various goods was established. Registration of medicines and medical products were also simplified with faster approval processes for distribution. Medicines used for heart and circulatory diseases were put into a high priority procurement and supply category. Free supply of medicines was provided to the victims of COVID-19 even for ambulatory (outpatient) treatment.

Regulatory provisions for credit institutions and non-banking financial institutions were relaxed, and provision of extra liquidity to banks as part of support for organizations of national importance was taken at the macro level for ensuring the availability of ready money in the system. Further, in this context, disposal of capital items through electronic transactions were allowed in order to facilitate the crediting of the funds. Specific measures for affected industries were also enacted, especially for the tourist and transport industries.

10.4 Discussion

The three-tier architecture of the Russian health system follows a 2-year planning period for different expenditures at all levels of governance.

The distribution is driven by the goals and the objectives of the state policy, as well as special decisions of the President of the Russian Federation and the government of the Russian Federation. The present top-down approach often ignores local needs which can, in turn, lead to inequalities in outcome.

In order to eliminate regional and territorial inequalities, federal authorities have created two state programs: "Zemsky Doctor" (local doctor) and "Zemsky Feldsher" (local paramedic), aimed at attracting qualified medical personnel to rural areas through financial incentives. However, the differences in state health expenditure across different Russian regions are the major impediments to these programs: Central Russia and the Far North regions are traditionally characterized by higher funding. The country's 10 wealthiest regions receive almost double the healthcare funding compared to the 10 poorest regions (Ulumbekova, 2019).

While Russia's strong centralized control has contributed to the coordination of COVID-19 responses across the country, the institutional frameworks, set up by countless laws, decrees, and instructions, have also contributed to the phenomenon of an "over-regulated state" (Paneyakh, 2013), combining a very high density of poor-quality state regulations with the sweeping discretion of regulatory agencies and state watchdogs. This has created increasing dysfunctionality in courts, police, and other state organizations (Volkov *et al.*, 2013; Paneyakh, 2014). Although the constitution confers the rights of regions to govern independently within a policy field, the position of the Governors has been turned into an office of the President for executing the federal policies, ignoring the specific needs of the local geography and undermining the preferences of the population groups within these regions.

The appointed governors face few constraints and little accountability for their actions. This, in turn, encourages blatant corruption and the mismanagement of resources (Sharafutdinova, 2009). Governors in the Russian Federation more often lose their jobs due to a failure to deliver votes and secure political support than for poor economic performance or for failing to secure the welfare of their respective populations. The cause of exacerbated inequity in health outcomes during COVID-19 is clearly a consequence of the governance process. The present system of governance through presidential decrees does facilitate the harmonization of processes for the execution of public policies, but it does so with clear costs at that impede the availability of resource efficiency at the regional level.

The effective implementation of priority projects and programs in the Russian Federation has been driven more by top-level political patronage than by a process of policy entrepreneurship effected through ministers, governors, and mayors or through academic leadership. Although political demand for success stories provides certain incentives for policy entrepreneurs, the system of political patronage often undermines incentives for them. While this rigid hierarchy did permit a focused top-down response to the pandemic, the ubiquitous corruption endemic in the system meant that policy decisions were based on rent-seeking behavior rather than responses to regional need. The rigid top-down mode of governance also meant that the ability of the public health system to respond nimbly to the shifting manifestation of COVID-19 (and to a changing understanding of the pathogen itself) was severely constrained.

"Policy entrepreneurship" is an important mechanism that facilitates systemic changes that better meet the demands of a policy system. Policy entrepreneurs are individuals who have a deep understanding of how systems work, what constraints they face, and novel ways of meeting the system demands. However, the combination of high density and low quality in the regulation of various sectors and policy fields on the one hand, and its arbitrary and selective enforcement by the state apparatus on the other, is clearly not conducive to policy entrepreneurship. In Russia, "pockets of efficiency" are found in some priority projects with the patronage of political leaders. However, as the political leadership is interested in success stories primarily to legitimize the political status quo and, secondarily, to facilitate rent-seeking goals (Muller, 2014; Orttung & Zhemukhov, 2014), the effect and reach of policy entrepreneurs in healthcare is generally limited.

Informal deals between political leaders and policy entrepreneurs require priority resource endowment and a high level of freedom for policy entrepreneurs on virtually all initiatives in their respective fields in exchange for quick and highly visible successes. However, the number of top priorities in Russia is limited, forcing policy entrepreneurs to compete with each other for scarce resources and meaningful attention from political leaders. Any change in the leaders' policy priorities (let alone a change of leaders themselves) can quickly put an end to projects and programs.

There is a common belief in Russian culture that without top-down pressure, the lower layers of the governance hierarchy (understood as the "power vertical") do not invest enough effort for the effective implementation of state policies. This has conferred wide-ranging and sweeping powers on regulatory agencies responsible for monitoring and auditing every organization in various sectors, including severe sanctions for noncompliance at all levels of governance (Gel'man, 2016). This, in turn, induces managers at all layers of the power vertical not to focus on policy entrepreneurship and improved performance in the respective domains but to be risk averse and to avoid possible punishment for any formal or informal violation of the rules.

COVID-19 loosened up this rigid vertical governance structure to a small degree. The Federal Service for Surveillance on Consumer Rights Protection and Human Well-being (Rospotrebnadzor), with its representative offices at the regions, has the authority to integrate health with other sectors like agriculture, pharmaceuticals, and environment actions. It has done so through mechanisms, such as the "Coordination Council" (for combating the new coronavirus infections), a "Crisis Centre" for coordinating measures preventing the introduction and further spread of the infection, another "Crisis Centre" for economic issues, which was responsible for the development of measures to support local businesses and organizations affected by the pandemic, and an "Information Centre" (for monitoring the coronavirus situation). This structure did ensure multilevel and interagency communication across the country, establishing synergy with the websites of all federal, regional, and municipal healthcare authorities and with the broadcasting channels of TV and radio, print media, social networks, and hotlines.

To the extent that these pandemic agencies effected a slight "deconcentration" of federal power, it was able to present a coordinated action to the immediate threats posed by COVID-19. However, this approach has not resulted in a robust system of pandemic management over a longer period of time. The top-level political patronage, the immediate priorities of political leaders, and some very limited policy entrepreneurship (under special regulatory conditions and with positive incentives) have contributed, in a limited and inconsistent way across regions, to the management of the pandemic. However, these positive outcomes are limited in both time and space (Gel'man, 2021): as DiMaggio and Powell (1983) suggest, "pockets of efficiency" under these conditions will become full of holes quickly without any dissemination of best practices of policy diffusion.

The Russian healthcare system has not been resilient to the demands placed on it by COVID-19. Due to the shortage of hospitals in neighborhood locations, patients with COVID-19 could only be hospitalized in repurposed hospitals located in large cities, mainly in regional centers. The obvious need to transport patients often over a distance of more than 100 km led to the denial of needed emergency medical care for the population of rural settlements and small towns. Also, the waiting time for the arrival of an ambulance for many COVID-19 victims amounted to hours or even days. Random and unplanned (without competence mapping) deployment of healthcare workers (often without substantive medical training) in COVID care facilities led to both a decrease in the effectiveness (often with avoidable uncertainty) of treatment of patients with COVID-19 and a significant reduction in the possibility of needed medical care for patients of other diseases. Furthermore, a shortage of many drugs in most regions did lead to both the growth of self-medication and the media advertisement of certain "miraculous" drugs without any proven scientific merit (Ivanov & Suvorov, 2022).

The overall funds for pandemic management allocated by the federal government and the regional governments could not compensate for the loss of income from provision of services for other specialties at the health facility level. The allocation measures aimed to ensure the prioritized provision of medical care for patients with COVID-19 (through the repurposing of treatment facilities designed for other ailments) resulted in a substantial decrease of earnings from the payments at the point-of-service for the health facilities. This caused an additional strain on the investment capacity of health facilities.

Most of the additional pandemic funding was for a relatively narrow list of tasks for organizing the treatment of patients with new coronavirus infections (i.e. deploying and equipping a dedicated bed, purchasing personal protective equipment, running diagnostic testing systems, and providing incentive payments to healthcare workers). The allocation for long-term investments in permanent intensive care beds, equipment for laboratory testing, and radiological diagnostics facilitating the improvement of the quality and availability of medical care in the overall health system was small in this additional flow of funds.

COVID-19-induced crisis has redefined resilience. There is, in theory, now more potential to initiate reforms aimed at protecting and diversifying health system revenue generation and financing mechanism for different levels of health facilities, to build a high level of "social capital" (institutional trust, cooperation capacity, and public awareness of health risks), and to design and institutionalize a well-functioning health system performance monitoring practice. And the public financing of healthcare, in theory, not only ensures universal access to healthcare but also allows more efficient use of health resources. But the present model of financing in the Russian health system does not provide greater efficiency of medical care in the Russian Federation. Also, despite the declared transition to universal compulsory health insurance, the main source of public funding for healthcare is still the state budget rather than individual insurance premiums for each insured person. Private funding of healthcare expenses, including contribution to voluntary health insurance, is about 35% of total health expenditure in the Russian Federation and is consistent over the last one decade. This is substantially high compared to the OECD country average (21% in 2022). Inequity in public financing is obvious: the 10 wealthiest regions receive almost double the public funding in healthcare compared to the 10 poorest regions. Intraregional inequality is primarily attributable to the macroeconomy of the region exacerbated by the strong federal approach of policy uniformity across the country.

Social capital includes trust and solidarity, collective action and cooperation, and civic responsibility and community responsiveness. In communities with a higher level of social capital, the degree of compliance affecting individual choice is generally higher and confers a positive impact on mitigating the risk of infection. The vulnerability of a region significantly depends on population density, air quality, the proportion of elderly people, and the level of education of the population. People less burdened by morbidity are better protected from and less likely to spread infection, while longer life expectancy entails an increased number of older people most vulnerable to disease. Therefore, an appropriate health system that is dynamically responsive has a long-term bearing on the well-being of the population. This responsiveness could be developed with an institutionalized system of monitoring and review that both established synergies among different interventions and clarified the tradeoffs and negative externalities resulting from policy initiatives.

10.5 Conclusion

Health governance in the Russian Federation does not recognize the limits of the state. The Soviet-style bureaucratic control that remains at the level of regional elites created a cohort of regional officials manifestly loyal to the President at the expense of good governance and the efficient implementation of federal and regional policies. The authoritarian and paternalistic mode of governance in Russia challenges policymaking in key areas like healthcare. Administrative domination (the hierarchical logic of rule for securing obedience and loyalty from the population) is not limited to any routine enforcement practices. Non-compliance is often criminalized, and the politics of threat operate through the "shadow of hierarchy," where the implicit threat of government action underlies ostensible freedom on the part of regional authorities. Policy entrepreneurs do not aim to establish new pockets of efficiency without strong support and patronage from the political leadership. The problem is that the availability of patronage is inherently limited, and the pool of potentially successful policy entrepreneurs is shrinking over time.

In this way, Russia has exhausted the potential of its infrastructural and personnel resources for creating success stories that are resilient over time and across geography. The key analytical question is thus the extent to which the Russian political leadership are amenable to changing the very paradigm of development, i.e. away from an orientation focusing a small number of extraordinary and highly visible achievements that impedes the overall development of better health policy. The common denominator across Russia, and across policy fields, is that power is of a personified nature where administration is organized vertically. For this reason it is impossible to change the Russian authorities through elections even as control on the part of the political elite is increasing. The governors ensure social stability, economic development, and law and order in the regions, but they perform these functions without a robust basis of political legitimacy.

The federal pandemic measures, supported by legislation and accompanied by expanded social support and sector specific measures, did have some effect on reducing the overall impact of COVID-19 in general, but the potential full effect of such measures specific to the population groups in their respective regions could not be realized primarily due to the focus on the regional harmonization of actions, the political hegemony of the regional governors, and, ultimately, the alienation of common people from state initiatives.

The subjects of the Russian Federation are extremely heterogeneous in regard to socioeconomic development, population need, and healthcare provisions (including accessibility and affordability). Because of this, a rigid top-down approach limits the efficacy of state action. The high mortality rate during the pandemic was due not so much to COVID-19 itself but rather to the imperfection of the entire healthcare system coupled with the governance deficit. The ideological basis of the Russian regime is a form of conservatism that ensures the stability of the regime. For ordinary Russians, conservatism is presented as a set of rules requiring them to conform to the authorities and to societal norms. At the same time, Russian conservatism is synonymous with ostentatious patriotism. Social stability is necessary for delivering correct voting results. "Managing" democracy and "engineering" elections define gubernatorial selection, and so any potential reform of the public health system may only emerge from a strong network of regional leaders with a proven ability to maintain socioeconomic stability and to use administrative resources effectively for delivering high levels of electoral support to the President. Because the public health system is so embedded in this larger system of governance, changes to the way in which public health is conceived or exercised will otherwise remain highly constricted.

References

Davos Agenda (2021). Online forum organized by the World Economic Forum, January 27, 2021, Moscow, Kremlin. http://www.kremlin.ru/events/president/transcripts (Accessed on April 27, 2023).

Di Maggio, P. and Powell, W. (1983). The "Iron Cage" revisited: Institutional isomorphism and collective rationality in organizational analysis. *American Sociological Review*, *48*(2), 147–160.

Food and Agriculture Organization (FAO) (2022). Regional conference for Europe, ERC/22/INF/18. https://www.fao.org/3/nj054en/nj054en.pdf (Accessed on April 27, 2023).

Galayants, S. (2020). Doctors of private clinics can be recruited to work in state medical institutions during epidemics. *Vademecum*, June 18. https://vademec.ru/news/2020/06/18/vracheychastnykh-kliniki-mogut-privlech-k-rabote-v-gosmeduchrezhdeniyakh-v-period-epidemiy/ (Accessed on September 9, 2022).

Gel'man, V. (2016). The vicious circle of post-Soviet neopatrimonialism in Russia. *Post-Soviet Affairs*, *32*(5), 455–473.

Gel'man, V. (2021). Exceptions and rules: Success stories and bad governance in Russia. *Europe-Asia Studies*, *73*(6), 1080–1101.

Healthcare Development Concept (2020). http://www.zdravo2020.ru/concept (in Russian) (Accessed on September 9, 2022).

Ivanov, V. N. and Suvorov, A. V. (2021). Modern development problems of Russian healthcare (Part 1). *Studies on Russian Economic Development*, *32*(6), 631–639.

Ivanov, V. N. and Suvorov, A. V. (2022). Modern development problems of Russian healthcare (Part 2). *Studies on Russian Economic Development*, *33*(1), 29–35.

Kravchenko, N. A. and Ivanova, A. I. (2021). Spread of the COVID-19 in Russia: Regional peculiarities. *Regional Research of Russia*, *11*(4), 428–434.

Muller, M. (2014). Higher, larger, costlier: Sochi and the 2014 Winter Olympics. *Russian Analytical Digest*, *143*, 2–4.

Nadskakuła-Kaczmarczyk, O. (2017). Sources of the legitimacy of Vladimir Putin's power in today's Russia. *Politeja*, *4*(49), 335–349.

Orttung, R. and Zhemukhov, S. (2014). The 2014 Sochi Olympic mega-project and Russia's political economy. *East European Politics*, *30*(2), 175–191.

Our World in Data (2023). COVID-19 deaths. https://ourworldindata.org/covid-deaths.

Outbound tourist trips of Russian citizens to foreign countries in the 1st quarter of 2020. https://www.gks.ru/free_doc/new_site/business/torg/tur/tab-tur1-2.htm (Accessed on May 4, 2023).

Paneyakh, E. (2013). Zaregulirovannoe gosudarstvo. *Pro et Contra*, *13*, 1–2.

Paneyakh, E. (2014). Faking performances together: Systems of performance evaluation in Russian enforcement agencies and production of Bias and privilege. *Post-Soviet Affairs*, *30*, 2–3.

Rosstat. (2022). https://rosstat.gov.ru/ (Accessed on September 9, 2022).

Sharafutdinova, G. (2009). Subnational governance in Russia: How Putin changed the contract with his agents and the problems it created for Medvedev. *The Journal of Federalism, 40*(4), 672–696.

Ulumbekova, G. E., Ginoyan, A. B., Kalashnikova, A. V., and Alvianskaya, N. V. (2019). Health care financing in Russia (2021–2024). Facts and suggestions. *Vestnik VSHOUZ* (HEALTH CARE MANAGEMENT: News, Views, Education. Bulletin of VSHOUZ). *5*(4), 4–19 (in Russian). https://cyber leninka.ru/article/n/finansirovanie-zdravoohraneniya-v-rossii-2021-2024-gg-fakty-ipredlozheniya (Accessed on September 9, 2022).

Volkov, V., Grigoriev, I., Dmitrieva, A., Moiseeva, E., Paneyakh, E., Pozdnyakov, M., Titaev, K., Chetverikova, I., and Shklyaruk, M. (2013). Kontseptsiya kompleksnoi organizatsionno-upravlencheskoi reformy pravookhranitel'nykh organov RF (St. Petersburg, Institute for the Rule of Law, European University at St. Petersburg). http://www.enforce.spb.ru/images/Issledovanya/IRL_KGI_Reform_final_11.13.pdf (Accessed on May 6, 2023).

World Health Organization (2020). Life expectancy and healthy life expectancy. https://www.who.int/data/gho/data/themes/mortality-and-global-health-estimates/ghe-life-expectancy-and-healthy-life-expectancy#:~:text-Globally%2C%20life%20expectancy%-20has%20increased,reduced%20years%20lived%20with%20disability (Accessed on September 9, 2022).

WTO (2021). Trade policy review, WT/TPR/G/416. https://www.wto.org/english/tratop_e/tpr_e/g416_e.pdf (Accessed on February 12, 2022).

Index

World Scientific Series in Global Health Economics and Public Policy

(Continued from page ii)

World Scientific Series in Global Health Economics and Public Policy

(Continued from page ii)